TOPS Club, Inc.

# A NUTRITION MONOGRAPH

# for

# Taking Off Pounds Sensibly

*Second Edition*

by

Ronald K. Kalkhoff, M.D.

TOPS Club, Inc., Milwaukee, Wisconsin 53207

Published 1980. Second Edition 1992
Printed in the United States of America

PUBLISHER'S NOTE:
Very rarely do different sources agree completely on the calorie content of specific foods, whether they are natural or processed. The precise number of calories can only be determined by chemical food analysis and even this will vary from one batch of a certain food to another. However, in most cases, the variances are not all that striking and are not going to make the difference in successful meal planning and weight loss.

This publication is designed to provide accurate and authoritative information in regard to the subject matter covered, but with the understanding that TOPS Club, Inc. does not endorse or recommend one brand over another and with the understanding that TOPS Club, Inc. is not engaged in rendering medical or other professional service. The services of a competent physician or professional person should be sought for medical advice or other assistance. The appearance of any trade name in this publication is not an endorsement or recommendation of that product.

# Table of Contents

# List of Figures

# List of Tables

## ABOUT THE AUTHOR

Ronald K. Kalkhoff, M.D., an internationally recognized expert in diabetes and obesity, was professor of medicine at the Medical College of Wisconsin in Milwaukee and had been chief of the endocrinology and metabolism division there from 1974 to 1988. Dr. Kalkhoff had served as director of the TOPS Club, Inc. Obesity and Metabolic Research Program since its inception in 1967 until his sudden death in December 1990. He had just completed the manuscript for the second edition of this monograph at the time of his death.

*Illustrations by Jo Anna Poehlmann*

# Foreword

Since the first edition of this monograph there have been remarkable changes in our understanding of the biology of weight gain, its impact on health, and the various options for achieving and maintaining weight reduction. In this second edition Dr. Ronald K. Kalkhoff has admirably assembled this information and presented it in the most professional way that is easy to comprehend.

It is estimated that approximately 35 million Americans are overweight, and the trend of increasing numbers of overweight subjects continues unabated. We have also learned that obesity is not simply a disorder of overeating and that genetic and several environmental factors interact in a complex fashion to enhance the individual's capacity to store calories as fat. We also have become aware of why not all obese subjects are likely to develop health complications such as diabetes, hypertension, heart disease and stroke. Indeed, research from the Medical College of Wisconsin, supported by funds from the TOPS Club, Inc. Metabolic and Obesity Research Program and by volunteering members of this organization, pioneered the view that location of the excessive fat along the body frame is a major predictor of the health impact of obesity. Centrally located fat around the waist and inside the abdominal cavity has serious consequences in terms of morbidity and mortality. Fat located in the thighs and buttocks, though cosmetically and mechanically inconvenient, has minimal impact on health.

After a long wait government agencies, including the office of the Surgeon General, the United States Department of Health and Human Services, the Centers for Disease Control, and the National Institutes of Health, are beginning to recognize the known fact that obesity is a significant public health problem which impacts on the quality of life, causes morbidity and mortality, and involves massive costs both in monies and loss of life. These agencies are beginning to request the experts' opinion on how to educate the public and how to prevent and treat this problem.

Ironically, the majority of overweight individuals who decide to reduce their excess weight either self-treat or seek storefront programs of quick weight loss. Unfortunately, the treatment history of the 40- to 55-year-old overweight person is characterized by approximately 10 to 20 unsuccessful short-term attempts to lose and stabilize weight. The TOPS Club, Inc. program, through its chapters and members' experiences, has long recognized the shortcomings of such attempts and has adopted the principles that weight gain is a chronic, progressive disorder and weight loss should be attained by Taking Off Pounds Sensibly. Leaders of their nationwide chapters have also learned through experience that weight-loss choices should be individualized and that appropriate expectations should be set for the individual.

We have now learned that repeated bouts of weight loss and regain are dangers to health and, hence, should be avoided. Taking Off Pounds Sensibly dictates the acquisition of up-to-date knowledge with respect to the biology of obesity, who should benefit from losing weight, who is likely to succeed and maintain this loss, what to lose and from where, and, finally, how to attain personal discipline and strong motivation in order to guarantee the long-term benefits. The goal of the Medical College of Wisconsin research group is to address these specific and crucial questions. This goal continues the efforts begun when TOPS Club, Inc. established the Obesity and Metabolic Research Program under the directorship of Dr. Ronald K. Kalkhoff in 1967.

Dr. Kalkhoff, professor and chief of the division of endocrinology and metabolism at the Medical College of Wisconsin, devoted over 20 years of his scientific and professional career seeking the mysteries of obesity and providing the leadership unraveling the biology of this disorder. Until his untimely death on December 20, 1990, he continued to contribute new directions to many of his students, fellows and colleagues. He served as consultant to the National Institutes of Health and the National Academy of Sciences on matters related to obesity, diabetes and their complications. He was the recipient of many honors, including the Distinguished Service Citation from the American Diabetes Association and an award from the Berzelius Society of Yale University, where he received his undergraduate degree. He was named best teacher of the Medical College of Wisconsin's department of medicine. This monograph reflects his outstanding professionalism and art. His contribution to the field of obesity will be sorely missed.

*Ahmed H. Kissebah, M.D., Ph.D.*
*Professor of Medicine and Pharmacology,*
*Chief, Division of Endocrinology,*
*  Metabolism and Clinical Nutrition,*
*Director, Clinical Research Center*
*Medical College of Wisconsin*

# Preface to First Edition

In 1967 TOPS Club, Inc., established its Obesity and Metabolic Research Program at the Medical College of Wisconsin in Milwaukee, Wisconsin. Relationships between the membership, the board of directors and the faculty of the medical school have been unique. Medical scientists were given the opportunity to investigate both basic and clinical problems associated with overweight. The outcome of these multidisciplinary studies has been productive during this period of time, including the publication of several papers in recognized professional journals on the subject. Many TOPS members participated in these investigations and greatly aided the research teams in understanding the goals of TOPS Club, its fundamental group approach to overweight and many individual, personal problems its members face on a day-to-day basis.

It was through this interaction and communication that the TOPS Club, Inc., board of directors elected to sponsor a series of monographs to aid chapters in their efforts to achieve weight control. It was a logical step to translate research findings gained from the program and general medical knowledge about obesity back to the members. It also was a reaffirmation of TOPS to align its objectives with those of the medical profession to promote sensible methods for weight reduction.

Shedding excess pounds isn't easy. It requires a great deal of personal sacrifice and self-discipline. Successful individuals in the organization are not only strongly motivated but also have a system to achieve their goals. Optimally, it represents the advice and management of a close personal physician, assistance of trained nurses, dietitians and other allied health professionals, the very important group support of TOPS chapters and personal determination.

The present monograph on nutrition is a supplement to this system of Taking Off Pounds Sensibly. It does not replace what already should and does exist but provides the TOPS member with some basic information on nutrition. It serves the membership in defining present levels of obesity, desirable weight goals, and acceptable methods for meal planning and personal aids to achieve those goals.

And speaking of goals—if the ensuing chapters help the TOPS member distinguish between ill-advised and sensible approaches to weight control and help close the communication gap between the medical profession, public health agencies and the obese individual, it will have served its major purpose.

*Ronald K. Kalkhoff, M.D.*

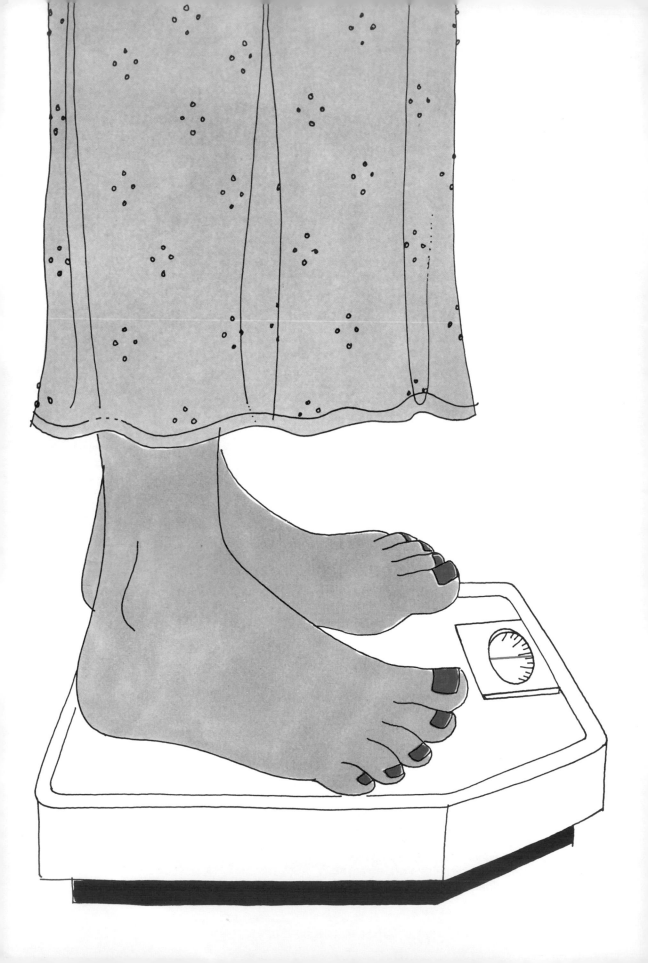

# PART ONE:
# What Is Obesity and What Are Its Risks?

Chapter 1: What Is Obesity?

Chapter 2: Risks of Obesity: Why Do
            Anything about It?

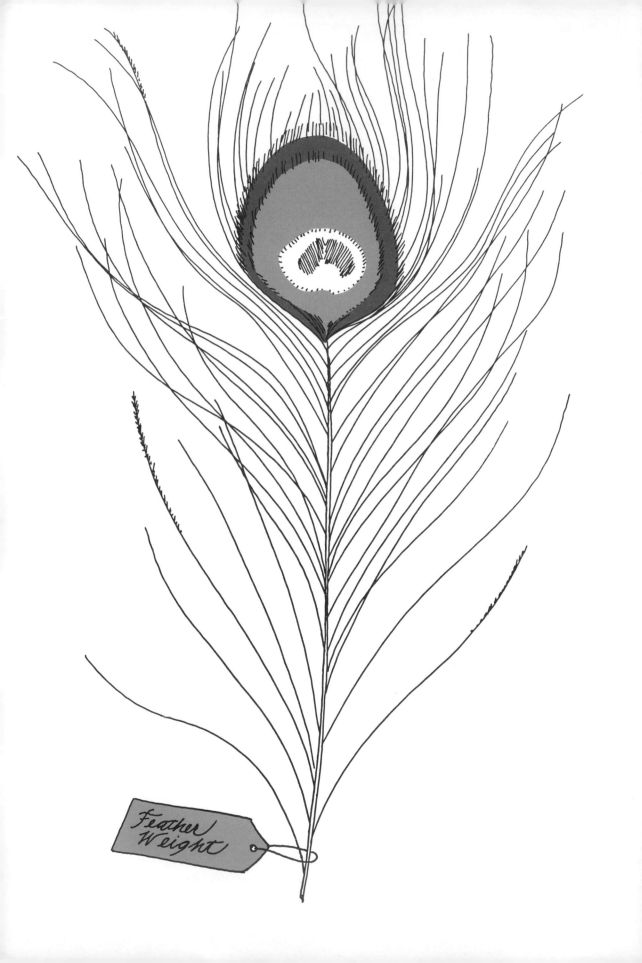

Feather
Weight

# Chapter 1: What Is Obesity?

Obesity is simply an excessive accumulation of body fat. Obesity usually means one is overweight for height and age, but not all overweight people are obese, and not all obese people are overweight. Examples of these various situations appear in table 1.

Table 1 indicates how both muscularity and adiposity contribute to body weight. Most overweight adults fall under category 5.

## How Obese Are You?

In normal adult men, 15 to 20% of total body weight is due to body fat. In normal adult women, 20 to 25% of total body weight is body fat. Values in excess of these percentages define obesity. In severe obesity, 50% or more of total weight is fat tissue.

The most accurate ways to measure obesity levels are those which determine fat mass relative to body weight. Scientific methods for doing this include: (1) multiple skin-fold thickness measurements with a caliper in different regions of the body; (2) underwater weighing that allows calculation of body volume and density; (3) distribution of specific radioisotopes in different body tissues that provides an estimate of lean (muscle) and fat tissue mass; (4) measurements of body impedance or resistance to conduction of low-level electrical currents which correlate with degrees of obesity; and (5) radiologic CT scanning of subcutaneous and intraabdominal fat layer thicknesses.

None of these methods is a practical, easy way to determine total body fatness. For this reason, standard tables for acceptable weights are most commonly used.

## Metropolitan Height and Weight Tables

In 1959 actuarial statistics from the Metropolitan Life Insurance Company indicated what weight-for-height in adult women and men had the lowest mortality rates. In 1983 these tables were revised. They are among the most commonly used criteria for obesity today. Table 2 defines the range of acceptable weights for men and women above the age of 25 years based on these statistics. They further subdivided the ranges according to size of body frame.

Most TOPS members should select the medium frame size. Individuals with large frames have broad shoulders and chest cages, a wide pelvis and large wrists. Small frame describes individuals with narrow shoulders, small chest cages, a narrow pelvis and small wrists. These designations are very subjective and arbitrary and were not described in detail by the Metropolitan Life Insurance Company.

It is emphasized that table 2 lists heights *without shoes*, whereas the original 1983 table allowed one inch for shoes. Secondly, these weights include *indoor clothing*. Weights without clothing are estimated to be 5 pounds less for men and 3 pounds less for women. Women and men who are between the ages of 18 and 24 ordinarily should choose desirable weights in the lower ranges for their respective body frames.

A good starting point for the TOPS member is to obtain an accurate height without shoes, select

## TABLE 1:
## RELATIONSHIPS BETWEEN OBESITY LEVEL AND BODY WEIGHT

| CATEGORY | CHARACTERISTICS | | | EXAMPLE |
| | Overweight? | Obese? | Muscular? | |
|---|---|---|---|---|
| 1 | No | No | No | Normal adults |
| 2 | Yes | No | Yes | Body builders, certain athletes |
| 3 | Yes | Yes | Yes | Japanese sumo wrestlers |
| 4 | No | Yes | No | Sedentary office workers with poor physical development |
| 5 | Yes | Yes | No | Typical obese individuals |

the correct frame size (usually medium) and obtain the desirable weight from table 2. If you wish to calculate how overweight you are, the following simple equations are used:

(1) Pounds overweight =
Actual weight – Desirable weight

(2) Percent above desirable weight =
$\frac{\text{Pounds overweight}}{\text{Desirable weight}}$ x 100

For example, if an individual weighs 200 pounds

and the desirable weight is 160, the calculation would be:

(1) 200 – 160 = 40 pounds above desirable weight

(2) $\frac{40}{160}$ x 100 = 25% above desirable weight

**Childhood Obesity**

Chapter 28 deals specifically with childhood obesity and includes normal heights and weights for children of different ages.

## TABLE 2: DESIRABLE WEIGHTS FOR ADULT MEN AND WOMEN

| HEIGHT | WEIGHT (pounds) | | |
| --- | --- | --- | --- |
| | Small Frame | Medium Frame | Large Frame |
| MEN | | | |
| 5' 1" | 128-134 | 131-141 | 138-150 |
| 5' 2" | 130-136 | 133-143 | 140-153 |
| 5' 3" | 132-138 | 135-145 | 142-156 |
| 5' 4" | 134-140 | 137-148 | 144-160 |
| 5' 5" | 136-142 | 139-151 | 146-164 |
| 5' 6" | 138-145 | 142-154 | 149-168 |
| 5' 7" | 140-148 | 145-157 | 152-172 |
| 5' 8" | 142-151 | 148-160 | 155-176 |
| 5' 9" | 144-154 | 151-163 | 158-180 |
| 5' 10" | 146-157 | 154-166 | 161-184 |
| 5' 11" | 149-160 | 157-170 | 164-188 |
| 6' 0" | 152-164 | 160-174 | 168-192 |
| 6' 1" | 155-168 | 164-178 | 172-197 |
| 6' 2" | 158-172 | 167-182 | 176-202 |
| 6' 3" | 162-176 | 171-187 | 181-207 |
| WOMEN | | | |
| 4' 9" | 102-111 | 109-121 | 118-131 |
| 4' 10" | 103-113 | 111-123 | 120-134 |
| 4' 11" | 104-115 | 113-126 | 122-137 |
| 5' 0" | 106-118 | 115-129 | 125-140 |
| 5' 1" | 108-121 | 118-132 | 128-143 |
| 5' 2" | 111-124 | 121-135 | 131-147 |
| 5' 3" | 114-127 | 124-138 | 134-151 |
| 5' 4" | 117-130 | 127-141 | 137-155 |
| 5' 5" | 120-133 | 130-144 | 140-159 |
| 5' 6" | 123-136 | 133-147 | 143-163 |
| 5' 7" | 126-139 | 136-150 | 146-167 |
| 5' 8" | 129-142 | 139-153 | 149-170 |
| 5' 9" | 132-145 | 142-156 | 152-173 |
| 5' 10" | 135-148 | 145-159 | 155-176 |
| 5' 11" | 138-151 | 148-162 | 158-179 |

NOTES: Heights are *without* shoes. Weights are *with indoor clothing*. Weights without clothes are 5 pounds less for men and 3 pounds less for women.

SOURCE: Modified from Metropolitan Life Insurance Tables, 1983.

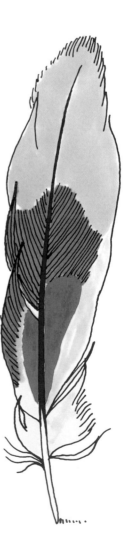

# Chapter 2: Risks of Obesity: Why Do Anything about It?

## Prevalence of Obesity

Studies of large populations reported by the National Center for Health Statistics in its National Health and Nutrition Examination Survey II[1] estimate that:

- Over 30 million adult Americans are obese.
- 10 million adult Americans within this group are severely obese.
- Obesity in adult women (24%) is more prevalent than in adult men (22%), and approximately one-third of these women and men are severely obese.

Other analyses indicate that the average weight of Americans has gradually risen over the past 25 years. Whether this is due to an increasing prevalence of obesity remains to be determined. Obesity tends to be more pronounced with advancing age and is more common in certain ethnic groups than in others. For example, black women have a two-fold greater incidence of obesity than do white women. People of Western European extraction are less obese as a population than people having Eastern European ancestry. Individuals of low socioeconomic status have a greater tendency to be obese than those of higher socioeconomic status. Some recent investigations also suggest that obesity varies in prevalence in different regions of the United States.

Genetic influences on the development of obesity are suggested by studies of adopted children who have body weights more similar to their birth parents than their foster parents. Others have shown that identical twins, separated and raised in different locations as children, have similar obesity levels when compared as adults.

All these observations emphasize that the prevalence of obesity in America is staggering. There is no single cause. Obesity appears to be a product of a number of complex hereditary and environmental factors that interact to promote body fat accumulation.

## Health Risks of Obesity

One of the first projects in the TOPS Club, Inc., Obesity and Metabolic Research Program was to determine what the health risks of obesity are among TOPS members. In the late 1960s, Dr. Alfred Rimm, professor and chief of the Division of Epidemiology and Biostatistics at the Medical College of Wisconsin, devised a questionnaire with his colleagues. TOPS chapters throughout the country were mailed 86,000 questionnaires. Over 73,000 were returned!

The analysis focused on that part of the questionnaire that dealt with medical ailments. Those TOPS women between the ages of 40 and 59 years were subdivided into five obesity levels ranging from nonobese to severely obese. Approximately 7,000 to 8,000 TOPS members were included in each of the five groups. Average ages and heights were similar at each level. Table 3 is a very abbreviated summary of this work, which was published in detail elsewhere.[2]

Medical conditions that were significantly greater in incidence in obese TOPS members are listed in table 3. For the most part, the risks sharply increase in the severely obese group (85% above desirable weight) as compared with the moderately obese women (38% above desirable weight).

### Diabetes Mellitus

The incidence of this disease was 1.5-fold greater in moderately obese and 4.5-fold greater in severely obese TOPS members as compared with nonobese TOPS women. This confirms several studies documenting the much higher risk of diabetes with increasing body fatness. In the United States approximately 40% of all maturity-onset or Type II diabetic subjects, both male and female, are obese. This complication of obesity is discussed in greater detail in chapter 26.

### High Blood Pressure (Hypertension)

When obesity develops, blood volume often increases and major blood vessels become more sensitive to factors that promote their constriction. This combination and other unknown factors promote hypertension. It has been known for some time that degrees of obesity run in parallel with degrees of blood pressure elevation. If untreated, hypertension has damaging effects on the heart and kidneys and may cause arterial disease that results in heart attacks, stroke and other vascular accidents. It is not surprising that our TOPS survey (see table 3) revealed a 1.9- and 3.3-fold greater incidence of hypertension in moderate and severely obese subjects.

[1]S. Abraham, M. Carroll, and M.F. Naijar, "Trends in Obesity and Overweight Among Adults Age 20-74 Years: United States 1960-1962, 1971-1974, 1976-1980," in *Vital and Health Statistics*, series 11 (Hyattsville, Maryland: National Center for Health Statistics, 1985).

[2]Alfred A. Rimm et al., "Relationship of Obesity and Disease in 73,532 Weight-Conscious Women," *Public Health Service Reports* 90 (1973):44-51.

## Gallbladder Disease

Bile metabolism is disturbed in obesity and leads to excessive accumulation of cholesterol-containing stones in the gallbladder. Stones may cause chronic irritation and acute inflammation (cholecystitis) and often result in the need for surgical removal of the gallbladder.

## Gout

Blood uric acid concentrations steadily rise with increasing levels of obesity. If excessive, uric acid crystals may deposit in joints, and acute and chronic inflammation may result. An attack of acute gouty arthritis is often very painful and favors the toes and other joints in the feet. Fortunately, there are medications available to control blood uric acid and prevent attacks.

## Heart Disease

Atherosclerotic heart disease is associated more often with overweight obese Americans. In the TOPS membership, this was most pronounced in the heaviest group (see table 3). This condition is even more common among those obese individuals who also have diabetes, hypertension, and disturbances of blood cholesterol and triglycerides. Cigarette smoking is an added risk factor.

## Arthritis

Degenerative joint disease (osteoarthritis) is a major complication of being overweight. Heaviness places an added stress on the back, hip and knee joints, and feet. Cartilage lining the joints is damaged, and tissue reactions lead to pain and stiffness. Eventually, severe limitations of joint movement may result.

## Blood Triglyceride and Cholesterol Abnormalities

There is a statistical relationship between weight gain and elevation of blood cholesterol levels. Obesity also results in disturbed triglyceride metabolism, and blood triglycerides also are more frequently increased. Higher cholesterol and triglyceride concentrations in the circulating blood do relate to a higher incidence of atherosclerosis (hardening of the arteries) and vascular diseases that are associated with heart attacks, strokes and peripheral vascular disease (see chapter 30).

## Gynecologic Disturbances and Cancer

Significant obesity in adult women is often associated with menstrual irregularities, lack of menstruation and infertility. Excessive facial and body hair also may occur. For reasons that are unclear, overeating and obesity disturb pituitary hormones that control ovulation. Lack of ovulation leads to irregular periods, which ultimately may become quite heavy when they do occur. Infertility is also a consequence. Weight loss frequently corrects the problem.

Because obesity is combined with menstrual irregularities or lack of menstruation, the endometrium or lining of the uterus is chronically and abnormally stimulated by estrogens. This may be responsible for the higher incidence of endometrial (uterine) cancer in obese females. Several epidemiological studies have documented this. Our TOPS survey suggests that women who develop endometrial cancer frequently have a lifelong history of obesity. In a group of 56,111 TOPS women, this form of cancer had its highest incidence among individuals whose weight problems began as teenagers.[3]

## TABLE 3:
## MEDICAL COMPLICATIONS IN 22,000 TOPS WOMEN, 30 TO 49 YEARS OLD

| CATEGORY | Age (years) | Weight (pounds) | % Above Ideal Wt. | MEDICAL CONDITION AND RELATIVE RISK* | | | | | |
| --- | --- | --- | --- | --- | --- | --- | --- | --- | --- |
| | | | | Diabetes | High Blood Pressure | Gallbladder Disease | Gout | Heart Disease | Arthritis |
| Level 1 (nonobese) | 38 | 132 | 10% | 1.0 | 1.0 | 1.0 | 1.0 | 1.0 | 1.0 |
| Level 3 (moderate obesity) | 40 | 165 | 38% | 1.5 | 1.9 | 1.6 | 2.4 | 1.1 | 1.2 |
| Level 5 (severe obesity) | 40 | 228 | 85% | 4.5 | 3.3 | 1.7 | 2.7 | 1.7 | 1.6 |

*Relative risk in Level 3 and Level 5 obese women is the times greater incidence of a disease relative to the incidence in the nonobese Level 1 group. For example, the risk of developing diabetes in the severely obese Level 5 women is 4.5 times greater than in Level 1 nonobese women.

SOURCE: Modified from data published by A.A. Rimm and co-workers.[2]

Obese women are also at greater risk for the development of breast cancer. Again, the reasons are not well defined, but it is possible that hormonal disturbances that occur during years of weight gain may contribute to this higher prevalence.

### Pregnancy

Both obesity and pregnancy promote diabetogenic stress, and when they coexist, elevated blood sugars and other metabolic abnormalities may emerge. This occurs during the latter half of gestation and, if unrecognized, may have devastating effects on the outcome of pregnancy (see chapter 29).

Other problems, including pre-eclampsia and eclampsia (hypertension with kidney complications) and heavy babies with prolonged, traumatic deliveries, are encountered more often in obese pregnant women.

### Lung and Vein Disorders

Certain lung problems are more likely to afflict obese than nonobese individuals. Breathing may be impaired mechanically by excessive fat tissue overlying the chest and abdomen. Irregular gas exchange in the lungs can lead to retention of carbon dioxide and reduction of oxygen. If severe and prolonged, there is a tendency toward sleepiness and impaired thinking (Pickwickian syndrome). This also places added strain on the heart as blood pressure within the lungs rises. These complications are usually seen only in very obese subjects.

Overweight people also are more likely to have poor vein function in the legs. Blood flow through the veins is often slowed. Varicose veins may develop. Legs and feet often swell, and with slowing of blood flow, blood clots may form. Acute inflammation of veins (phlebitis) can result from this, and blood clots may break loose and travel to the lungs (pulmonary embolus). These are potentially very serious complications.

## Summary

Obesity itself is a relatively simple process of accumulating excessive body fat. On the other hand, its cause is a product of many genetic and environmental factors. Its prevalence is at an alarmingly high level in the United States.

The most important reasons for doing something about obesity are the associated health problems that occur. Our TOPS research survey of the membership clearly demonstrates the importance of weight control from a medical standpoint. Results of other numerous studies of obese adult populations performed by reputable governmental and university-based research groups support our conclusions.

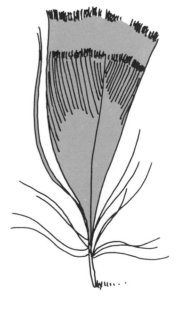

[3]Peter H. Blitzer, Eleanor C. Blitzer, and Alfred A. Rimm, "Association Between Teenage Obesity and Cancer in 56,111 Women: All Cancers and Endometrial Carcinoma," *Preventive Medicine* 5 (1976):20-31.

Milk
Noodles
Tea
Zucchini
Flour
Margarine
Oatmeal
Cottage Cheese
Parsley
Lemons
Cereal
Pickles

Yogurt
Oranges
Decaf
Bread
Chicken

# PART TWO:
## Nutrition

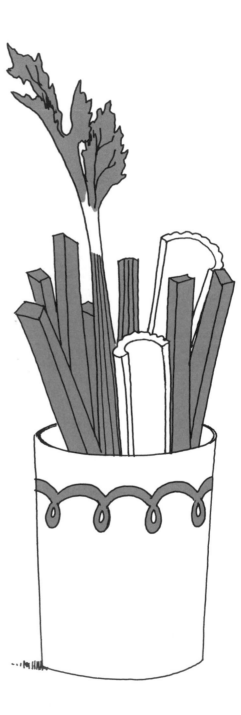

# Chapter 3: Calories, Carbohydrate, Protein and Fat

## Calories

Calories (actually kilocalories) are units of heat energy. One kilocalorie raises the temperature of one liter of water one degree centigrade. Science also uses the calorie to express the amount of energy in food and the amount of energy man requires to maintain cellular metabolism, body heat and physical activity. Excess calories that are not used for these processes are stored for later use in times of need between meals or during more prolonged starvation.

Adipose or fat tissue is the largest reservoir of accessible, stored calories in the body. During times of overeating, extra calories are stored primarily in individual fat cells as triglyceride or neutral fat. The cells actually expand, and in obese people their average size exceeds measurements of fat cells in lean subjects of similar age. During times of low-calorie feeding, the cells release their stored fat as fatty acids into the blood to provide the balance of energy not supplied by the diet. Fat cells shrink in size and body fat mass is reduced. The rate of reduction of fat tissue depends on the degree of caloric restriction and is most rapid during total starvation. These relationships can be summarized by three simple statements.

(1) If food calories eaten are greater than calories "burned" or expended, fat tissue weight is gained.
(2) If food calories consumed equal expended calories, fat tissue weight is unchanged.
(3) If food calories consumed are below expended calories, fat tissue weight is lost.

Table 4 reveals the approximate number of calories required each day to maintain various levels of body weight in normally active adults. The values may be adjusted downward for inactive normal people but usually not more than 5 to 15%. It is inserted in this section to emphasize that obesity is the result of excessive caloric intake. For example, those TOPS members who weigh 200 pounds (about 2,700 calories of food per day) but who should weigh 140 pounds (1,900 calories per day) are exceeding their desirable weight-maintaining requirements by 800 calories daily. Just 200 extra calories with each of three meals and a nighttime snack over a prolonged period of time are enough to push body weight up 60 pounds!

Calories do count, and in all foods. Two hundred calories as oranges, apples or grapefruit are the same as 200 calories as meat, potatoes, milk or candy. The foods are different but the caloric price is the same. On the other hand, calories do vary from one food to another on a weight basis:

```
Carbohydrate . . . . . . . . . . . .4 calories/gram
Protein  . . . . . . . . . . . . . . . .4 calories/gram
Fat . . . . . . . . . . . . . . . . . . . .9 calories/gram
```

## Carbohydrate

According to nutritionists, a healthy diet should contain about 50% of its calories as carbohydrates. Natural sources of this nutrient are mostly fruits and vegetables. Processed foods contain carbohydrate in the form of flour, added table sugar and other ingredients.

Carbohydrate provides fuel for sustaining the central nervous system, circulating blood cells and exercising muscle. It is essential for cellular metabolism in virtually every tissue of the body.

Carbohydrates can be subdivided into (a)monosac-

## TABLE 4: DAILY CALORIC INTAKE FOR WEIGHT MAINTENANCE

| WEIGHT (Pounds) | ESTIMATED DAILY CALORIC NEEDS (Calories) | WEIGHT (Pounds) | ESTIMATED DAILY CALORIC NEEDS (Calories) |
|---|---|---|---|
| 300 | 4,100 | 160 | 2,200 |
| 250 | 3,400 | 140 | 1,900 |
| 220 | 3,000 | 120 | 1,600 |
| 200 | 2,700 | 100 | 1,400 |
| 180 | 2,500 | | |

NOTES: These are estimations to the nearest 100 calories for adults with average physical activity. The figures are 15% lower for very inactive people and 15% or more higher for very active people.

charides, (b)disaccharides and (c)polysaccharides (see figure 1). The most familiar monosaccharides are simple sugars such as glucose (dextrose) or fructose (levulose), which are found naturally in many fruits, as well as mannose and galactose. Disaccharides, as the name implies, are two monosaccharides chemically linked together. Examples are sucrose or table sugar (glucose-fructose), lactose or milk sugar (glucose-galactose), and maltose from partial digestion of starch (glucose-glucose).

The principal digestible polysaccharide in our diets is starch. Natural, unprocessed foods containing starch include potatoes, corn, wheat, oats and barley. Flour produced from grains provides the primary source of starch in processed foods like bread and other bakery products. Figure 1 illustrates that starch is a series of repeating glucose units in branching chains. Starch as well as disaccharides require digestive breakdown to simple sugars before intestinal absorption. How-

ever, this process is very rapid. Monosaccharides require no digestion.

There are some polysaccharides in our diets that are not digestible. These are structural components of fruits and vegetables that give them support and resilience to withstand the elements of nature. Many of them are defined as food fiber or "roughage" and are also composed of repeating glucose units. Because the intestine of man does not have the enzymes required to break down these polysaccharides, they pass completely through the gastrointestinal tract and are eliminated.

Cellulose and other fibers in natural food give bulk to a diet and are an extremely important component of every meal plan. Many vegetables with substantial fiber, like lettuce, are calorie-free and have use in weight-reduction diets familiar to all weight-conscious individuals. The specific value of food fiber in meal plans is discussed in greater detail in chapter 5.

## FIGURE 1: POLYSACCHARIDES, DISACCHARIDES AND MONOSACCHARIDES

# DIETARY CARBOHYDRATE
## (DIAGRAMATIC)

I. EXAMPLES OF MONOSACCHARIDES

●      O      ■
GLUCOSE      FRUCTOSE      GALACTOSE
(Dextrose)      (Levulose)

II. EXAMPLES OF DISACCHARIDES

●—O      ●—■      ●—●
SUCROSE      LACTOSE      MALTOSE
(Glucose + Fructose    (Glucose + Galactose    (Glucose + Glucose
as in table sugar)    as in milk sugar)    from partial digestion
of starch)

III. EXAMPLE OF POLYSACCHARIDE

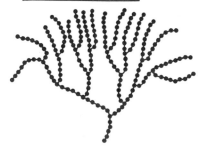

STARCH
(note repeating glucose units in
branching chains)

### Protein

Rich sources of protein include meats, dairy products, poultry, fish and, to a lesser extent, certain vegetables like nuts and beans. Protein resembles starch, since it represents a storage form of another basic nutrient, *the amino acid*. It, too, is composed of chains of different amino acids held together in peptide linkage.

Protein must be digested in the intestinal tract and broken down into its component amino acids before absorption and entrance into the bloodstream can take place. The amino acids, then, can gain entrance into tissues, where new protein is made into such things as hair, nails, connective tissue, skeletal and heart muscle, and structural components of many cells and tissues. Amino acids also form the building blocks for certain hormones and for blood proteins that carry vital trace minerals throughout the circulation to various organs. Amino acids may also serve as an energy source and are freely converted to sugars, like glucose in the liver, particularly when carbohydrate intake is poor. Adequate intake of protein is especially important during periods of growth in children and during pregnancy for proper fetal development.

Nonessential amino acids can be made in the body and are not necessarily obtained from food. However, approximately eight amino acids must be derived from food and are required for maintaining lean tissue. These so-called "essential" amino acids, if not present in a diet, can lead to malnutrition and body wasting. The importance of high-quality dietary protein deserves emphasis from this standpoint alone.

### Fat

Fat in our diets resembles the type found in human adipose tissue. Most of it is triglyceride or neutral fat composed of glycerol linked to three free fatty acid molecules (see figure 2). Dietary fat is found in nonlean meat and some poultry; cooking oil and margarine; dairy products, like cream, butter, whole milk, eggs and cheese; some fruits, such as avocado and olives; and all nuts and seeds.

FIGURE 2: DIETARY FAT AND FREE FATTY ACIDS

# DIETARY FAT
## (DIAGRAMATIC)

I. FATTY ACIDS

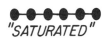
"SATURATED"
A fatty acid fully saturated with hydrogen.

"UNSATURATED"
A fatty acid with one or more sites of incomplete hydrogen saturation.

II. TRIGLYCERIDE (a principal form of dietary fat)

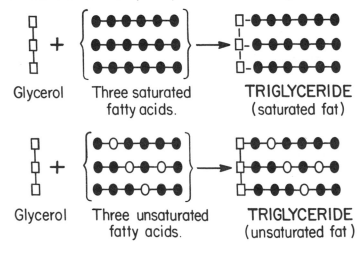

Glycerol — Three saturated fatty acids. → TRIGLYCERIDE (saturated fat)

Glycerol — Three unsaturated fatty acids. → TRIGLYCERIDE (unsaturated fat)

Dietary triglyceride finds its way through the intestine into the lymphatic system and ultimately into the blood circulation, where it is broken down into fatty acids and glycerol and taken up by various tissues, including body fat. Free fatty acids are the simplest form of fat and are the primary source of energy in the body (recall that fat has over twice as many calories per gram as carbohydrate and protein).

A normal person eats intermittently. Between meals or during periods of starvation, free fatty acids released from fat tissue supply fuel for work organs like the heart and muscles. Free fatty acids are also utilized in the formation of phospholipids, which are found in membranes of all human living cells. They also form parts of sphingolipids and glycolipids, many of which are components of tissue in the brain and peripheral nerves.

### Saturated and Unsaturated Fat

The terms "saturated" and "unsaturated" refer to the amount of hydrogen in the fatty acid molecule. A "saturated" fatty acid contains maximum amounts of hydrogen. "Monounsaturated" and "polyunsaturated" fatty acids have one or more sites where hydrogen is not present (see figure 2).

Saturated fat is more abundant in food from animal sources (cream, butter, meat, cheese, whole milk, etc.). This form has a higher melting point and tends to be solid or hard in the refrigerator. Unsaturated fat, derived mostly from plants and seeds, has a lower melting point and usually retains a liquid or "soft" form in the refrigerator. Examples of fat containing an abundance of unsaturated fatty acids include corn, cottonseed, linseed, sunflower, safflower and soybean oil. By way of contrast, cocoa butter, solid shortenings, coconut oil, palm oil and chocolate are relatively low in polyunsaturates and high in saturated fat.

Housewives ordinarily would not purchase a liquid oil as a spread. There is usually a compromise. Industry will "harden" or "hydrogenate" liquid fats like corn oil by putting some hydrogen into them in order to give them a more solid consistency as a margarine. This sacrifices some of their content of unsaturated fat, of course.

### Essential Fatty Acids

Normally the body can tailor-make many fatty acids from simple sugars and amino acids. However, there are two fatty acids contained in dietary fat that are not made by human tissues. These are *linoleic* and *linolenic acid*, both of which are unsaturated. Experimentally, feeding laboratory animals a diet nutritionally complete except for these two essential fats leads to impaired growth, scaliness of the skin around the feet and tail, kidney damage, fatty liver and impaired reproduction. A form of infantile eczema has also been traced to essential fatty acid deficiency.

### A Word about Cholesterol

Cholesterol is another form of fat or lipid that is present in foods of animal origin. Dietary intake of cholesterol and dietary fat generally have a major impact on blood levels of cholesterol. The metabolism of cholesterol is discussed elsewhere (see chapter 30).

### Summary

Calories are units of energy present in food. The number of calories consumed relative to body needs determine the amount of body fat. Obesity is a product of excessive caloric intake.

This chapter stresses the importance of carbohydrate, protein and fat in a healthy meal plan by explaining their sources, types and roles in body metabolism.

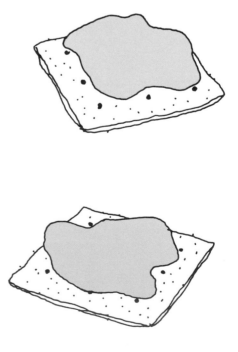

# Chapter 4: Vitamins and Minerals

Obesity, in some instances, is an example of malnutrition. Often abnormal eating patterns with emphasis on the wrong kinds of food and unbalanced meals lead to a marginal intake of important vitamins and minerals. A common myth is that vitamins and minerals actually promote obesity. Nothing could be further from the truth, since they have no caloric value of their own.

Vitamins and minerals are catalysts or cofactors that are necessary for many important biochemical reactions to occur in our bodies. Certain minerals, like calcium and phosphorus, also are critical for proper mineralization of bones and teeth. Deficiencies can lead to serious health problems. However, excessive intake of some vitamins and minerals may be more dangerous to health than previously realized.

Recommended daily dietary allowances for children and adults are listed in table 5. Under normal circumstances there is no need to take vitamin and mineral supplements if proper nutrition exists. In adults, the one exception is pregnancy, because there are additional needs for iron and folacin and other supplements that cannot be met by a nutritious diet alone.

## Fat-Soluble Vitamins

Vitamins A and D, E and K are insoluble in water but do dissolve in fat. For this reason, they are classified as fat-soluble.

### Vitamin A

Vitamin A is found only in animal tissues. Rich concentrations exist in the liver of most animals and saltwater fish. In fact, polar bear liver has extremely high levels, and it is now presumed that some polar explorers died of vitamin A poisoning as a result of subsisting on cooked liver from these animals. Vitamin A also can be obtained indirectly from a variety of fruits and vegetables because they contain a family of pigments known as *carotenes*. These substances impart some of the characteristic color seen in these foods, such as the yellow-orange color of carrots. Carotene, when consumed in the diet, also can be converted into vitamin A by the gastrointestinal tract and stored in the liver.

The daily requirements for vitamin A or its equivalent in carotene can easily be met by normal intakes of vegetables and fruits, especially carrots, sweet potatoes, spinach, greens of beets, chard, mustard, turnips, as well as parsley, broccoli, pumpkin, winter squash and tomatoes. Beef and chicken or other animal liver is also a good source. Dried peaches, prunes or apricots have moderate concentrations as do butter and margarine. Some foods, like margarine and milk, are fortified with the vitamin.

*Vitamin A deficiency* is a rare occurrence in most developed countries because of the ample dietary sources. When the deficiency is seen, the characteristic changes attack the eye, skin, and lining of the respiratory tree, gastrointestinal tract, etc. Vitamin A enters into the formation of rhodopsin, an important light-sensitive pigment in the retina of eyes. Without the vitamin, night blindness may occur. This deficiency also leads to reduced secretions from tear, salivary and sebaceous glands, which, in turn, can cause chronic dryness and damage to eyes, skin and body hair. Resistance to infection is diminished because of similar effects on delicate linings of the lung and other tracts where moist secretions are important.

### Vitamin D

Vitamin D is important for gastrointestinal absorption of calcium and phosphorus and for normal bone formation. Vitamin D can be made in the skin after sufficient exposure to sunlight. The dietary requirement, then, would be least in fair-skinned individuals living in tropical climates. In more cold regions and industrial areas where heavy clothing and indoor employment are common, additional sources from food are required. The potential problem of vitamin D deficiency is largely prevented by fortifying milk and other food products with it. One quart of fortified milk per day supplies the minimum daily requirements. Natural sources of the vitamin are concentrated in fish liver oils of cod and halibut and are found in ocean fish, like herring, sardines, mackerel, salmon, tuna, shrimp and similar seafoods.

*Vitamin D deficiency* is seen in children as rickets and in adults as osteomalacia. Both conditions are due to defective mineralization of bone. In children, marked deformities can occur, especially in the legs. Teeth are often malformed. In adults, severe bone pain and thinning of bones can occur.

### Vitamin K

Vitamin K is necessary for normal blood clotting. Vitamin K exists throughout nature, and the minimum daily requirement is not known. It is extremely rare for vitamin K deficiency to occur even in severe forms of malnutrition.

### Vitamin E

Vitamin E, also known as alpha tocopherol, has enjoyed prominence in the lay press in recent years. Many claims of its curative effects for many ills have not been supported by nutritional re-

# TABLE 5: FOOD AND NUTRITION BOARD, NATIONAL ACADEMY OF SCIENCES–NATIONAL RESEARCH COUNCIL RECOMMENDED DIETARY ALLOWANCES[a] (Revised 1989)

Designed for the maintenance of good nutrition of practically all healthy people in the United States

| CATEGORY | Age (years) or Condition | Weight[b] (kg) | Weight[b] (lb) | Height[b] (cm) | Height[b] (in) | Protein (g) | FAT-SOLUBLE VITAMINS Vitamin A (µg RE)[c] | Vitamin D (µg)[d] | Vitamin E (mg α-TE)[e] | Vitamin K (µg) | WATER-SOLUBLE VITAMINS Vitamin C (mg) | Thiamin (mg) | Riboflavin (mg) | Niacin (mg NE)[f] | Vitamin B6 (mg) | Folate (µg) | Vitamin B12 (µg) | MINERALS Calcium (mg) | Phosphorus (mg) | Magnesium (mg) | Iron (mg) | Zinc (mg) | Iodine (µg) | Selenium (µg) |
|---|---|---|---|---|---|---|---|---|---|---|---|---|---|---|---|---|---|---|---|---|---|---|---|---|
| Infants | 0.0–0.5 | 6 | 13 | 60 | 24 | 13 | 375 | 7.5 | 3 | 5 | 30 | 0.3 | 0.4 | 5 | 0.3 | 25 | 0.3 | 400 | 300 | 40 | 6 | 5 | 40 | 10 |
|  | 0.5–1.0 | 9 | 20 | 71 | 28 | 14 | 375 | 10 | 4 | 10 | 35 | 0.4 | 0.5 | 6 | 0.6 | 35 | 0.5 | 600 | 500 | 60 | 10 | 5 | 50 | 15 |
| Children | 1–3 | 13 | 29 | 90 | 35 | 16 | 400 | 10 | 6 | 15 | 40 | 0.7 | 0.8 | 9 | 1.0 | 50 | 0.7 | 800 | 800 | 80 | 10 | 10 | 70 | 20 |
|  | 4–6 | 20 | 44 | 112 | 44 | 24 | 500 | 10 | 7 | 20 | 45 | 0.9 | 1.1 | 12 | 1.1 | 75 | 1.0 | 800 | 800 | 120 | 10 | 10 | 90 | 20 |
|  | 7–10 | 28 | 62 | 132 | 52 | 28 | 700 | 10 | 7 | 30 | 45 | 1.0 | 1.2 | 13 | 1.4 | 100 | 1.4 | 800 | 800 | 170 | 10 | 10 | 120 | 30 |
| Males | 11–14 | 45 | 99 | 157 | 62 | 45 | 1,000 | 10 | 10 | 45 | 50 | 1.3 | 1.5 | 17 | 1.7 | 150 | 2.0 | 1,200 | 1,200 | 270 | 12 | 15 | 150 | 40 |
|  | 15–18 | 66 | 145 | 176 | 69 | 59 | 1,000 | 10 | 10 | 65 | 60 | 1.5 | 1.8 | 20 | 2.0 | 200 | 2.0 | 1,200 | 1,200 | 400 | 12 | 15 | 150 | 50 |
|  | 19–24 | 72 | 160 | 177 | 70 | 58 | 1,000 | 10 | 10 | 70 | 60 | 1.5 | 1.7 | 19 | 2.0 | 200 | 2.0 | 1,200 | 1,200 | 350 | 10 | 15 | 150 | 70 |
|  | 25–50 | 79 | 174 | 176 | 70 | 63 | 1,000 | 5 | 10 | 80 | 60 | 1.5 | 1.7 | 19 | 2.0 | 200 | 2.0 | 800 | 800 | 350 | 10 | 15 | 150 | 70 |
|  | 51+ | 77 | 170 | 173 | 68 | 63 | 1,000 | 5 | 10 | 80 | 60 | 1.2 | 1.4 | 15 | 2.0 | 200 | 2.0 | 800 | 800 | 350 | 10 | 15 | 150 | 70 |
| Females | 11–14 | 46 | 101 | 157 | 62 | 46 | 800 | 10 | 8 | 45 | 50 | 1.1 | 1.3 | 15 | 1.4 | 150 | 2.0 | 1,200 | 1,200 | 280 | 15 | 12 | 150 | 45 |
|  | 15–18 | 55 | 120 | 163 | 64 | 44 | 800 | 10 | 8 | 55 | 60 | 1.1 | 1.3 | 15 | 1.5 | 180 | 2.0 | 1,200 | 1,200 | 300 | 15 | 12 | 150 | 50 |
|  | 19–24 | 58 | 128 | 164 | 65 | 46 | 800 | 10 | 8 | 60 | 60 | 1.1 | 1.3 | 15 | 1.6 | 180 | 2.0 | 1,200 | 1,200 | 280 | 15 | 12 | 150 | 55 |
|  | 25–50 | 63 | 138 | 163 | 64 | 50 | 800 | 5 | 8 | 65 | 60 | 1.1 | 1.3 | 15 | 1.6 | 180 | 2.0 | 800 | 800 | 280 | 15 | 12 | 150 | 55 |
|  | 51+ | 65 | 143 | 160 | 63 | 50 | 800 | 5 | 8 | 65 | 60 | 1.0 | 1.2 | 13 | 1.6 | 180 | 2.0 | 800 | 800 | 280 | 10 | 12 | 150 | 55 |
| Pregnant |  |  |  |  |  | 60 | 800 | 10 | 10 | 65 | 70 | 1.5 | 1.6 | 17 | 2.2 | 400 | 2.2 | 1,200 | 1,200 | 320 | 30 | 15 | 175 | 65 |
| Lactating | 1st 6 months |  |  |  |  | 65 | 1,300 | 10 | 12 | 65 | 95 | 1.6 | 1.8 | 20 | 2.1 | 280 | 2.6 | 1,200 | 1,200 | 355 | 15 | 19 | 200 | 75 |
|  | 2nd 6 months |  |  |  |  | 62 | 1,200 | 10 | 11 | 65 | 90 | 1.6 | 1.7 | 20 | 2.1 | 260 | 2.6 | 1,200 | 1,200 | 340 | 15 | 16 | 200 | 75 |

[a] The allowances, expressed as average daily intakes over time, are intended to provide for individual variations among most normal persons as they live in the United States under usual environmental stresses. Diets should be based on a variety of common foods in order to provide other nutrients for which human requirements have been less well defined.

[b] Weights and heights of Reference Adults are actual medians for the U.S. population of the designated age, as reported by NHANES II. The median weights and heights of those under 19 years of age were taken from Hamill et al. (1979). The use of these figures does not imply that the height-to-weight ratios are ideal.

[c] Retinol equivalents. 1 retinol equivalent = 1 µg retinol or 6 µg β-carotene.

[d] As cholecalciferol. 10 µg cholecalciferol = 400 IU of vitamin D.

[e] α-Tocopherol equivalents. 1 mg d-α tocopherol = 1 α-TE.

[f] 1 NE (niacin equivalent) is equal to 1 mg of niacin or 60 mg of dietary tryptophan.

search. Nevertheless, science has established that vitamin E protects many vital nutrients, vitamins and cofactors from oxidative destruction in the body; promotes normal maturation of blood cell elements; and is essential for normal reproduction. Its greatest concentrations are found in vegetable oils obtained from corn, soybeans, cottonseeds and peanuts and in margarines made from them. A variety of cereals, fruits and vegetables also supplies enough of the vitamin, since the requirement is relatively low.

## Water-Soluble Vitamins

Water-soluble vitamins include vitamin C, the B vitamins, biotin, pantothenic acid, choline and folic acid. Since no human deficiencies of biotin, pantothenic acid and choline occur naturally in man, they will not be discussed.

### Vitamin C

Vitamin C or ascorbic acid is essential for normal wound healing and prevention of infection and is involved in a variety of metabolic reactions. Vitamin C is found in many fruits, especially of the citrus type, and in many vegetables. Because processed foods and beverages are often fortified with this vitamin, its deficiency is extremely rare in industrialized nations.

Vitamin C deficiency leads to scurvy. This condition begins with pinpoint bleeding around hair follicles on the body and progresses to larger "bruise-like" hemorrhages in other areas. Gums become soft and infected and bleed. Bleeding within muscles and joints, chronic anemia, weakness, low blood pressure, fainting and vomiting are other symptoms. In the United States, very young children are vulnerable if pediatric care and nutrition are poor.

### B Vitamins

B vitamins are catalysts for many biochemical pathways that use basic fuels for combustion and energy release, for making certain important compounds for metabolism within cells, and for the production of new cells, including blood elements.

Thiamine (vitamin $B_1$), riboflavin (vitamin $B_2$) and niacin are frequently discussed together because deficiencies of all three may exist in the same individual. The commonest illness associated with lack of thiamine in North America is chronic alcoholism and its accompanying malnutrition. Heart failure, fluid accumulation and peripheral nerve damage (Beriberi) as well as psychiatric disturbances (Korsakoff's psychosis), impaired walking, mentation and eye motility (Wernicke's syndrome) are consequences of thiamine deficiency. Pellagra develops from chronic niacin deficiency and is characterized by marked inflammation of skin exposed to sunlight, sore tongue and mouth, diarrhea and bizarre emotional episodes. Pellagra is most commonly seen as a separate entity in regions where corn is the principal food eaten, since corn is low in niacin compared with other natural grains. Riboflavin deficiency eventually causes inflammation and soreness around the lips, tongue, mouth and eyes with acne-like lesions on the face and skin inflammation elsewhere.

The rarity of this B complex deficiency in most modern countries, like the United States, reflects good food supplies and enrichment of many processed food and flour with these vitamins. Cereals, bread and other bakery products contain them as do liver, certain fish and meats, nuts and vegetables like dried peas.

A true deficiency of vitamin $B_6$ is extremely rare and may be responsible for some forms of anemia in adults. It is present in many of the foods containing the other B vitamins mentioned above.

One hears about vitamin $B_{12}$ in connection with pernicious anemia. This condition does not evolve because of poor vitamin intake but because of lack of a key substance, an "intrinsic factor," which is made in the stomach. This factor is necessary for proper absorption of vitamin $B_{12}$ in the small intestine. Dietary $B_{12}$ deficiency is distinctly rare except among those who are strict vegetarians and who also do not take vitamin supplements. It also may be a complication of surgical removal of the stomach or follow chronic inflammatory conditions of the small intestine in regions where $B_{12}$ is absorbed. $B_{12}$ is not present in plants to any extent but is amply supplied in most meats, especially liver, where it is normally stored. A chronic lack of this vitamin results in severe anemia and peripheral nerve damage with marked disturbances in position sense, particularly in the lower extremities.

Folacin and folic acid deficiencies are being recognized with increasing frequency even though this important vitamin is present in most green leafy vegetables, organ meats, like liver, yeasts, and many other foods of animal and plant origin. True dietary lack occurs most often among alcoholics and recluses who subsist on fast, easy foods like sandwiches and who rarely consume high-quality, balanced meals. Pregnancy sharply increases this requirement as will any condition that accelerates destruction and turnover of red blood cells or impairs intestinal absorption of these vitamins. The principal complication of this deficiency is profound anemia similar to that observed in conditions of low vitamin $B_{12}$ availability.

## Minerals and Trace Elements

Because nutritional deficiencies of many minerals and trace elements are rare in the United States, they will only be mentioned and not discussed: copper, zinc, chromium, cobalt, manganese, molybdenum and selenium.

## Iron

This mineral is required for normal hemoglobin production in red blood cells, and its insufficient supply is a frequent cause of iron deficiency anemia. Iron is not well absorbed in the intestinal tract, but normal losses are quite small, also. Normal diets supply sufficient quantities in most instances. However, menstruating women are particularly vulnerable to this deficiency owing to variable losses of iron in menstrual blood. Pregnant and lactating women as well as infants have increased requirements.

Yearly checkups with physicians include complete blood counts, and iron deficiency anemia is easily diagnosed. If warranted, iron can be prescribed and the anemia followed properly. Lesions of the gastrointestinal tract, like a peptic ulcer or cancer, may present initially as anemia because of chronic low-grade bleeding. The diagnosis may be missed if the patient has been taking enough iron to mask the disease. For this reason, self-treatment with over-the-counter iron remedies is not recommended without a doctor's approval.

## Iodine

This element was formerly of widespread interest because of its deficiency associated with thyroid enlargement or goiter. Iodine is an important component of thyroid hormone. In regions like the Great Lakes where soil iodine content is poor, the thyroid may enlarge to compensate for low availability of this element. Today, however, iodine is added to many foods, including bread, bakery goods and table salt. This has greatly relieved this problem. Individuals are encouraged to use iodized salt, for example, to meet daily requirements.

## Calcium, Magnesium and Phosphorus

True deficiencies of these elements are also rare and are most apt to occur in chronic alcoholics and in individuals who have severe intestinal ailments with diarrhea and malnutrition. As explained earlier, vitamin D deficiency may also upset calcium and phosphorus balance.

All three minerals have important roles in proper muscle function, and their lack results in irritability and profound weakness of this tissue. Severe phosphate depletion may also result in anemia and abnormal psychiatric behavior. Convulsions can accompany very low calcium and magnesium blood levels.

There is also concern about proper dietary intake of calcium and phosphorus during a lifetime to prevent reduction of bone mass. Osteoporosis or thinning of bones is commonly observed in the elderly. Some scientists speculate that it may be a complication of years of poor intake of foods like dairy products rich in these minerals. Postmenopausal women appear to be especially prone to this condition.

## The Megadose Vitamin C Craze: Beneficial or Harmful?

In recent years there has been a fanatic compulsion by many to take vitamin C in huge amounts that are often several-fold greater than the recommended adult daily allowance (50 to 60 milligrams per day). Because so many processed foods and beverages are fortified with the vitamin and because so many natural fruits and vegetables contain it, the daily requirements are easily met with sensible food intake. Nevertheless, it is not uncommon for loyal enthusiasts to take 100 to 500 milligrams or more of vitamin C supplements each day.

Is megadose vitamin C intake beneficial? Probably not. Most scientific studies reviewed to date have failed to prove that high-dose vitamin C reduces the incidence of upper respiratory infections. Until there is clear-cut evidence, there appears to be no health advantage for its use in large amounts. Research continues.

Is megadose vitamin C harmful? Yes, there may be adverse side effects. Gastrointestinal upset is not uncommon. Others report that vitamin C in large amounts may destroy certain B vitamins when the two are mixed in the gastrointestinal tract. A small percentage of individuals who are predisposed to forming kidney stones from oxalate may aggravate the condition by high-dose vitamin C intake.

Some case reports suggest that excessive use of vitamin C increases dependency on the vitamins. Adults may develop signs of vitamin C deficiency (scurvy) when megadoses are stopped. Pregnant women who take excessive amounts may bear children who develop scurvy because of increased dependence on the vitamin.

Diabetic patients who regularly test their urine for glucose may show false positive or false negative results because of chemical interference by urinary vitamin C if large amounts are taken.

## Vitamin A and D Poisoning

Fat-soluble vitamins, unlike water-soluble vitamins, can be stored in the body to a much greater extent. Chronic overdose can lead to dangerously high body levels with time. This most commonly occurs with vitamins A and D.

Many well-meaning parents believe that more vitamins are better. This probably accounts for the higher incidence of vitamin toxicity in children. The U.S. Food and Drug Administration is concerned about the ready availability of high-dose vitamin preparations that may be purchased without prescription.

A single high toxic dose of vitamin A causes headache, drowsiness and vomiting. Prolonged, less severe overdoses induce anemia and stimulate abnormal bone growth, loss of hair, and enlargement of the liver and spleen. Blood calcium levels may also increase to very high levels.

Vitamin D toxicity primarily results in elevation of blood calcium. Weakness, poor mentation and deposition of abnormal amounts of calcium in soft tissues, arteries, kidneys, joints, lungs and eyes may result.

## Vitamins and the Dieter

The monograph includes diet plans in the range of 1,200 to 1,800 calories per day. Lower caloric intakes reduce the amount of available vitamins to threshold levels. For this reason, it is recommended that vitamin supplements should be taken with meal plans below 1,500 calories per day. The supplement should be a simple, conservative preparation containing vitamins A, C, D, E, B complex and folic acid. Iron may be added to the supplement if the dieter is a menstruating woman. A physician should advise the individual about this. Each tablet should not exceed the recommended daily allowance of each vitamin by more than 150%. The label should confirm this. A pharmacist can help. Therapeutic vitamin preparations that contain "shotgun" amounts of vitamins as well as minerals should be avoided.

## Common Sense Conclusions

Proper amounts of vitamins and minerals are essential for good health. Almost all recommended daily allowances are met with sensible eating. Normal individuals who require additional supplemental vitamins are infants, pregnant women and lactating women. Therapeutic doses of vitamins are given to people with illnesses that cause deficiencies: starvation, alcoholism, extensive burns, gastrointestinal ailments, anemia, etc.

There is no advantage for healthy people to take high doses of vitamins daily. In fact, adverse side effects may occur, particularly with vitamins A and D as well as C. Approximately 4,000 new cases of vitamin poisoning occur annually in the United States alone. Unfortunately, the majority afflict children as a result of ill-advised administration of excessive vitamins by parents.

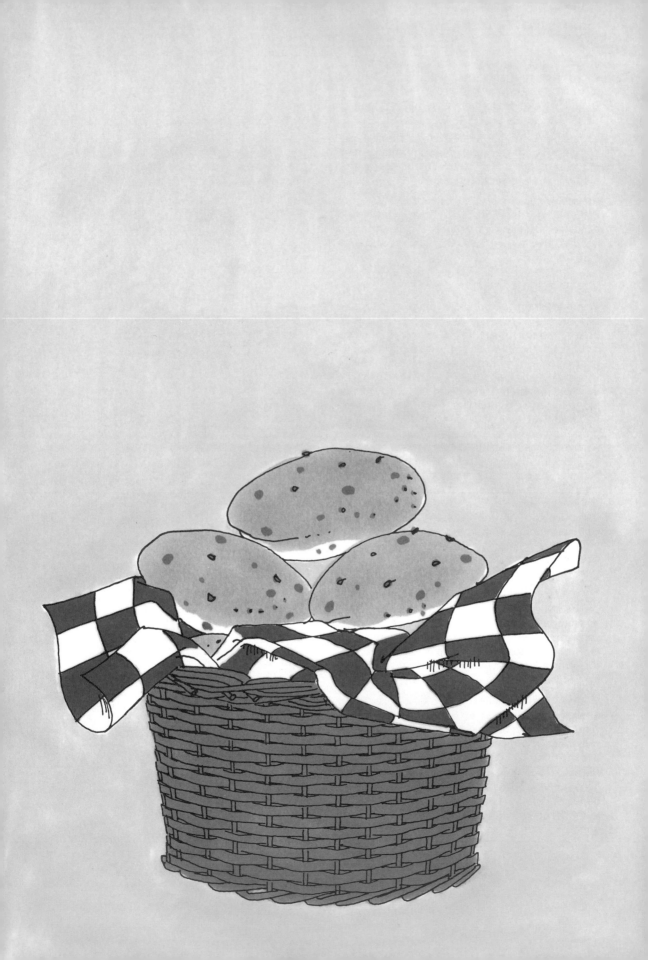

# Chapter 5: Food Fiber

In recent years there has been much interest in food fiber because it may have several health benefits to consumers. Food fiber is found exclusively in the plant world and is subdivided into five different types.

| Food Fiber | Examples of Food Source |
|---|---|
| Insoluble: | |
| 1. Cellulose | Wheat |
| 2. Hemicellulose | Cereals, vegetables |
| 3. Lignins | Vegetables |
| Soluble: | |
| 1. Gums | Legumes, oats, barley |
| 2. Pectins | Citrus fruit |

As discussed in chapter 3, insoluble food fiber provides structural components of outer coverings and the interior of fruits and vegetables to give them support and resilience. They are not digestible and not soluble in water. Gums and pectins are forms of plant polysaccharides that do dissolve in water. The different types of dietary fiber have different effects on gastrointestinal function.

**Actions of Insoluble Food Fiber on the Gastrointestinal Tract**

Because fiber increases the volume or bulk in food, there is a greater feeling of fullness in the stomach when high-fiber foods are eaten. In the small and large intestine, cellulose and hemicellulose fiber absorbs water and adds to stool weight. Passage through the intestines is faster and more smooth and regular. This latter effect is also accentuated by lignins. The benefits of these effects are:

(1) Greater satisfaction of appetite
(2) Prevention of constipation and hemorrhoids
(3) Reduced incidence of colon cancer
(4) Reduced incidence of diverticulosis and diverticulitis

Many authorities believe that the laxative action of food fiber decreases back pressure on rectal veins during bowel movements. This helps to prevent rectal varicose veins (hemorrhoids). The laxative effect also reduces the time of exposure of the colon to cancer-producing chemicals (carcinogens) and, on this basis, may decrease the incidence of colon cancer. More primitive countries in the world which have much higher intakes of unprocessed food and food fiber have a lower incidence of colon cancer. These nations also have a lower intake of dietary fat than Western populations. The combinations of reduced fat (a possible source of colon carcinogens) and high food fiber consumption are probably important factors in this protection.

Diverticula are weaknesses or out-pouchings of the intestinal wall. If they become inflamed (diverticulitis), infection and bleeding may result. Gastroenterologists generally agree that high-fiber foods may prevent the frequency of diverticulitis by promoting faster intestinal passage of softer stool.

**Benefits of Soluble Food Fiber**

Gums, pectins and, to some extent, insoluble lignins have other effects of potential benefit. In the small intestine, these fibers coat the inner surface. This may delay rates of glucose absorption in patients with diabetes and reduce the height of blood sugar concentrations after a meal. These types of fibers also bind cholesterol-rich bile acids in the small intestine. Such binding prevents their reabsorption back into the blood stream. Blood cholesterol levels may be reduced by this action.

**General Comments**

The average American consumes about 15 to 20 grams of food fiber daily. This is approximately one-half the amount taken in by people in underdeveloped countries. In chapter 13 the recommended level is up to 35 to 40 grams per day. This increase should be done gradually to give the intestinal tract the chance to adjust. A sudden increase often leads to too much intestinal gas and abdominal distension and discomfort.

Purchase of food fiber tablets or other similar supplements is neither necessary nor desirable. They usually do not contain all five fiber types, they are often expensive, and they do not have the nutritive value, including vitamins and minerals, present in natural food sources of fiber.

Individuals with preexisting intestinal ailments should consult their physicians before changing to high-fiber diets. There may be adverse side effects in some situations. Obese subjects on low-calorie diets must be careful not to take in too much food fiber, since there may be impaired absorption of vital nutrients. This may be exaggerated when food intake is cut down. To avoid this problem, the American Diabetes Association recommends that *no more than 25 grams of food fiber be consumed per 1,000 calories of a weight reduction meal plan* (see table 6).

Much more research needs to be done on food fiber. Present knowledge suggests that we need more of it in our diets and that it is beneficial to

both nonobese and obese individuals. A comprehensive list of fiber content in various foods appears in later sections of this monograph.

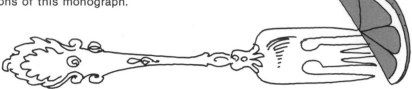

## TABLE 6: DIETARY RECOMMENDATIONS FOR ADULTS BY THE AMERICAN HEART ASSOCIATION, AMERICAN DIABETES ASSOCIATION AND NATIONAL RESEARCH COUNCIL/NATIONAL ACADEMY OF SCIENCES (NRC/NAS)

| FOOD CONSTITUENT | AMERICAN HEART ASSOCIATION[a] | AMERICAN DIABETES ASSOCIATION[b] | NRC/NAS[c] |
|---|---|---|---|
| Carbohydrate | At least 50-55% of total calories with emphasis on increased complex carbohydrates. | Up to 55-60% of total calories. Emphasis on unrefined carbohydrate with fiber. | Eat more high-fiber foods such as whole grain cereals, fruits and vegetables. |
| Fat | Total fat intake should be less than 30% of total calories. Saturated fat should be less than 10% of total calories. Cholesterol not to exceed 300 mg/day. | Ideally total fat should be less than 30% of total calories, and cholesterol <300 mg/day. Saturated fat should be <10% of total calories, polyunsaturated fat 6-8% and the remainder as monounsaturated fat. | Reduce fat intake to 30% of total calories. |
| Protein | 15% of total calories. | 0.8 g/kg body weight (0.36 g/pound). | _____ |
| Sodium | Not to exceed 3,000 mg/day. | 1,000 mg per 1,000 Kcalories of food, not to exceed 3,000 mg/day. | Eat moderately of salt-cured, smoked and nitrate-cured foods. |
| Food Fiber | Select foods providing soluble and insoluble food fiber. | Up to 40 g/day. 25 g/1,000 Kcalories for persons on low-calorie diets. | 20-30 g/day, not to exceed 35 g/day. |

[a]Nutrition Committee, American Heart Association, "Dietary Guidelines for Healthy American Adults," *Circulation* 77 (1988):721A-724A.

[b]Committee on Food and Nutrition, American Diabetes Association, "Nutritional Recommendations and Principles for Individuals with Diabetes Mellitus," *Diabetes Care* 10 (1987):126-132.

[c]Committee on Diet, Nutrition and Cancer. Assembly of Life Sciences National Research Council, National Academy of Sciences. *Diet, Nutrition and Cancer.* Washington, D.C.: National Academy Press, 1982.

# Chapter 6: What Is the Ideal Diet?

## The Ideal Diet: A General Definition

What is the ideal diet? Everyone agrees that it should provide enough calories to sustain a desirable weight. It should be nutritious with appropriate amounts of vitamins, minerals and protein. It should be pleasant, tasty and not monotonous. Above all, it should not be injurious to one's health.

Table 5 lists recommended dietary allowances for total calories, protein, vitamins and certain minerals for children, adults, and pregnant and lactating women. This information is revised periodically by the Food and Nutrition Board, National Academy of Sciences–National Research Council. There is no controversy over these figures, and they do compare favorably with published recommendations of similar groups in Canada and many European countries. Most adults in developed countries have no difficulty meeting these requirements.

What, then, is wrong with the American diet? Nutritionists and epidemiologists continue to tell us that we are not eating right.

## Criticism #1: Too Much Refined Sugar

A typical American meal contains about 46% of total calories as carbohydrate, 12% as protein and 42% as fat. What's astounding is that one-half of the carbohydrate calories is in the form of refined sugar (sucrose). In the United States, the per capita consumption of sugar is three-tenths of a pound daily or 100 pounds per year! Much of it is found in soft drinks, bakery goods, candy and other desserts. However, substantial amounts also are contained in modern cereals, toppings, sauces, canned soups and fruits, frozen dinners and other processed foods.

### The Case Against Refined Sugar

There is no question that excessive intake of sugar promotes tooth decay. No other health problems can be directly linked to its use. On the other hand, too much refined sugar becomes a substitute for other forms of dietary carbohydrate that are superior from a nutritional standpoint. The potential disadvantages of this are:

(1) Calories in refined sugar are concentrated in a small volume and satisfy appetite less well than a comparable amount of calories as carbohydrate in fruits and vegetables and starches, such as breads and cereals.
(2) Refined sugar offers no additional sources of vitamins and minerals in contrast to natural, unprocessed fruits and vegetables.
(3) Refined sugar has no dietary food fiber unlike many natural carbohydrate-containing foods.

Although there is no scientific justification for banning refined sugar from our diets, there is a strong argument for reducing its consumption in favor of substituting dietary carbohydrate contained in other foods of greater nutritive value.

## Criticism #2: Too Much and the Wrong Kind of Dietary Fat

It is estimated that 125 pounds of fat are eaten by each American each year. Not only is too much fat consumed (often over 40% of total daily calories) but the percentage of saturated fat derived from animal sources is too high relative to unsaturated fat from vegetables. We are also told that along with too much fat consumption cholesterol intake is too high.

### The Case Against Too Much Dietary Fat

Health experts now believe that too much and the wrong kind of fat in diets may be a major factor contributing to disease and death from atherosclerosis in the Western World. Atherosclerosis (hardening of the arteries) eventually restricts or blocks blood flow through a major vessel. In the case of myocardial infarction, stoppage of circulation through coronary arteries that supply heart muscle leads to heart attacks and often death. Strokes are frequently the consequence of occlusion of arteries supplying blood to the brain, whereas similar lesions involving the kidney may result in hypertension and kidney failure. Diabetics are especially prone to these problems as well as to peripheral obstruction of vessels to the lower extremities, a situation that predisposes to gangrene.

The atherosclerotic process begins as a streak or plaque on the inner surface of an artery, which then progresses to more thickening until the lumen within the vessel is totally obliterated. The composition of these lesions is primarily fat, including cholesterol and triglyceride. There is now good evidence that some, if not most, of this fat comes from the blood and lodges in these arterial sites where the damage occurs.

Although the atherosclerotic plaque is the product of a very complex series of events, there is now evidence that dietary manipulations can influence its progression. Studies of nonhuman primates, like the monkey, as well as man himself have shown the reduction of total dietary fat content and restriction of food cholesterol intake can reverse early atherosclerosis. It also has been documented that increasing the proportion of unsaturated fat relative to saturated fat helps to reduce blood cholesterol. Thus, it appears that good arguments for changing the amount and composition of fat in the average American diet are emerging.

## Criticism #3: Too Much Sodium

This is a most controversial area, and there is no uniform agreement among nutrition experts. The Food and Nutrition Board, National Academy of Sciences–National Research Council, recommends that between 1,100 and 3,300 milligrams of sodium intake daily is safe and adequate for most human needs (see table 6). The American Medical Association considers a moderate consumption of sodium to be 4,800 milligrams per day.[1]

Sodium is everywhere in our diets. Approximately one-third is added to food by consumers as common table salt or sodium chloride. One teaspoon containing 6 grams or 6,000 milligrams of salt is 40% sodium (2.4 grams or 2,400 milligrams). Another one-third is added by industry to processed food as salt, meat tenderizers, monosodium glutamate, etc. Another one-third occurs naturally in unprocessed food.

The average American has a widely varying intake of sodium, but estimates range between 2,300 and 6,900 or more milligrams per day. Thus, portions of our population are exceeding the upper limits of adequate or moderate amounts as recommended above.

### Too Much Concern Over Too Much Sodium?

Sodium is a very important component of body fluids and helps to maintain plasma volume, cell membrane electrical activity, and a variety of chemical reactions. In healthy individuals, there is a great capacity to rid the body of excess sodium and to conserve it when intake is low or losses are excessive.

Limitation of sodium intake is appropriate in individuals with heart disease (congestive heart failure), advanced forms of kidney failure, certain forms of liver disease, and hypertension. Dietary guidelines are focusing primarily on the possible link between excessive sodium intake and hypertension. This is where the controversy primarily exists.

As reviewed elsewhere,[2] some researchers have documented a relationship between levels of sodium consumption and incidence of hypertension in the United States. About 15% of Americans are afflicted with high blood pressure. The proponents of greater salt restriction suggest that this prevalence may fall with reduced sodium intake. The conservative experts take the position that individuals without hypertension need not reduce their salt consumption.[2] As we shall see, there is a prudent way to approach this controversy and provide sensible guidelines for use of sodium in our diets.

## Dietary Goals for the United States

In 1977 the Select Committee on Nutrition and Human Needs of the U.S. Senate issued a report entitled "Dietary Goals for the United States."[3] Several prominent senators on this committee deliberated several months while obtaining input from health officials, nutritionists and other scientists. Six objectives were developed to improve eating habits and the health of the nation in an effort to reduce nutrition-related disease. Briefly, they include the following:

(1) Increase carbohydrate consumption from the present 40% of total caloric intake to 55 to 60%. This carbohydrate should be obtained mostly from fruit, vegetables and natural grain products (starches and natural fruit sugars in foods with a higher-fiber content).

(2) Reduce total dietary fat from 40% to 30% of the total caloric intake.

(3) Reduce saturated fat intake to 10% of total calories and provide 20% of total calories as unsaturated fat.

(4) Reduce cholesterol consumption to 300 milligrams per day (Note: One egg contains approximately 250 milligrams.)

(5) Reduce refined sugar from 25% to 15% of total calories in the diet.

(6) Decrease salt consumption from the present range of 6 to 18 grams per day to 3 grams daily.

(Author's note: Point 6 was confusing to some reviewers of these objectives. The recommended salt intake did not take into account salt contained naturally in unprocessed foods.[2] This adds an additional one-third or a total recommended daily intake of about 4½ grams of salt or 1,800 milligrams of sodium.)

## Further Refinements of Dietary Goals

In more recent years three prominent groups have given the public their specific positions on what good dietary goals should be. They are presented side by side in table 6. The American Heart Association emphasizes its dietary recommendations in order to reduce cardiovascular disease. A similar goal is implicit in the recommendations

[1]Council on Scientific Affairs, American Medical Association, *Journal of the American Medical Association* 242 (1979):2335.

[2]M.J. Fregley, "Sodium and Potassium," in *Present Knowledge in Nutrition*, 5th ed. (Washington, D.C.: Nutrition Foundation, Inc., 1984), pp. 439-58.

[3]Catalog No. Y 4.N95:D 63/3. (Washington, D.C.: Government Printing Office).

by the American Diabetes Association. In addition, improved metabolic control of the diabetic patient is an objective. The third set of guidelines, published by the National Academy of Sciences–National Research Council, focuses on the potential value of a high-fiber, low-fat diet in preventing cancer of the colon. Not only are the dietary recommendations of the three groups similar, but they appear to be in very good agreement with those of the U.S. Senate Committee on Nutrition and Human Needs published in 1977. All these guidelines have been considered in the meal plans formulated for weight reduction as well as weight maintenance for the TOPS membership (see part 4).

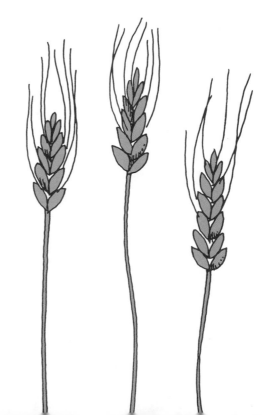

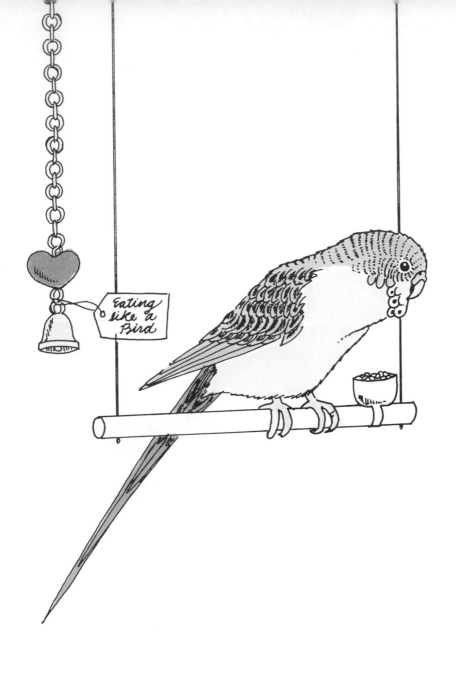

# PART THREE:
# Problems with Quick Weight-Loss Schemes

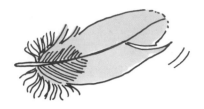

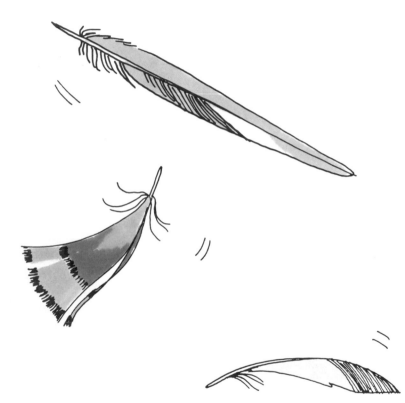

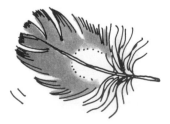

# Chapter 7: Facts and Fancy about Quick Weight-Loss Diets

During the past several years a great number of diets have been thrown to the public in a sensational fashion. They find their way into books, magazines, newspapers, television and radio. Most have catchy titles and claims that are appealing to the desperately obese. After a brief period they fall into obscurity only to be reshuffled under a different name and offered again to the public as a new final word in weight control.

There are so many fad diet schemes that space does not permit an individual discussion of each. Instead, the various types are defined together with opinions regarding their safety and effectiveness.

## Very Low Calorie Diets

These meal plans restrict calories to 300 to 500 calories per day and are usually in the form of a liquid formula administered three times daily. In one type, amino acids derived from protein are the sole source of calories, the so-called "protein-supplemented fast." An example is *The Last Chance Diet* (R. Linn; New York, Lyle Stuart, Inc., 1976). In another type, smaller amounts of amino acids are combined with carbohydrate in the formula. Examples are Optifast,® introduced in 1974 by The Delmark Co., Inc. (now Sandoz Nutrition), Minneapolis, and the Cambridge Diet, released by the Cambridge Diet Plan, Monterey, California, in 1980. They emphasize a high fluid intake together with vitamin and mineral supplements.

## Risks vs. Benefits of Very Low Calorie Diets

The strategy behind this approach is to promote a faster rate of fat tissue breakdown by severely limiting calories. These plans promote ketosis. Fatty acids released by fat tissue at this brisk rate are circulated to the liver, where they are converted to betahydroxybutyric and acetoacetic acids (ketone bodies). When this conversion is exaggerated, ketones pile up in the blood and eventually appear in the urine. Ketosis supposedly suppresses appetite and the craving for food.

Most experts agree that this form of dieting has no place in the routine management of obesity. Recommendations are to restrict their use to very obese individuals whose health risks for maintaining their weight outweigh the risks of adverse side effects that may occur with severe caloric restriction. Ideally, these plans should be implemented in a hospital, and patients should be followed by physicians and medical personnel who are familiar with the potential dangers.

Unfortunately, this was not done in the 1970s when these types of diets reached peak popularity in the United States. The Food and Drug Administration (FDA) estimated that millions of Americans were following protein-supplemented fasts with little or no medical supervision. Many commercial products were nutritionally poor in essential amino acids. By 1978 over 50 deaths were reported in association with their use.[1] Results of 13 autopsies were made available to the FDA, and in eight cases either degeneration or inflammation of heart muscle was found.

Supporters of the very low calorie diets containing both carbohydrate and protein argue that their diet plans cannot be compared to protein-supplemented fasts. They claim blood acid (ketones) buildup is less, physical endurance is better, and rates of weight loss are comparable. This remains controversial, however. To their credit, researchers who developed formulations that were subsequently marketed as Optifast or the Cambridge Diet evaluated long-term success rates. As reviewed by Howard,[2] they were disappointing. After discontinuing the very low calorie regimens, very few maintained their lost weight and the majority regained most of what they lost. To what extent a more intense follow-up with behavior modification and nutrition education can improve the success rate remains to be determined.

Regardless of the composition of very low calorie diets, side effects do occur and are reviewed below for the benefit of the reader.

(1) *Dehydration.* Very low calorie diets promote a brisk water and salt loss from excessive urination. This leads to a reduced, contracted blood volume. The initial quick weight losses observed are illusionary, since much of it is due to increased water excretion and not tissue weight reduction.

(2) *Light headedness, dizziness and occasionally fainting.* Because of reduced blood volume, circulation is impaired to the head, particularly during changes in posture or exercise. Blood

[1]"Protein Diets," *FDA Drug Bulletin* 8 (January-February 1978): 1-4. Catalog No. Y 4.N95:D 63/3. (Washington, D.C.: Government Printing Office).

[2]A.N. Howard, "The Historical Development, Efficacy and Safety of Very-Low-Calorie Diets," *International Journal of Obesity* 5 (1981):195-208.

pressure may become quite low. This can be very hazardous to individuals with preexisting heart or peripheral vascular disease in whom circulation to heart, brain or limbs may be already reduced.

(3) *Fatigue and difficulty carrying out daily tasks.*

(4) *Blood salt imbalances.* Excessive losses of sodium, potassium and calcium may occur. Bone mineral may be reduced. Excessive acid accumulation from fat tissue breakdown (ketosis) may occur, particularly in severely dehydrated subjects.

(5) *Gout.* This form of arthritis may occur rarely in those whose blood uric acid levels rise too high when ketosis is established and uric acid excretion in the urine becomes impaired.

(6) *Scalp hair loss and dry skin.* This usually reverses when normal eating patterns are resumed.

(7) *Nausea and constipation.* In addition, acute gallbladder attacks or inflammation of the pancreas may afflict those who resume normal or excessive eating too quickly after following very low calorie diets.

(8) *Muscle cramps and wasting.* This is due to water and electrolyte disturbances and the low calorie intakes.

(9) *Heart rhythm disturbances.* Cardiac effects like these have not been common.

While it is fortunate that most of these side effects are not frequent, the sensitivity to very low calorie diets varies a great deal from one person to the next. No one can predict when and in whom they will occur.

The FDA and others warn that children, pregnant women, and individuals with heart, blood vessel, kidney and lung disorders as well as those with liver disease should not follow these diets. Patients taking water and blood pressure pills, lithium, insulin or oral agents for diabetes, asthma medicines or significant doses of cortisone are also at high risk for harmful effects.

## Unbalanced Low-Calorie Diets

These meal plans are less restricted in calories (often 1,000 calories or more per day) but are very severely reduced in one or more food types. Low-carbohydrate diets are among the most commonly promoted in this class.

For example, *The Doctor's Quick Weight Loss Diet* (I.M. Stillman and S.S. Baker, Englewood Cliffs, N.J., Prentice Hall, 1967) and *Dr. Atkins' Diet Revolution* (R.C. Atkins, New York, David McKay Publishers, 1972) lower carbohydrate to less than 10% of total calories. This is in contrast to a 50 to 55%

proportion of carbohydrate in balanced meal plans. In the Stillman diet, protein and fat both exceed 40% of total calories, while in Atkins' regimen over 70% of calories is fat.[3]

Because of the marked carbohydrate restriction, these plans also promote ketosis. The "quick weight loss" is also primarily due to excessive water elimination. Side effects are similar to those found with the use of very low calorie diets that were discussed earlier. The principal criticism of this approach is that it is an abnormal departure from good eating habits and does not provide a long-term example for sensible nutrition or weight control. In the case of the Atkins and Stillman diets, the high fat content is contrary to current national recommendations for fat intake of less than 30% of total calories. In many instances, the transition back to normal eating is difficult. As soon as carbohydrate content is raised, water is retained, appetite returns, and both water and fat weight may be rapidly regained.

Since there are no scientific evaluations to indicate that these diets are either sensible or successful for long-term weight control, there is little to recommend low-carbohydrate ketogenic diets.

## Other Unbalanced Meal Plans

*The Beverly Hills Diet* (J. Mazel, New York, Berkley Books, 1982) is an example of a fruit diet. The sole emphasis of one food group deprives the individual of any meaningful fat and protein intake, and almost all calories are derived from fruit carbohydrate (over 80%).[3] Thus, over a long period of time a serious protein deficiency could result. From a nutritional standpoint this is another meal plan that also has been severely criticized by experts in the field. Other examples of unbalanced meal plans that deemphasize basic food groups are numerous, ill-advised and frequently appear in the lay press.

## Balanced Low-Calorie Diets

Most meal plans that exceed 1,000 calories per day and have ample amounts of carbohydrate, protein and fat are generally regarded as safe to follow. In this monograph only balanced weight-reduction diets in the range of the 1,200 to 1,800 calories per day are recommended and described. Appropriate proportions of carbohydrate, protein and fat assure good nutrition. When a weight goal is reached, the same proportions continue at higher caloric level to maintain ideal weight. In this way, good eating habits over the long term can be established.

[3]M.C. Fisher and P.A. LaChance, "Nutrition Evaluation of Published Weight-Reducing Diets," *Journal of the American Dietetic Association* 85 (1985):451-55.

## Recommendations to TOPS members

(1) Very low calorie diets (600 calories per day or less) are not recommended for the routine treatment of obesity. The risks of adverse side effects outweigh the short-term benefits of rapid weight loss. These regimens are reserved for individuals with massive obesity in whom deterioration of health demands an urgent, drastic approach. Only physicians experienced with this type of treatment should be involved in the management of such cases.

(2) Unbalanced weight-reduction diets that severely restrict basic nutrients such as carbohydrate or protein should be avoided.

(3) Meal plans that contain over 1,000 calories per day and which are balanced in high-quality carbohydrate, protein and fat are the most desirable and sensible plans to follow.

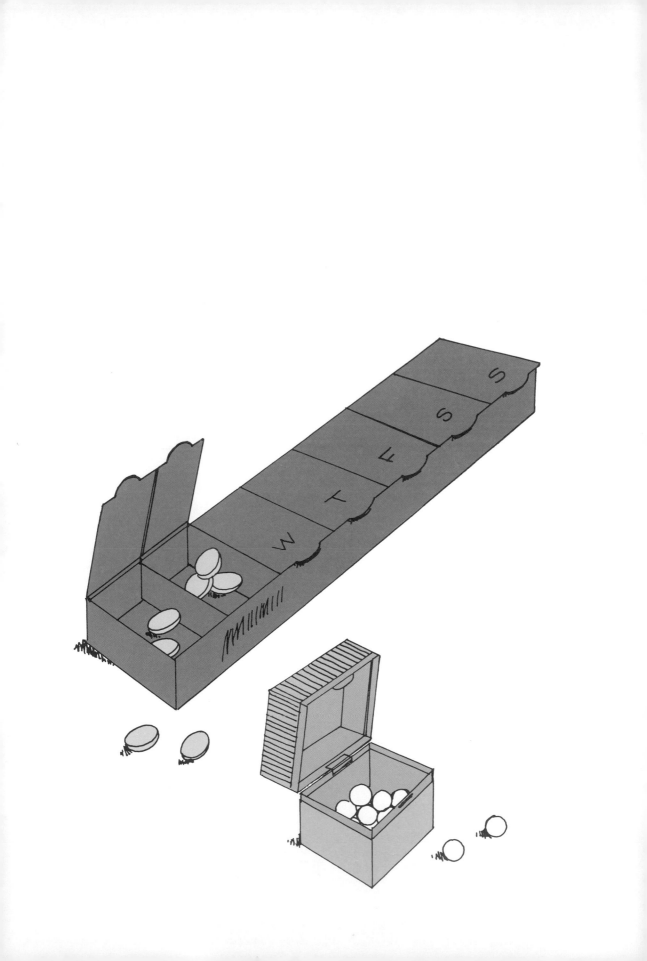

# Chapter 8: Drugs, Gadgets and Surgery

## Drugs

### Amphetamines

These are the so-called pep pills that were used for years to control appetite and promote weight reduction. As central nervous system stimulants, however, they also had a great many undesirable side effects, including addiction. The FDA banned their use in weight control for these reasons.

### Over-the-Counter Diet Pills

Nonprescription diet pills are a big business, are advertised extensively and are sold under a variety of trade names in pharmacies. They include Acutrim,® Dexatrim,® Stay Trim,® etc. All contain phenylpropanolamine (PPA). The FDA allows it to be sold without prescription if the total daily dose is 75 milligrams or less.

What is PPA? PPA is related to amphetamine but, unlike the latter, it is not addictive. These amine compounds are central nervous system stimulants, increase heart rate, constrict blood vessels and open air passages. PPA is also found in a large number of cold remedies because it is a decongestant. Although they have weak appetite suppressant properties, they do not promote weight loss over and above diet alone.

There are problems with PPA. Although there may be some short-term effects on appetite, tolerance rapidly develops and safe doses are no longer effective. Other problems include adverse side effects. In certain sensitive individuals, these agents may increase blood pressure and heart rate to abnormally high levels. They should not be taken by individuals who already have high blood pressure, diabetes or cardiovascular disease. PPA in diet pills may accidentally increase exposure to the drug if someone is taking a cold remedy or nasal decongestant that also contains PPA. If someone is considering them, a physician should be consulted first, especially if other medications are being taken. Ill effects from interactions of PPA with other drugs can occur.

The American Medical Association has taken the position that over-the-counter diet pills have no important role in weight reduction.

### Water Pills

Water pills or diuretics with significant action can only be prescribed by a physician. Some are more potent than others. Unfortunately, this class of medications is among the more commonly abused among obese people who want to show a weight loss.

The weight loss is actually false and relates to water elimination and not to true fat tissue weight reduction. If taken too aggressively, dehydration, low blood pressure, excessive salt losses, weakness and many other ill effects can occur. Weight is rapidly regained once salt and water losses are replenished to a normal level.

There are legitimate reasons for physicians to administer diuretics to individuals. They are useful agents for controlling edema or swelling that is a complication of heart, kidney and liver failure. They are also useful in the control of high blood pressure. However, they should never be used by individuals with obesity who are otherwise healthy and who simply want to register a temporary weight loss.

### Thyroid

It is easy to understand why so many people believe that obesity is a problem of low metabolism or sluggish burning of calories. Since thyroid hormone controls our metabolic rates, they reason that obesity should be treated with thyroid medications. Rev up the metabolism, so to speak. Nothing could be further from the truth even though some overweight individuals continue to abuse its use.

Thyroid hormone (thyroxine) and related derivatives (triiodothyronine) are manufactured by several pharmaceutical firms and have many trade names. The only indication for their use is the treatment of hypothyroidism (low thyroid function) and certain types of enlarged thyroid glands (goiters). No competent physician would prescribe thyroid unless these conditions are documented by examination and appropriate laboratory tests. Most physicians also are aware that people with obesity have no greater incidence of thyroid problems than does the general population.

If any obese person is concerned about her or his thyroid status, a physician should be consulted and testing done. We emphasize that thyroid hormone should never be used in the treatment of obesity. It does not work and may be toxic if excessive amounts are taken.

### HCG Treatments

For many years it was popular for women with weight problems to seek physicians who administer injections of HCG (human chorionic gonadotropin) and place patients on low-calorie diets. This regimen was devised by a physician in the 1950s. It often is quite expensive and has no scientific basis whatever.

The TOPS research program extensively evaluated this treatment and found that HCG had no effect on weight loss over and above that achieved with diet alone.[1] Subsequently, the FDA took the position that HCG should not be used for weight control and requires all package inserts that come with the hormone to make that statement. HCG, a hormone made by the placenta of pregnant women, does have a place in the treatment of infertility problems but not obesity.

### Future Drug Therapy of Obesity

There is reason to be optimistic about the future development of safe medications that may control appetite. Current research is unraveling the very complex regulation of many vital centers in the brain, including those influencing appetite, mood and behavior. This involves the identification of several chemicals (neurotransmitters) and hormones that act alone or in combination to stimulate or suppress appetite. When this regulation is understood, safe, effective medications may be devised to set one's appestat at a level that insures weight reduction. At present it is unfortunate, but true, that there are no reliable, safe ways to control appetite and obesity through prolonged drug therapy.

## Obesity "Remedies"

These approaches as cure-alls for obesity appear and disappear from the scene at such an astonishing rate that it is difficult to keep up with the parade of products. The reason for their rapid rise and fall in popularity is that none of them works. If weight loss is achieved, it is due to the diet and/or exercise program that is followed and not the remedy.

Most of them are introduced through television, newspaper or magazine ads. Many are supported by articles or accompanying brochures written by "doctors" or "nutritionists" whose backgrounds in science, medicine and nutrition are marginal at best. It is difficult for a lay person to discriminate between their persuasive, misleading scientific jargon and statements made by legitimate experts in the field.

The list of worthless remedies is endless. Some of them appearing in recent years include obscure herbs, teas or potions imported from foreign lands, algae-protein tablets, amino acid tablets, coenzyme pills, other special vitamin and mineral preparations, a variety of plant extracts, patches that are soaked in solutions and applied to skin, etc. Many more will appear as the years go by and as long as there are people to buy them.

If these remedies are not very effective, why are they allowed to be sold with the claims they carry? As long as the product is harmless, its usefulness in the treatment of obesity is usually unchallenged. It would take an enormous amount of manpower (which the FDA does not have) to screen and evaluate every item like this that comes along. If harmful side effects do occur, the FDA moves swiftly to ban them. A case in point recently was the starch blocker pill, an inhibitor of intestinal starch digestion and absorption. Serious gastrointestinal ailments that related to its use resulted in prompt removal from store shelves.

## Gadgets

If a device that supposedly melts fat away sounds too good to be true, it probably is another gimmick to lure the public pocketbook. For example, neck-to-ankle plastic suits worn for long periods of time may cause a minimal, short-lived weight loss through excessive perspiration. When the suit is removed and liquids are drunk, the weight returns. Similarly, one cannot massage or pound fat away with exotic machines while a person reclines passively on a table. If some sort of mechanical approach to weight control is appealing to an individual, an investment in a good bicycle, rowing machine or other quality equipment that requires physical exertion is the only sensible solution. Any gadget that is claimed to take pounds off without exercise or dieting is ineffective and joins the ranks of ill-advised remedies discussed earlier.

## Medical Devices and Surgery

### Gastric Balloons

Qualified physicians in multicenter trials have been evaluating balloon devices in recent years. This technique requires the passage into the stomach of a balloon-like device which is subsequently inflated to partially fill the stomach. This prevents the obese subject from consuming large amounts of food at any given time.

However, preliminary experience with this method has been disappointing. Inflammation of the stomach, obstruction and other serious side effects have been reported. Rapid regaining of lost weight after the balloon is removed is another drawback. As a consequence, this approach to weight control is waning in popularity.

### Intestinal and Gastric Bypass Surgery

These procedures are reserved for massively obese individuals in whom all other attempts at weight reduction have failed and in whom obesity threatens health.

Jejunoileal bypass short-circuits the ileum of the small intestine. This removes a substantial portion of food-absorbing surface in an effort to decrease absorption of food. Although success

[1]Kaup R. Shetty and Ronald K. Kalkhoff, "Human Chorionic Gonadotropin (HCG) Treatment of Human Obesity," *Archives of Internal Medicine* 137 (1977):151.

has been reported with this operation, mortality rates average 4%, and post-operative as well as long-term complications are significant. They include infection, diarrhea, malabsorption of nutrients, vitamins and minerals, kidney stones, liver failure and intestinal obstruction.

An alternative procedure focuses on the stomach. Gastric bypass excludes 90% of the stomach. The upper 10%, which accepts food, is small and is connected through a small opening into the small intestine. A variation of this operation is gastroplasty. The upper 10% of the stomach is isolated and connected to the remainder of the stomach through a small channel. It has the advantage of being the easiest to reverse and restore the stomach to its normal anatomy if necessary.

Gastric bypass and gastroplasty have fewer complications than ileal bypass if the skill of the surgeon is comparable. The patient eats less because the gastric size has been reduced and cannot accommodate as much food. However, in all of these procedures the patient rarely drops below an obesity level of 50% above ideal body weight. For a morbidly obese patient, this still represents an achievement. Additional dieting and exercise are necessary if ideal weight goals are to be reached.

None of these surgical approaches is appropriate for individuals with uncomplicated obesity.

## Summary

An enormous amount of money is needlessly spent each year by obese adults in their endless search for an easy path to weight loss. There are none at present. There may be major breakthroughs in the future which will lead to better medical methods to control overweight.

Before spending money on what sounds like a great diet, drug, remedy or device, consult your physician or representative of your local county medical society.

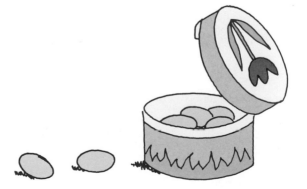

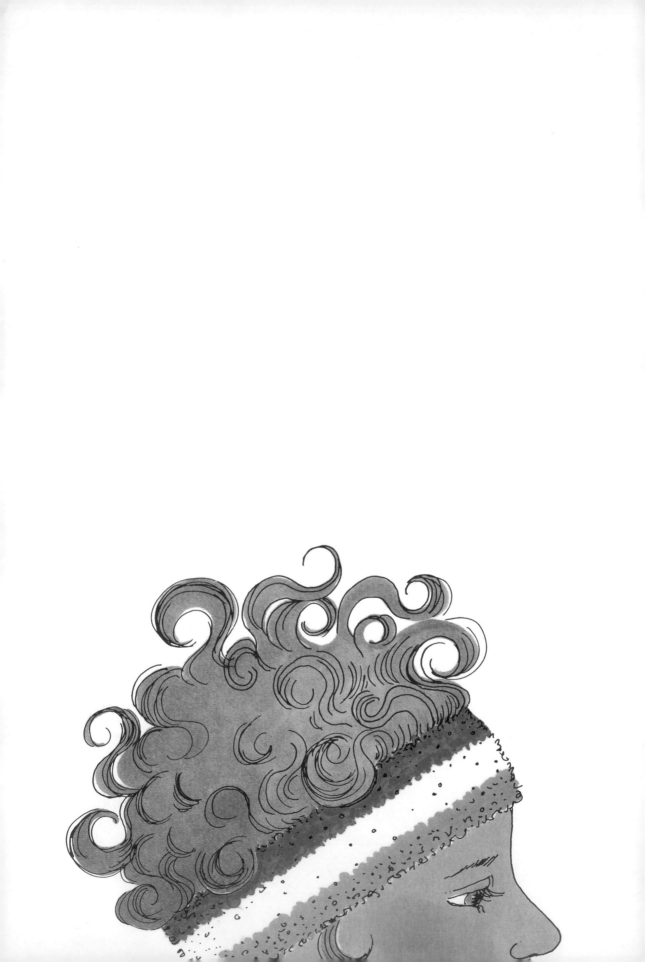

# PART FOUR:
## Taking Off Pounds Sensibly I:
## Steps To Take before Dieting

# Chapter 9: Four Important Steps To Take Before Dieting

It takes a long time to become very obese. It also takes a long time to lose those extra pounds. The excessive body fat expresses a lifestyle of over-eating relative to physical activity. Both eating and exercise habits have to be examined and corrected if any success story is going to emerge.

To accomplish your goal:

• You must want to lose weight. This requires a new attitude and motivation that must come from within. Don't start a long-term weight-reduction program unless your motivation level is strong. On the other hand, don't put off a serious try at weight reduction forever.

• Your problem with obesity is your responsibility. If you succeed, take full credit. If you do not succeed, don't blame failure on someone or something else.

• You will need help—from your physician and his or her professional colleagues, and from family, friends and TOPS.

• You should analyze your present lifestyle. By knowing what you are doing wrong, you can take steps to correct your mistakes.

• This also means becoming more informed about how to lose weight. That's what this monograph is all about.

• Once you know yourself and your mistakes and become more informed, you must become very objective and develop a new lifestyle to follow for the rest of your life and for a more healthy way to live.

• Changing your lifestyle consists of four basic steps:

Step 1: A medical evaluation and an on-going follow-up with your physician and other health professionals

Step 2: Developing a program of exercise

Step 3: A self-analysis of bad eating habits and ways of changing them

Step 4: Knowing what foods to avoid and what foods to consume

The chapters that follow discuss each of these four steps. If you take them in order and don't omit any one of them, your chances of success will be much greater. This will put you in a much better position to follow a meal plan and lose weight (see Part 5: Taking Off Pounds Sensibly II) and to maintain your desirable weight once your goal is reached (see Part 6: Keeping Off Pounds Sensibly).

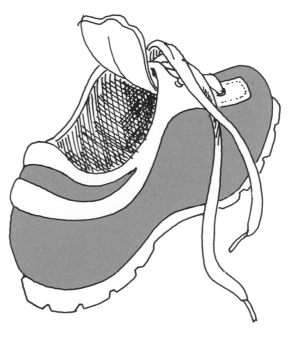

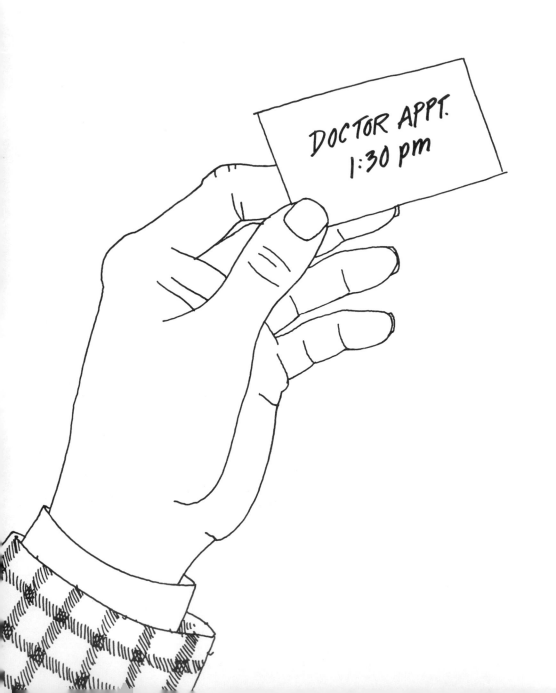

# Chapter 10: Step One: Consulting a Physician

## The Medical Evaluation

Correcting obesity should begin with a thorough medical evaluation by a physician. Obesity is associated with a number of health disorders that may be unrecognized without a physical examination and appropriate laboratory tests. Unless relative health is defined, a sensible program for meal planning and exercise cannot be prescribed.

A competent physician combines a detailed medical history with an extensive physical examination. Blood pressure measurements on obese individuals should always be done with a large cuff. Regular size wraparound cuffs frequently give an erroneously high reading on fleshy arms. Body weight and height as well as other vital signs also are recorded. The ensuing examination, including eye and nervous system assessments, should be thorough.

All women should have breast and pelvic examinations each year. The physician also may request mammograms. This is particularly important in obese women, since the incidence of breast and uterine cancer is higher than in the general population (see chapter 2). All men should have a prostate examination on a yearly basis.

## Laboratory Tests

The laboratory evaluation usually includes:

(1) Complete blood counts and a urinalysis
(2) A screening test for traces of blood in the stool
(3) Blood chemistries that measure glucose, triglycerides, cholesterol, uric acid, certain blood salts, creatinine and urea nitrogen (These are usually done after an overnight fast.)
(4) A two-hour, oral 75-gram glucose tolerance test, particularly in substantially obese people and/or patients with positive family histories of diabetes mellitus
(5) A chest film and electrocardiogram

Other tests may be ordered by the physician based on the assessment. If medical conditions are uncovered, they can be treated before or during the medical management of weight loss.

## Allied Health Professionals

Most TOPS members know of local clinics or community hospitals where additional help may be obtained for their weight-reduction program. Personal physicians can refer patients to them for specific problems.

(1) *Registered Dietitians (R.D.):* The term "registered" is important, since it signifies that these professionals are college-trained in all aspects of nutrition and are familiar with the exchange system. They can help individuals familiarize themselves with meal plans and answer questions about them. If necessary, they can make dietary readjustments for certain medical illnesses or help trouble-shoot problem areas. Avoid consultations with nutritionists and dietitians who are not registered.
(2) *Physical Therapists:* These individuals are usually hospital-based. Since exercise is a very important component of any weight management program, the physician may refer a patient to them for exercise training. In some instances a physical therapist may work with a heart specialist to help patients exercise within the limits of their heart disease. They are especially useful to overweight persons who have limited mobility because of arthritis, partial paralysis and related disorders. Special exercises can be taught to help trim and tone the body without undue stress to the patient.
(3) Other health professionals:

   *Pharmacists* can answer questions about medications you may be taking.

   *Registered Nurses* who often work with your personal physician may help you with problems that arise, particularly when your physician cannot be reached.

   *Psychologists (Ph.D.)* and *Psychiatrists (M.D.)* are available as consultants when emotional disorders are recognized by your doctor. By gaining insight into their cause and with appropriate psychotherapy, obese patients with mental stresses can face the challenges of weight reduction much better.

   *Social Workers* affiliated with your community hospital or local health agency are often valuable for seeking solutions to problems that arise in the home (marriage, family, economics) or at work. They help physicians to define the nature of the problem and guide patients to ways of resolving them.

TOPS Club, Inc., has always aligned itself with the medical profession. After the initial evaluation by a physician, it is a good idea to return to him or her at regular intervals for follow-up care. The medical team is an important component of weight management for all TOPS members.

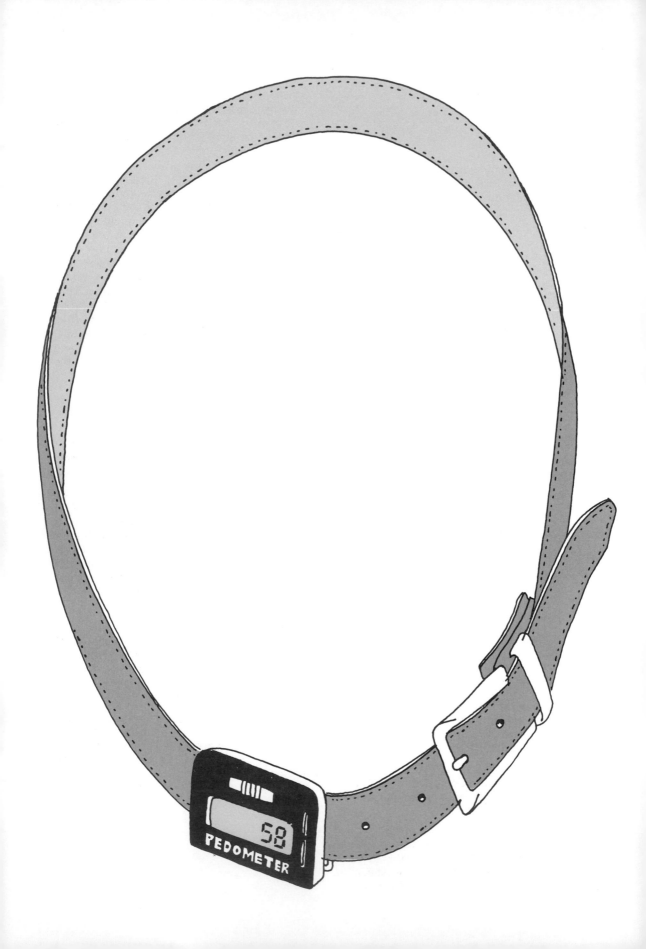

# Chapter 11: Step Two: Developing a Program of Exercise

Physical fitness is important to one's health. A regular exercise program is also a very valuable part of weight reduction when combined with sensible meal planning and caloric restriction. Once a desirable weight is reached, exercise also helps to preserve health and prevent regaining lost pounds.

For example, if one eats the same for one year but burns 300 extra calories during daily exercise, up to 20 additional pounds of weight may be lost during that time.

## Aerobic Exercise

A good aerobic exercise program requires use of most major muscles in the body. The physical exertion must be intense enough to raise pulse rate and breathing rate and cause some sweating. Examples of preferred aerobic exercises include walking, jogging, bicycling, calisthenics, aerobic dancing, swimming and cross-country skiing. The term "aerobic" implies exercising vigorously enough to breathe in more oxygen and burn the necessary calories to meet the energy needs of the physical activity.

Note: To gain any benefits from an exercise program, it should be done at least three times per week for a minimum of 20 minutes. If it is done only three times each week, it is preferable to workout every other day rather than on three consecutive days.

The advantages of an aerobic exercise program go beyond simply controlling weight and include:

• increased muscle tone and physical endurance
• improved strength of ligaments and bones
• improved heart and lung function
• improved feeling of well-being, self-confidence and alertness
• reduced nervous tension

## Preliminary Steps to Exercising

Before starting an exercise program it is best to consult a physician and have the medical evaluation outlined in chapter 10.

Based on these findings, a type of exercise tolerance test or "stress" electrocardiogram may be requested. This is essential in any individual with preexisting heart disease and is often requested in obese individuals who are over 40 years of age and have not exercised for long periods of time. This allows the physician to monitor the EKG tracing, pulse and breathing rates, and blood pressure during graded, well-controlled walking or running on a treadmill. In this way, safe limits of exercise can be defined.

## How To Begin

Select an exercise or exercises that are the most convenient and the most fun for you. Exercises that are boring or not attractive are doomed to failure. Reserve a regular time for the exercise in your daily routine. Also select the proper clothing. It should be comfortable, loose-fitting and light enough for warm months. During colder days, if exercise is done outside, it is better to wear two or more layers of lighter clothing than a single heavy layer.

For those who choose walking or jogging, footwear is very important. It is wise to invest in quality jogging or walking shoes (not tennis or deck shoes) that have cushioned soles, good arch supports and a soft, padded interior. There should always be ample room for the toes without tightness from above or the sides. The shoes should not slip over the back of the heel. The tops should be made of good material that allows the feet to "breathe" and ventilate. Be certain that both feet are carefully measured and fitted to the shoes you are buying.

## How To Exercise

Physical fitness experts recommend that regular exercise sessions begin with a mild, 5-minute "warm-up" or stretching session. This prepares muscle groups for the exercise and helps to prevent cramps, muscle pulls and other discomfort. Figures 3 to 7 illustrate various types of stretching maneuvers that are recommended.

As you begin your workout, do it gradually over the first few minutes until you reach full intensity. Then, as you approach the end of the exercise period, gradually reduce the intensity for the last few minutes. This is another way to prevent undue strain on working muscle groups. After the exercise is over, repeat the mild, 5-minute stretching routine during the "cooling off" interval.

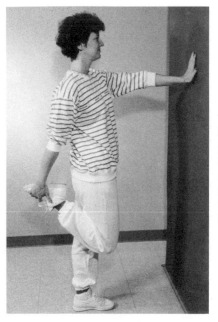

## FIGURE 3: FRONT THIGH STRETCH

This exercise stretches the front thigh muscles. Stand erect on one foot and balance yourself by placing one outstretched hand against a wall. Grasp the other foot with the opposite hand and slowly pull the leg upward towards your backside while keeping the knee pointing down towards the floor. Hold for 20 seconds. Repeat once more; then switch sides.

## FIGURE 4: CALF STRETCH

This exercise stretches the calf muscles. Place both outstretched hands against a wall at eye level. Bend one leg at the knee and place it near the wall. Extend the opposite leg straight back with the heel on the floor and bear most of your weight on it. Next, lean into the wall with your forehead coming close to your hands as you bend your elbows. Hold for 20 seconds. Repeat a few times and do the opposite side.

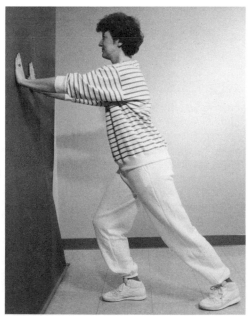

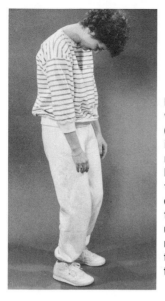

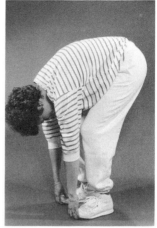

## FIGURE 5: ROLL DOWN

Begin by spreading the feet apart to shoulder width with knees bent slightly and head down (left panel). Slowly bend down in steps, starting with the shoulders and upper back, middle back and lower back as you bend your knees. Eventually bring your hands close to the side of your shoes with your head tucked down (right panel). Hold for 20 seconds and then slowly roll up again (with the knees flexed) until you reach the starting position. Stay as relaxed as possible. This exercise stretches the shoulder, back, buttocks and posterior thigh muscles.

## FIGURE 6: LOWER BACK AND SPINE STRETCH

Lie on the floor. Curl arms around the legs behind the knees. Pull knees toward your chest with legs flexed and head on the floor. Then gradually curl the head toward the knees. Repeat several times to loosen the back muscles.

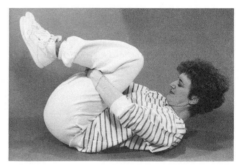

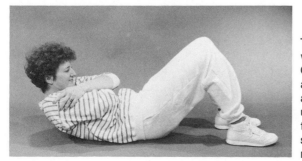

## FIGURE 7: ABDOMINAL CURL-UP

To stretch the abdominal muscle, lie on the floor with legs flexed and both feet flat on the floor. Cross the arms across the chest. Raise your head and place chin as close to your chest as possible and hold it there. Raise your shoulder blades and upper back off the floor on a 30 degree angle and then curl back down. Do this several times. You should feel muscle stretching in the upper abdomen and upper back.

## Target Heart Rates

No matter what exercise is done, target heart rates should be determined. Unless you achieve a certain range of heart rate, the aerobic exercise is not nearly as meaningful, and true physical conditioning and caloric expenditure may not be very significant.

To measure heart rate, one takes the radial pulse in beats per minute. Figure 8 shows you how to find the radial pulse on the wrist. To practice, count the number of pulse beats for 10 seconds. Multiply this number by 6 and you will have your heart rate in beats per minute. For example, if your radial pulse is 12 beats in 10 seconds, that is equivalent to 12 x 6 = 72 beats in 60 seconds or 1 minute. Your heart rate is 72 per minute. This is approximately the average heart rate for an adult at rest.

Keep track of your resting heart rate. As physical conditioning takes effect, this value decreases to ranges as low as 50 to 60 per minute. Indeed, long distance runners may have values under 50 per minute. Major changes in resting heart rates frequently take several weeks to achieve and only after consistent exercising. A lower resting heart rate indicates that your heart is stronger and pumping more efficiently.

Most people do not know how fast their heart rate should be during good aerobic exertion. Experts advise that people should achieve a rate that is somewhere between 60% and 80% of maximum heart rate. The maximum heart rate is an estimate of what is achieved during extreme exercise near a point of exhaustion in an individual who is breathing in maximal amounts of oxygen. This value is estimated according to one's age, and an example is given below:

(1) Individual's age is 40 years old.

(2) Maximum heart rate is 220 minus age.
    (220 – 40 = 180 beats per minute)

(3) 60% (or 0.6) of 180 is 108 beats per minute.
    80% (or 0.8) of 180 is 144 beats per minute.

(4) Therefore, the desirable range for heart rate is 108 to 144 beats per minute during peak exercise in a 40-year-old person. The 10-second pulse rate range would be one-sixth of these values or 18 to 24 beats.

Table 7 gives the desirable or "target" heart rates per minute and their equivalent in 10-second rates for healthy subjects in various age groups. Select the age level that is closest to your own. If you are 53, pick the 55-year old values. If you are 62, select the 60-year old level, etc. These ranges represent the 60 to 80% fraction of maximum heart rate you should achieve during exercise.

### TABLE 7: DESIRABLE HEART RATES AND 10-SECOND PULSE RATES DURING AEROBIC EXERCISE

| AGE | HEART RATE RANGE (beats/min.) | 10-SECOND COUNT |
|---|---|---|
| 8-20 | 120-160 | 20-27 |
| 25 | 117-156 | 20-26 |
| 30 | 114-152 | 19-25 |
| 35 | 111-148 | 19-25 |
| 40 | 108-144 | 18-24 |
| 45 | 105-140 | 18-23 |
| 50 | 102-136 | 17-22 |
| 55 | 99-132 | 16-22 |
| 60 | 96-128 | 16-21 |
| 65 | 93-124 | 16-21 |
| 70 | 90-120 | 15-20 |

SOURCE: *Forward to Fitness: Wisconsin Governor's Council on Fitness and Health. September 1986. Document POH 4015, Madison, Wisconsin.*

*Note:* Individuals who are taking allergy or sinus medicine, blood pressure or heart medicine, and other types of medication may have increases or decreases in their resting heart rate. Their responses to exercise also may be different. Before using the desirable heart rate table, check

## FIGURE 8: RADIAL PULSE COUNT

Your wristwatch should be on the opposite wrist. To obtain a 10-second pulse count, place two fingers on the inner side of the opposite wrist at the level of the thumb. Count the number of pulse beats during a 10-second period on the wristwatch while exercising. Refer to table 7 for your desirable heart rate.

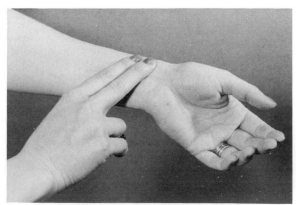

with your physician to see if any adjustments to your heart rate range are necessary.

It is a good idea to keep records of your resting heart rate, rates before exercise, and rates at peak exertion as well as after the "cooling down" period. The 10-second pulse rate is useful in this regard, since it may be obtained quickly while exercising by timing the number of pulse beats during any 10-second interval on your wristwatch. After a time you will have a better feel for how intense your exercise must be to reach the desirable range.

### Some Additional Suggestions

Those who are older and not in very good physical shape should begin their program slowly. Select the lower range of the "target" heart rate and limit your peak exercise to a brief period, perhaps 5 to 10 minutes. From there one can gradually prolong the period and raise the range of the heart rate. Eventually, try to sustain your exercise at least 20 minutes. If it is more comfortable, it is permissible to perform two 10-minute or four 5-minute exercises consecutively during one session to reach the minimum goal. Again, the exercises should be done no less than three times per week, preferably on alternate days.

• Do not exercise to the point of exhaustion. If weakness, chest pain, light headedness or other symptoms overcome you, stop the session.
• Avoid exercising out-of-doors in extreme temperatures such as very hot, humid weather or extremely cold weather.
• Do not hesitate to drink water before, in between or after exercising, especially during prolonged exertion when there is much perspiring.
• Allow at least two hours to elapse after eating a meal before you exercise.

If the program includes walking, jogging, bicycling or cross-country skiing, you might like an idea of the distances you are covering. In that way you can calculate your speed in miles per hour. If you have no idea about mileage, you can drive your car along the same route and take mileage from the odometer.

### Where To Exercise

It makes little difference where exercise is done as long as it is convenient, accessible and not expensive. Individuals who wish to exercise at home can use stationary bicycles, rowing machines and similar aerobic exercise equipment. Calisthenics or aerobic dancing can be done with or without direction from an exercise program on television. If the weather is bad, the walkers may wish to go to enclosed shopping malls, where they are often welcome. Local community parks, public schools, YMCAs and similar institutions often provide

adults their facilities for exercising of all types for a nominal fee.

### Walking

This form of exercise is probably the most popular among people of all ages and is particularly attractive to people over the age of 40 with weight problems. Any form of walking is beneficial, but if you are going to reach your target heart rates, a certain degree of intensity or briskness is required. Don't forget to do the same warm-up and cooling-down stretch exercises before and after your walks.

Walk erect, looking ahead, and swing your arms. Walk on a level surface at first and avoid bumpy, soft earth. Take long strides and maintain an even pace. A slow walk is 2 miles per hour. Begin with that if you are just starting. Eventually, if you are able, increase your speed to 3 miles per hour. True fitness walking is in the range of 4 miles per hour and should be your goal if you are physically able. At that rate you will burn twice as many calories as you would at 2 miles per hour if the distance is the same. Physical exertion is even greater and more calories are expended if hills are included in the walk.

Remember, the longer you walk, the faster you walk and the more hills you walk over, the greater your loss of calories will be. But don't overdo and keep within your target heart rate!

### How To Estimate Calories "Burned" During Exercise

This is difficult and is an estimate at best. Heavier persons will burn more calories doing the same exercise than lighter people, because it takes more work to move their bodies. The other big factor is the intensity and consistency of exercise. Golfing while riding on a cart and not carrying golf clubs represents much less physical effort than walking and carrying one's clubs. Certain sports like bowling are more intermittent and do not represent sustained aerobic exercise. They are less beneficial for that reason.

Table 8 lists calories burned for various types of physical activity. Look upon them as crude estimates with a great deal of individual variation.

### Those Other Activities: Don't Ignore Them!

Physical fitness experts also stress the importance of other forms of exercise that can be a part of the daily routine. Work around the home is the best example. Mowing the lawn, polishing the car, gardening, trimming the bushes, washing the windows, household repairs all contribute to physical well-being and burning calories.

For short distances, walking rather than driving

in a car can be substituted. Taking stairs rather than riding an elevator up a floor or two also helps.

Start thinking about all the ways you can become physically more active. It will pay many additional dividends in weight control.

## TABLE 8:
## CALORIES EXPENDED DURING COMMON EXERCISES

| ACTIVITY | CALORIES/MINUTE | CALORIES/HOUR |
|---|---|---|
| Sleeping or reclining | 1 | 60 |
| Sitting or standing | 1-2 | 60-120 |
| Light housework | 2-2½ | 120-180 |
| Level walking, 2 miles/hour | 2½-4 | 150-240 |
| Moderate housework<br>Bowling<br>Bicycle riding, 6 miles/hour<br>Walking, 3 miles/hour | 4-5 | 240-300 |
| Heavy housework<br>Golf, carrying clubs<br>Many calisthenics<br>Aerobic dancing<br>Walking, 3½ miles/hour<br>Bicycle riding, 8 miles/hour<br>Badminton and volleyball | 5-6 | 300-360 |
| Skating<br>Walking, 4 miles/hour<br>Bicycling, 10 miles/hour<br>Aerobic dancing, moderate | 6-7 | 360-420 |
| Tennis<br>Walking, 5 miles/hour<br>Bicycling, 11-12 miles/hour<br>Aerobic dancing,<br>   moderate to heavy<br>Cross-country skiing, moderate | 7-8 | 420-480 |
| Jogging, 5 miles/hour<br>Bicycling, 12 miles/hour<br>Sustained swimming<br>Rowing<br>Downhill skiing | 8-10 | 480-600 |
| Running, 6 miles/hour<br>Hardball<br>Squash<br>Basketball, football<br>Bicycling, over 12 miles/hour<br>Heavy rowing | Over 10 | 600 + |

NOTE: These are estimates and are influenced by the weight of the patient and the intensity of the exercise.

# Chapter 12: Step Three: A Self-Analysis of Bad Eating Habits and Ways of Changing Them

Take some time to decide what undesirable eating pattern best describes your present lifestyle. It may be a combination of those described below.

## The Daily Overeaters

### The Multimeal Overeater

This individual eats three square meals a day and may not be particularly prone to snacking between meals. Often the right kinds of foods may be consumed. The problem is eating too much, including generous desserts, at meal time. This type is frequently a "retired" athlete. At a younger age exercise and lots of physical activity were a daily routine. No weight was gained then. As the amount of physical activity declines and the food intake remains the same, weight is gradually gained and the bulges move in.

### The Nibbler

This person may eat properly at meal time. Between meals, however, small amounts of food are taken throughout the day and night—sometimes almost without thinking. The housewife or teenager grabs a cookie here and some candy there with each pass through the kitchen. Ditto for the man of the house at night or on weekends. At work it may be the tempting morsels placed next to the office coffee pot or the easily accessible small snacks in the vending machines or cafeterias. Whatever the source, the size of the snack may not be that great at any one time, but over a 24-hour period the number of nibbles can add up to that extra 300 or 400 calories that put on substantial amounts of new weight over a period of months or help to sustain too much weight in the first place.

### The Night-Eater

This individual has a more pronounced eating disorder. Overeating becomes a compulsion that begins in the late afternoon—after school or after work. It includes a heavy dinner and continuous snacking while sitting, usually in front of a television set, until bedtime. In the morning there is little desire to eat breakfast. A small lunch may be consumed. But as the end of the day approaches, the crescendo in appetite rapidly builds, and the pattern repeats itself. It is not uncommon to take in 2,000 or 3,000 calories or more during this four- to six-hour period at night by those who have significant weight problems.

## The Periodic Overeaters

### The Socializers and Other Weekly Goal-Missers

The socializers follow their weight-reduction programs most of the time. But one or two days out of the week social functions enter the picture. In its simplest form it may be eating out at a restaurant with family or friends. Among many women it is the clubs, bridge, church groups and other get-togethers where there is open competition for each hostess to serve the most elaborate and calorie-dense food. Among men there are similar social groups where food and beverage levels also run high. The difficulty is saying "no" to the caravan of calories.

Related situations find business men and women entertaining clients or being entertained by others at luncheons or dinners as part of their work. Or it may be a holiday season when good will, good food and drink are everywhere among relatives and friends.

There is nothing wrong with socializing. Unfortunately, the extra food exposure becomes too much to resist. Any headway made on a diet at home for that week may be totally reversed by these occasions "out on the town" if they occur often enough and too much food is eaten. Most socializers tend to overlook this kind of periodic overeating.

Other weekly goal-missers differ from the socializers only because their periodic diet indiscretions do not necessarily occur in a social setting. Going off of a diet can be done alone as well as in a crowd. Even socializers know that. They may do both!

### The Binge-Eater

The binge-eater is not unlike an alcoholic binge-drinker. For a time sensible eating is a part of his or her lifestyle for weeks or months. Weight may be lost. And then, much to the surprise of family and peers, this person slips into an interval of ravenous overeating for several days. Weight is rapidly regained. There is much remorse and feelings of guilt afterwards. A new resolution is made and a meal plan is followed once again until the binge period returns. This cycle may repeat itself several times with a weight loss-weight gain pattern over a year that resembles a yo-yo going up and down, up and down. This abnormal eating pattern and the obesity that is associated with it are among the most difficult to correct.

Before going any further in this chapter, take a pad of paper and pencil and start doing some self-analysis. Write down the answers to questions that appear here and elsewhere.

(1) How many meals do I eat each day on an aver-

age: one, two or three? The preferred answer is three.

(2) If I eat two to three meals each day, do I overeat during most of them? If the answer is yes, I am a daily *multimeal overeater*. I have to decide what excess foods and desserts I am overeating every day.

(3) Do I eat snacks (no matter what size) between meals each day? If the answer is yes, I am a *nibbler*. Before I can solve my problem, I have to tell myself what the situations are that lead me to snacking and what high-calorie foods I must avoid nibbling each day.

(4) Do I overeat at different meals as well as snack between meals? If so, I am both a *multimeal overeater* and a *nibbler*. I have to define the problems that exist for both.

(5) Am I one of those people who does not eat much for breakfast, if anything? Do I overeat mostly between late afternoon and bedtime? If the answer is yes, then I am a *night-eater*. I know I must focus my attention on what I eat for supper and how to avoid overeating during the evening hours. Also, what steps can I take to begin eating an appropriate breakfast while cutting way back on gorging at night?

(6) Do I overeat periodically rather than every day? Am I a person who follows a meal plan most of the week but ignores the diet on one or more social occasions during that same week? Then I am probably a *socializer*. Or at least I have some moments of indifference to dieting that happen often enough to prevent me from losing weight *(a weekly goal-misser)*. The solution to my problem is deciding what social or other events lead to my weekly lapses in following a meal plan. What can I do to control or avoid these lapses? How can I be more consistent?

(7) Am I a *binge-eater*? How long can I follow a weight-reduction program without bingeing on food? What causes me to binge? Do I have an underlying emotional or psychological problem that resurfaces from time to time? Do I need professional help to determine the cause and seek solutions?

## Social Factors That Contribute to Abnormal Eating Patterns

### Family and Ethnic Considerations

Many families have a built-in attitude that eating plenty of food is healthy regardless of the weight put on. This is often a tradition carried over generations from the "old" country. An abundance of food and mouths to enjoy it are symbols of security and well-being. To be pleasingly "plump" is a natural outcome of this culture despite the pressures of society and medicine to be at a desirable weight.

Those who have weight problems and who are members of this type of family will have a more difficult time unless there is an understanding reached in the household and support is given.

### Peer Pressures

This applies especially to "socializers." Peer pressure on children with obesity is obvious. To be one of the gang is to eat with them and like them after school and during the usual times out with them. The adult versions also are obvious and similar. Peer pressure to forget the weight problem, eat and be merry occurs in a variety of social situations. For these reasons strategies have to be worked out to control these situations when they arise.

## Personal Factors That Contribute to Overeating

### Food Cueing

Many people overeat because they confuse false cues or signals to eat with normal feelings of hunger. Or they may overshoot on how much they eat because they have lost their recognition of satiety or feeling full. The cause of this is unknown. It may be an inherited disorder of appetite control among people with lifelong weight problems. It may be an acquired response (out of habit) to a variety of situations.

There are many examples of eating inappropriately after a food cue. Some people are very vulnerable to the sight of or access to food. Just being in the kitchen with food in plain view is a signal to eat even in the absence of hunger. A bountiful buffet in a home or restaurant can lead to second or third helpings despite adequate satisfaction of hunger after the first go-around. Time of day may be a significant cue, since some obese individuals are inflexible about routine and will eat at specific times each day whether they are hungry or not. Watching television, working in the den, doing homework, and reading in bed may become situational cues to eat independent of appetite. Others are programmed to eat whenever they pass by a favorite delicatessen, drugstore, fast food restaurant or grocery store.

In your search of personal factors that contribute to overeating, ask yourself the following:

(1) How much willpower do I have to control my eating if too much food and desserts are served at meal time or if food is readily available between meals?

(2) What situations at home, school, work or social events are cues for me to eat even if I am not hungry?

### Idleness and Boredom

One of the biggest enemies to a weight-conscious person is idleness or boredom. This usually occurs when the individual is alone. Without active involvement in something, attention soon turns to eating. This ritual is very often linked to passive entertainment like television viewing.

In this regard, ask yourself:

(1) What are my free, idle times during the day?
(2) Do I usually snack during these periods?
(3) What can I do to occupy myself during these times to avoid turning to food?

*Fatigue*

Being tired from lack of sleep is a powerful stimulus to eat. If there is prolonged, daily fatigue, the body sends out signals to eat more. Anyone who wants to be successful at losing weight should have regular sleeping hours and adequate rest. These hours should be coordinated with other family members if possible. Needless late hours and sleeping late in the morning detract from meal planning and routine daily living with the rest of the family. If adequate amounts of sleep overnight are not possible, a nap should be worked into the day.

How many hours of sleep do you require to feel refreshed and alert the next day? Most people need seven to eight hours. Children need more.

*Eating without Thinking*

Believe it or not, following a meal plan requires a lot of thought. Without thinking about what you are eating, mistakes are often made without being aware of them.

Eating without thinking happens whenever distractions occur during meal time. The housewife may consume extra food while actually preparing the meal. One can overshoot on calories if one eats while watching television, while reading, while talking on the telephone or while doing desk work. Some eat without thinking while shopping for food. A very common cause for eating without thinking occurs when a person is in a hurry to get to work, school, a meeting or other event. The rush on eating often leads to a barrage of swallowing high-calorie foods.

Ask yourself the following questions to see if you eat while your mind is on something else:

(1) Do I eat meals in one place in the home or in several different places?
(2) Do I give myself enough time to eat my meals?
(3) Do I do desk work or homework while eating my meals? Do I read or watch television or anything else while I eat a main meal?

*Stress*

There are many who blame their failure to lose weight on stress. It may be within the family—a marital problem, a husband out of work, a maladjusted teenager, a personal illness or a dying relative, a serious financial problem, a lawsuit, etc. At school or work it may be extreme friction with fellow students, colleagues, teachers or bosses. For women it may be that time of the menstrual cycle (premenstrual tension). For men and women it may be too heavy a workload, long hours without rest or recreation, few vacations and so forth.

The relationship between stress and obesity is a complicated one. For some people there are legitimate stresses that drive them to overeat, to seek comfort in food. This is especially true of the binge-eater. For others, our psychology research group tells us that it is not always stress that causes overeating; it is the obese individual seeking a scapegoat or reason to overeat. It becomes a way to shift responsibility or blame away from self to other persons or events to justify the overeating. The blame is not only placed on stress. These same individuals often use pleasant scapegoats as well—weddings, holidays, vacations, reunions, birthdays. With this long list of causes for their weight problem, it is no wonder that they have few times to be conscientious about weight reduction. In reality, overeating is more important to them than losing weight. Something or someone else has to take the blame.

To gain some insight into this problem ask yourself:

(1) Is stress really causing me to overeat?
(2) If so, what stresses occur often enough in my life that I can identify? Where are they? At home, school, work or some other place?
(3) Is it a person or persons causing the stress? Or is it a situation?
(4) Can I take steps to avoid the stress completely? If not, can I find a way to handle the stress without becoming upset and overeating?
(5) If I cannot solve my problem with stress, to whom can I turn for good advice on ways to cope with it?

## Solving Abnormal Eating Patterns

*Before You Begin Dieting*

(1) In future chapters you will select a meal plan that is most appropriate for you. Seek approval from your physician and review it with a registered dietitian. Continue to study and review. Ask questions and return to your professional help until you understand it thoroughly.
(2) Let your family know what you are trying to do. Seek their support, especially a spouse's or parent's. If there are other obese members in the family, try to convince them to join you in your program of weight loss. If you live alone, enlist the aid of a friend or fellow TOPS member who may wish to help you or join you in your program as a partner.
(3) Review your plan for weight reduction at your TOPS chapter. There is no substitute for group support like this!

(4) Plan your menus several days in advance. Write them down and prepare your food shopping list from them. Buy only what is on the list. Shop after eating a regular meal. You will be less likely to purchase food that you are supposed to avoid.

(5) Keep records! The most successful weight losers keep a food diary. Write down everything you eat. Check the diary against your meal plan. This is an excellent way to keep you aware of what you should be doing. It also helps your physician and dietitian determine if mistakes are being made. Also keep records of your weekly weight changes and monthly body measurements. For example, buy a tape measure and determine your chest, waist, hips and thigh circumferences.

You may also wish to keep records of your exercise program. Put the dates you exercised in your book. Record the type, duration and what target heart rates you achieved.

### Dieting in the Home

(1) First and foremost, eat three regular meals each day. Your meal plan also provides a small nighttime snack. Do not skip a meal in order to justify eating a larger meal later. This simply doesn't work.

(2) Eat your meals at home in only one place. This is usually the kitchen, dinette or dining room. Do not eat elsewhere, such as the recreation or TV room, den, living room, bedroom, etc. Try to stay away from the kitchen unless it is meal time.

(3) Eat your meals without distractions. It is nice to converse with your family at this time. Apart from this, avoid watching television, listening to the radio, reading or anything else that takes your mind off your meal. If a particular meal time is tense due to noise, people in a hurry or anything else, either anticipate the problem and eat beforehand or wait until things quiet down.

(4) Keep extra helpings of food off the table. Put leftover food away before you begin eating. Use small plates. Your meal will appear larger.

(5) Eat slowly. Chew your food well. Put your fork or spoon down on your plate while you chew. This will give your stomach a chance to tell your appetite that it is catching up with hunger.

### For the Nibblers

(1) Keep high-calorie snacks out of sight (although tell the nonobese members of your family where they are). If there is no one that should consume them, keep them out of the house.

(2) To take the edge off your food cravings, keep low-calorie snacks available. Refrigerated cut celery or carrot sticks or other low-calorie fresh vegetables are ideal. Use your imagination for other low-calorie foods. Some are described in later sections of this monograph. There are many food products that also are low in calories: dietetic soft drinks, gelatins and other frozen desserts. Be sure to make allowances for them in your diet.

(3) Use your willpower at school or work. Consciously avoid the vending machines, cafeteria desserts, and office cookies and bakery. Pack your own lunch and low-calorie snacks if necessary.

### For the Idle, the Bored and the Night-Eaters

Free and idle time at home, particularly at night, should not be an automatic situation for eating. For those of you who tend to do this, it's time to change. Resurrect hobbies to keep busy. Do household chores or repair work. Go for walks or consider doing your daily exercises at the very times idleness and boredom are most likely to draw you to food.

The night-eaters, more than anyone else, have to avoid excessive evening television and sitting. Their late hours and late evening eating have to be converted to more physical activity and early retirement, earlier rising in the morning and ample time for breakfast.

### Eating Out

Know your restaurants and their menus ahead of time. A conscientious meal planner can easily work restaurant food into the diet. Concentrate on the main entree. It should be simply prepared and not drowned in high-calorie sauces or gravy. A salad with low-calorie dressing is a good partner to the main course along with a low-calorie vegetable. Go with baked or boiled rather than fried potatoes. Watch the dinner rolls, since they often are first on the table long before the meal is served. Pass up dessert unless a low-calorie version is available, such as fresh fruit, a small dish of ice cream or other food that is within the limits of your meal plan.

### For the Socializers

If it is time to party at someone's home, then there will be peer pressure to overeat with plenty of food cues and temptations. Try to find out ahead of time what food is going to be served. If there is not much that is on your diet, take low-calorie foods with you to add to the table. Include some low-calorie beverages. To avoid overeating, have part of your customary meal at home before you go. You will arrive less famished, especially if food is being served late.

If someone serves you, be pleasantly firm about how much you want. If more is given than you requested, leave what you do not need on your plate.

Avoid remaining too close to buffet tables. After you have what you need, move away and visit with guests elsewhere. Talk more and eat less!

*What about Stress?*

Many overweight people have not learned to handle major stress. One good reason is often the inability to express their true feelings to other people. They don't communicate. If a person or situation gives rise to a very uncomfortable feeling of being stressed, the individual may keep the emotion within, withdraw and overeat.

A number of strategies can be developed to overcome these problems. Control yourself and do not emotionally explode. On the other hand, do not hesitate to tell other people who are responsible for the stress that there is a problem. Talk it out in a civil fashion whether it is with a spouse, family, relatives, friends, boss, teacher, coach or fellow employee. Be firm, but listen to their side of the story and be reasonable. Very often an understanding and solution can be reached in this way.

Certain situations may be particularly stressful. If it does not have to involve you, try to avoid it altogether. Many stressful situations at home, work or school have to include you and cannot be avoided. That's part of living and frequently a responsibility you have to shoulder as a homemaker, a parent, a student, an employee or a boss.

How can you adjust to stress without overeating if you cannot avoid it or prevent it by communicating your feelings? It takes a great deal of concentration, because this response is like a reflex. You have to stop the reflex. The stress is a distraction and causes you to eat without thinking. You have to be firm, even angry with yourself to stay away from food. Say to yourself, "I will not eat. I will not eat." Wait 20 minutes and let the urge pass. Have a glass of water or diet soda while you are thinking about it. This also is a good time to go for a walk or do some other physical activity, if you can.

Some people with weight problems overreact to all stresses, mild or severe. They may be "touchy" or hostile with low self-esteem. Often they are depressed and withdrawn and don't know exactly what is causing them to feel this way. This is often the setting for binge eating or severe night eating. Filling up with food is not satisfying hunger, because there is none. Filling up with any and all types of food is out of desperation to find comfort. The compulsive overeater is frequently psychologically hurting and needs help.

The only solution to this kind of problem is to seek professional help. A physician can refer the person to a good psychologist or psychiatrist for psychotherapy. This helps one define what is causing the emotional problems. It also leads to positive solutions to turn things around. The TOPS chapter can reinforce the process by providing the group help and support these individuals need so very much.

**Rewards**

Whatever challenges people with weight problems face, a good program of meal planning, exercise and weight loss brings something very positive into their lives. A sense of accomplishment and a good feeling about one's self is deserving of non-food rewards—a trip or vacation, tickets to a major entertainment event, new clothing, new items for a hobby, or some other personal gift. Periodic mini-awards can mark each new weight goal that is reached. Just think about it. If all goes well, you may be one of those honored at TOPS' International Recognition Days with this kind of performance!

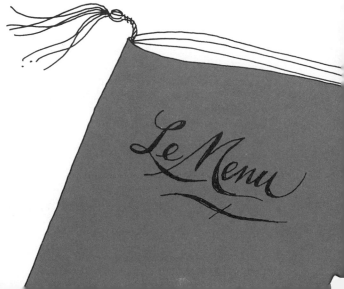

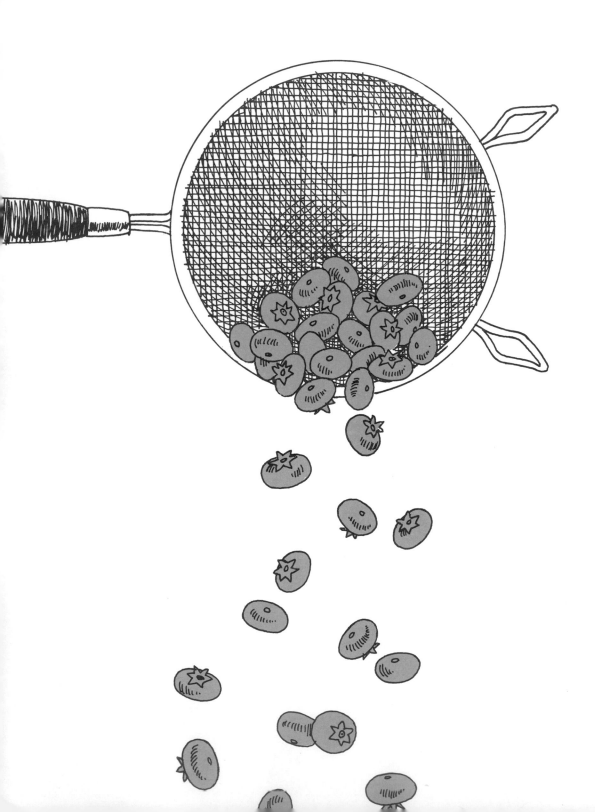

# Chapter 13: Step Four: Knowing What Foods To Avoid and What Foods To Consume

## General Comments

All the meal plans for weight reduction and weight maintenance that are described in subsequent chapters conform to many of the recommendations outlined in chapter 6 and to recent guidelines released by the National Cholesterol Education Program.[1]

(1) Carbohydrate content of each meal plan is at least 50% of total calories.
(2) Fat content is approximately 30% of total calories.
(3) Protein content represents the balance of calories.

## Carbohydrate

Although the amount of carbohydrate in each plan is guaranteed, the types consumed are up to the individual. The following guidelines are offered to deemphasize certain types of carbohydrate and emphasize others:

(1) Reduce consumption of foods containing high concentrations of sugar. They include:

| | |
|---|---|
| honey, molasses, syrup | sugar |
| jellies, jams, preserves and marmalade | doughnuts, crullers and coffeecake |
| candy | sweet rolls and Danish |
| candied fruit | soft drinks sweetened with sugar |
| sweetened condensed milk | cereals containing much added sugar |
| sundae toppings, frosting, malts and milkshakes | processed foods and dishes of unknown composition |
| pies, pastries, cakes | |

Note: Utilize low-calorie and no-calorie sweeteners in place of table sugar to sweeten cereals, beverages and other foods you prepare. Shop for low-calorie desserts, gelatins, frozen desserts, low-calorie syrup substitutes, jellies and jams, etc. Make free use of sugar-free, low-calorie soft drinks.

(2) Increase the amounts of simple sugars (glucose and fructose) found in fruits. These include any fresh, frozen, canned or dried fruits. Packaged or canned items should not contain added sugar or other sauces.

(3) Increase the proportions of complex carbohydrate (starch) from vegetables and certain processed foods.

Examples of vegetables with a high content of starch:

| | |
|---|---|
| barley | potatoes |
| beans | pumpkin |
| corn | sweet potatoes |
| parsnips | winter squash |
| peas | |

These may be canned, dried, fresh or frozen. Avoid packaged or canned vegetables with added sugar or fat-containing sauces.

Acceptable processed foods with a high content of starch:

| | |
|---|---|
| whole grain or enriched flour | whole grain cereals low in sugar |
| whole grain or enriched bread (low-fat, low-sugar) | crackers (low-fat, low-sugar) |
| bagels, buns, biscuits, rolls and muffins (low-fat, low-sugar) | macaroni, noodles, spaghetti, rice (plain) |
| | popcorn, pretzels (low-fat, low-salt) |
| | bread sticks |

Many commercial bakery goods, including crackers, are prepared with butter and cooking oils. Others contain hidden high sugar content. Certain items like biscuits and pretzels may be high in salt. Read labels before purchasing packaged goods. Some individuals may prefer to bake their own. Popcorn is best made in the home, since the amount of butter and salt normally added to the packaged variety can be eliminated or carefully controlled. Avoid starchy "junk food" snacks that are high in fat and salt.

## Fat

Although the fat content of our meal plans has been reduced to a range of 30%, an additional goal is to increase the proportion of fat calories as unsaturated fat and decrease the amount of saturated fat and cholesterol in this 30% allotment.

(1) Reduce saturated fat in the diet. Foods containing much saturated fat include:

fatty cuts of beef, lamb, pork, veal

regular cold cuts, sausage, spareribs, hot dogs, bacon

---

[1]National Heart, Blood and Lung Institute, National Institutes of Health, United States Public Health Service, Bethesda, Maryland. January 1988. *National Cholesterol Education Program: Report of the Expert Panel on Detection, Evaluation and Treatment of High Blood Cholesterol in Adults.* N.I.H. publication no. 88-2925.

whole milk, cream, half-and-half, most imitation nondairy creamers, whipped toppings, all natural cheeses, cream cheeses, sour cream, regular ice cream, whole milk yogurt, whole milk or creamed cottage cheese

chocolate, butter, coconut and coconut oil, palm oil, lard, shortening, bacon fat, dressings and sauces made with any of the preceding

fried foods

(2) Increase the proportions of foods that are lower in saturated fats. These include the following alternatives:

lean cuts of beef, lamb, veal and pork

fish, poultry without skin, certain shellfish

skim milk, 1% fat milk, buttermilk

low-fat cottage cheese (1% or 2%), low-fat cheeses, farmer or pot cheeses, low-fat yogurt

sherbet, sorbet

baking cocoa, unsaturated fat cooking oils (corn, olive, canola, safflower, sunflower, soybean or sesame oils), margarine or shortenings produced from these oils

mayonnaise, salad dressings made with unsaturated oils, low-fat dressings

seeds and nuts

## Cholesterol

By reducing saturated fat in the diet, blood cholesterol should decrease. In addition, certain foods high in cholesterol should be reduced. They include:

egg yolks and any food items, bakery, noodles, sauces or dressings prepared from them, and shellfish (shrimp and crayfish)

organ meats: liver, kidneys, brain and sweetbreads (pancreas)

Whenever possible, use egg whites (mostly protein) or cholesterol-free egg substitutes in place of egg yolks. Limit consumption of whole eggs to four per week. Daily cholesterol intake should average 300 milligrams or less.

## Protein

In the meal plans, red meats are subdivided into low-fat, medium-fat and high-fat categories. As suggested in the previous section on fat, choose lean cuts of beef, lamb, veal and pork whenever possible. Red meats should not be totally eliminated from the diet, because they are rich in a variety of nutrients, including iron.

Other good sources of protein are derived from poultry, fish and low-fat dairy products as indicated in the section on fat.

## Food Fiber

Based on recommendations outlined in chapter 6, a realistic goal for food fiber intake is 30 grams per day. This is approximately 10 to 15 grams higher than the present daily American average of 15 to 20 grams. The benefits of food fiber are discussed in chapter 5.

Most food fiber sources are in the starch/bread, vegetable and fruit exchange lists. The majority of items on these lists provide an average of 2 to 3 grams per serving. There are some foods that are much higher in fiber than others. They are listed in table 9.

An easy way to increase food fiber is to emphasize bran cereals for breakfast. On days when high-fiber cereals are not consumed, attempt to work into the meal plan one or more servings of vegetables and fruits on this list. Increase food fiber in your diet gradually. Excessively high intakes may cause bloating and intestinal gas.

## Oats, Food Fiber and Cholesterol

In recent years much emphasis has been placed on the beneficial effects on blood cholesterol of foods containing oats. Some nutritionists suggest that the relatively high proportion of soluble food fiber in whole or rolled oats as well as oat bran may lower blood cholesterol an additional 2 to 3% if one daily serving of a high oat bran cereal or similar food is consumed. The effect of soluble fiber on cholesterol was discussed in chapter 5. More refined or milled oat grain has less soluble fiber.

Oat cereals currently on the market have total food fiber content ranging between 1 and 6 grams per serving. Most are in the 2 to 3 gram range. Soluble food fiber is a smaller fraction of the total. It is important to read the food label on these products for several reasons. Higher food fiber usually means more sugar is added to improve taste. In addition, high fiber oat cereals may contain coconut oil as the fat source to improve consistency and taste. Coconut oil is a saturated fat that may offset some of the cholesterol-lowering action of the oat grain. Selection of oat cereals with more moderate fiber content (2 to 3 grams per serving) may be a better nutritional choice, because amounts of sugar and saturated fat are usually lower if not absent. It also is not sensible to consume large amounts of bakery goods containing oats if calories and levels of sugar, fat and salt are high. For example, some single oat bran muffins may contain as much as 200 to 300 calories.

The emphasis on oat bran in the diet is controversial for several reasons. Recent research suggests that oat bran may not reduce blood cholesterol directly. Instead, consumption of oat products may reduce intake of fat in the diet. It is the latter change that has cholesterol-lowering action.[2] Moreover, the attraction to oat bran food overlooks the fact that some wheat cereals are very high in food fiber (see table 9). Table 9 also indicates that grain products are not the only foods with high fiber content. One can plan a fiber-rich meal around a variety of fruits and vegetables as well. Many of these items have greater amounts of total and soluble food fiber in smaller serving sizes than do several grain products. It is best not to seek fiber from only one source. It is not only boring but prevents the individual from using all kinds of nutritious foods.

Most important of all, one must remember that food fiber is of little value in decreasing blood cholesterol unless (1) the meal plan is restricted in saturated fat and cholesterol and (2) desirable weight is achieved and maintained.

### Salt

It is difficult to give the TOPS membership a precise upper limit of sodium intake. As reviewed in chapter 6, the recommendations are as low as 1,800 milligrams per day (4½ grams of salt) from

## TABLE 9: FOODS WITH HIGH FIBER CONTENT

| EXCHANGE LIST | SERVING SIZE | TOTAL FIBER (grams) | SOLUBLE FIBER (grams) |
|---|---|---|---|
| Starch/Bread | | | |
| All Bran Cereal | ⅓ cup | 8.8 | 1.6 |
| Bran Buds Cereal | ⅓ cup | 7.8 | 1.5 |
| 40% Bran Flakes (Kellogg) | ½ cup | 3.1 | 0.5 |
| 40% Bran Flakes (Post) | ½ cup | 3.7 | 0.6 |
| Black-eyed peas | ⅓ cup | 8.2 | 3.7 |
| Beans, lima | ½ cup | 4.4 | 1.2 |
| Beans, kidney | ⅓ cup | 3.8 | 1.7 |
| Beans, white | ⅓ cup | 3.4 | 1.0 |
| Peas, split | ⅓ cup | 3.4 | 1.1 |
| Peas, garden | ½ cup | 5.4 | 2.7 |
| Corn | ½ cup | 6.0 | 2.6 |
| Squash, acorn | ¾ cup | 5.3 | 0.5 |
| Bread, pumpernickel | 1 oz. slice | 3.8 | 0.5 |
| Vegetables | | | |
| Asparagus, raw | 1 cup | 4.6 | 0.8 |
| Brussels sprouts | ½ cup | 3.6 | 1.5 |
| Carrots, raw | 1 cup | 3.6 | 1.5 |
| Onions, raw | 1 cup | 5.0 | 1.6 |
| Free Vegetables | | | |
| Chinese cabbage | 1 cup | 4.6 | 2.3 |
| Zucchini, raw | 1 cup | 3.9 | 1.8 |
| Fruits | | | |
| Blackberries, raw | ¾ cup | 6.7 | 1.0 |
| Raspberries, raw | 1 cup | 9.1 | 0.5 |
| Strawberries, raw | 1¼ cup | 4.1 | 1.5 |
| Dried apricots | 7 halves | 5.8 | 1.4 |
| Dried figs | 1½ cups | 5.2 | 1.2 |
| Prunes, uncooked | 3 med. | 4.0 | 1.2 |

[2]J.F. Swain et al., "Comparison of the Effects of Oat Bran and Low Fiber Wheat Germ on Serum Lipoprotein Levels and Blood Pressure," *New England Journal of Medicine* 322 (1989):147-152.

the U.S. Senate Select Committee on Human Needs and Nutrition to as high as 4,800 milligrams of sodium (12 grams of salt) per day by the American Medical Association. Intermediate levels not to exceed 3,000 milligrams of daily sodium intake (7 ½ grams of salt) were advocated by the American Heart Association and the American Diabetes Association.

Approximately one-third of sodium intake is controlled in the home and at the dinner table. To assure a reasonable level of consumption, it is recommended that:

(1) Use of table salt during meals should be sharply reduced and preferably eliminated.
(2) Heavy salting of foods during preparation and cooking of meals should be avoided.

The balance of sodium is supplied by foods in which sodium occurs naturally (one-third) and by processed foods to which sodium is added by industry (one-third).

These recommendations apply only to healthy individuals living in normal environments. Certain medical ailments may demand greater salt restriction but should be determined only by a physician. Salt needs may increase during acute illnesses accompanied by significant vomiting and diarrhea.

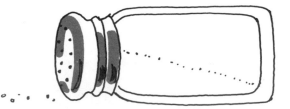

# PART FIVE:
## Taking Off Pounds Sensibly II: Meal Planning for Weight Reduction

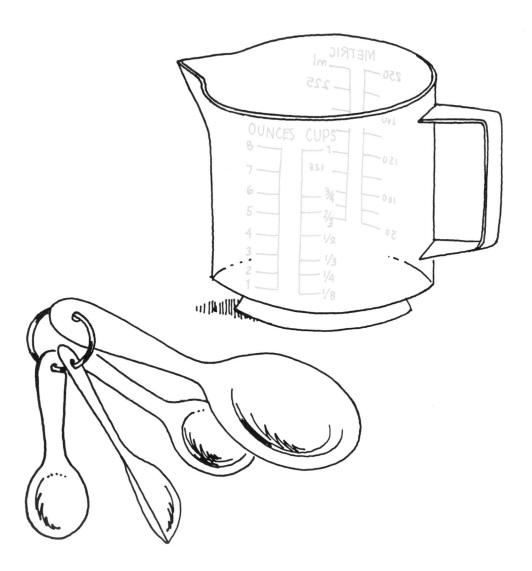

# Chapter 14: The Exchange System for Counting Calories

Several years ago the American Dietetic Association and the American Diabetes Association developed a system that greatly simplifies counting calories and menu planning. Today physicians prescribe this kind of diet for patients with diabetes as well as for individuals with weight problems. This system was selected for the TOPS monograph because it is well known to health professionals throughout this continent and is readily available in virtually all community hospitals and clinics where registered dietitians are employed.

Various foods are inserted into six different exchange lists. Each list contains foods that are similar in type and composition. They include:

• Starch/Breads
• Meats, including low-, medium- and high-fat meats
• Vegetables
• Fruits
• Milk
• Fats

## Learning To Use Exchange Lists

Examine each of the six lists that follow. Please note:

(1) At the top of each table the total calories as well as grams of carbohydrate, protein and fat contained in one exchange serving are stated. Food fiber is also indicated in the starch/bread and fruit exchange lists.
(2) Each table gives the type of food on the left. On the right, the amount of food or serving size is given. In other words, all the food serving sizes have the same number of calories and are equivalent to each other and to one exchange.
(3) Foods that are high in salt are marked with an asterisk. Items that have a relatively high fiber content are indicated by a dagger (†) sign.
(4) Other items of interest:

Foods for occasional use are at the bottom of the starch/bread list.

Meat substitutes are provided after the meat exchange list because of their relatively high protein content. However, their starch and fat content in terms of exchanges are also included and must be worked into all meal plans.

Vegetables that contain very few calories and

that can be consumed as desired are included at the bottom of the vegetable exchange list.

Free foods are also very low in calories and can be eaten at any time without counting them.

## Metric and English Weights and Volumes

In order to follow meal plans accurately, the conscientious TOPS member should be familiar with metric and English units of volume and weight. Table 10 provides this information. This is important when purchasing foods and when determining the amount of food required for the various exchanges.

A glass measuring cup with graduation markings on the side for ounces and milliliters (or cubic centimeters) is an invaluable measuring device. A set of measuring spoons that include tablespoon and teaspoon units is also preferred rather than household dinnerware spoons. With experience, weights of meats and other foods can be estimated by size, but some may find it easier to use a small weighing scale when there is a question. All these items are inexpensive, good investments.

---

Author's Note: The exchange lists in chapter 14 were reproduced with permission from the American Diabetes Association and the American Dietetic Association.

## TABLE 10:
## METRIC AND ENGLISH WEIGHTS AND MEASUREMENTS

| MEASURE | ENGLISH | METRIC |
|---|---|---|
| VOLUME | | |
| 1 gallon | 4 quarts | 3.8 liters |
| 1 quart | 2 pints | 0.95 liter |
| | 4 cups | |
| | 32 fl. ounces | |
| 1.06 quarts | 33.8 fl. ounces | 1 liter |
| 1 cup | ½ pint | 0.24 liter or 240 |
| | 8 fl. ounces | milliliters[†] |
| | 16 tablespoons | |
| 1 tablespoon* | 3 teaspoons | 15 milliliters[†] |
| | ½ fl. ounce | |
| 1 teaspoon* | ⅙ fl. ounce | 5 milliliters[†] |
| WEIGHT | | |
| 1 pound | 16 ounces | 0.454 kilogram or 454 grams |
| 2.2 pounds | 35.2 ounces | 1 kilogram or 1,000 grams |
| 1 ounce | 1/16 pound | 28.35 grams |

*Level measures only.

[†] Although not strictly correct, milliliters (ml) and cubic centimeters (cc) are often interchanged freely.

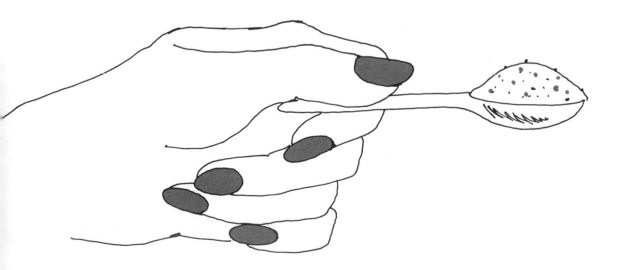

# LIST 1: STARCH/BREAD EXCHANGE

One exchange contains:
Carbohydrate . . . . . . . . . . . . 15 grams
Protein . . . . . . . . . . . . . . . . . . . 3 grams
Fat . . . . . . . . . . . . . . . . . . . . . . . . trace
Fiber . . . . . . . . . . . . . . . . . . . . 2 grams
Calories . . . . . . . . . . . . . . . . . . . . . 80

| FOOD ITEM | AMOUNT TO USE FOR ONE EXCHANGE | FOOD ITEM | AMOUNT TO USE FOR ONE EXCHANGE |
|---|---|---|---|
| Bagel, 1 oz. | ½ med. | Oyster | 24 |
| Barley, cooked | ½ cup | Ritz | 6 (also 1 fat exchange) |
| Barley, dry | 1½ T. | Ritz, cheese | 7 (also 1 fat exchange) |
| Bialy | 1 | Rusk | 2 |
| Biscuit, 2½″ dia. | 1 (also 1 fat exchange) | Ry-Krisp, 2″ x 3½″ | 4 |
| Bread: | | Saltines, 2″ squares | 6 |
| Enriched white, wheat, rye | 1 avg. slice | Soda, 2½″ squares | 3 |
| Boston brown | 1 slice | Triangle Thins | 12 (also 1 fat exchange) |
| Cocktail rye | 3 slices | Triscuit Wafers | 5 (also 1 fat exchange) |
| French, 3″ across x 1″ thick | 1 slice | Wheat Thins | 12 (also 1 fat exchange) |
| Italian | 1 slice | Zwieback | 3 |
| Pita | ½ | Croissant, small, 5″ x 2″ | 1 |
| Raisin, unfrosted | 1 avg. slice | | (also 2 fat exchanges) |
| Bread crumbs, dry, grated | ¼ cup | Croutons, low-fat | 1 cup |
| soft | ⅓ cup | Flour, enriched | 2½ T. |
| Bread sticks, 4″ long x ½″, ⅔ oz. | 2 | Macaroni, plain, cooked | ½ cup |
| Bread stuffing, prepared | ¼ cup | Matzoth, 6″ dia. | 1 |
| | (also 1 fat exchange) | Matzoth meal | 3 T. |
| Buns: | | Muffins: | |
| Frankfurter | ½ | English | ½ |
| Hamburger | ½ | Plain, 2″ dia. | 1 small |
| Cereal, cooked: | | | (also 1 fat exchange) |
| Bulgar | ½ cup | Noodles, cooked | ½ cup |
| Cornmeal | ½ cup | Pancakes, 4″ dia. | 1 (also 1 fat exchange) |
| Grits | ½ cup | Popcorn, popped (no fat added) | 3 cups |
| Other cooked | ½ cup | Popover | 1 (also 1 fat exchange) |
| Cereal, dry (not sugar frosted): | | Potato chips* | 15 (also 2 fat exchanges) |
| Bran, concentrated[†] | ⅓ cup | Pretzels | ¾ oz. |
| Bran flakes[†] (All Bran, Bran Buds) | ½ cup | Rice, cooked | ⅓ cup |
| Granola | ¼ cup | Rice cakes | 2 |
| | (also 1 fat exchange) | Rolls: | |
| Grape-Nuts | 3 level T. | Dinner-type, 2″ dia. | 1 |
| Puffed | 1½ cups | Hard-type | ½ large (4″ dia.) or 1 small |
| Shredded wheat | ½ cup | Spaghetti, cooked | ½ cup |
| Wheat germ[†] | 3 T. | Taco shells | 2 (also 1 fat exchange) |
| Other ready-to-eat | ¾ cup | Tapioca, dry | 2 T. |
| Chow mein noodles | ½ cup | Toast, melba | 5 oblong or 10 round |
| | (also 1 fat exchange) | Tortilla, 6″ dia. | 1 |
| Corn bread, 2″ cube | 1 | Vegetables: | |
| | (also 1 fat exchange) | Baked beans (no pork)[†] | ¼ cup |
| Corn chips* | ½ cup | Beans, dried (kidney, navy)[†] | ⅓ cup |
| | (also 2 fat exchanges) | Beans, lima[†] | ½ cup |
| Cornflake crumbs | 3 T. | Corn, 6″ ear[†] | 1 |
| Cornstarch | 2 T. | whole kernel[†] | ½ cup |
| Crackers: | | Onion rings | 2 oz. |
| Animal | 8 | | (also 1 fat exchange) |
| Graham, plain, 2½″ squares | 3 | Parsnips, diced | ⅔ cup |
| Hi-Ho | 6 (also 1 fat exchange) | | *(Continued on next page)* |

[†]Three or more grams fiber per serving.

*High in salt content.

## LIST 1: STARCH/BREAD EXCHANGE
## (continued)

| FOOD ITEM | AMOUNT TO USE FOR ONE EXCHANGE | FOOD ITEM | AMOUNT TO USE FOR ONE EXCHANGE |
|---|---|---|---|
| Peas, dried (black-eyed, cowpeas, split, lentils), cooked[†] | ⅓ cup | Hash browns | ¼ cup (also 1 fat exchange) |
| Peas, green, canned or frozen, cooked[†] | ½ cup | Mashed (no fat added) | ½ cup |
| Plantain[†] | ½ cup | Mashed (made from dry flakes according to box directions) | ½ cup (also 1 fat exchange) |
| Potatoes: | | Sweet (no sugar added) | ⅓ cup or ½ small |
| White, 2″ dia., 3 oz. | 1 | Tater Tots | 10 (also 2 fat exchanges) |
| Flakes, dry | ⅓ cup | Pumpkin | ¾ cup |
| French fries, 2″ x ½″ x ½″ | 10 (also 1 fat exchange) | Squash, winter | ¾ cup |
| | | Waffle, 4½″ square | 1 (also 1 fat exchange) |

[†]Three or more grams fiber per serving.

*High in salt content.

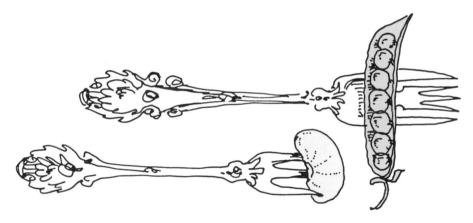

## FOODS FOR OCCASIONAL USE

| FOOD ITEM / AMOUNT TO USE | EXCHANGE VALUE |
|---|---|
| Angel food cake, no frosting, 1/12 cake | 2 starch/bread |
| Cake, no frosting, 1/12 cake or 3″ square | 2 starch/bread, 2 fat |
| Cookies: | |
| 3 gingersnaps | 1 starch/bread |
| 6 vanilla wafers | 1 starch/bread, 1 fat |
| Other cookies, 2 small | 1 starch/bread, 1 fat |
| Doughnut, plain without glaze or filling: | |
| 1 cake-type | 1 starch/bread, 1 fat |
| 1 yeast-type | 1 starch/bread, 1 fat |
| Gelatin, sweetened, ½ cup | 1 starch/bread |
| Granola bar | 1 starch/bread, 1 fat |
| Ice cream, ½ cup | 1 starch/bread, 2 fat |
| Ice milk, ½ cup | 1 starch/bread, 1 fat |
| Pudding, ¼ cup | 1 starch/bread |
| Sherbet, ¼ cup | 1 starch/bread |
| Yogurt, frozen, ⅓ cup | 1 starch/bread |

# LIST 2: MEAT EXCHANGES

Meat has various amounts of fat per ounce or exchange. Because the fat content varies so much, this group is divided into "lean," "medium-fat" and "high-fat." It is best to choose most of your servings from the "lean" and "medium-fat" group. Try to limit selections from the high-fat meat groups to three times or less per week.

## LEAN MEAT

One exchange contains:
Protein....................7 grams
Fat ......................3 grams
Calories ......................55

Lean meat is low in saturated fat.

| FOOD ITEM | AMOUNT TO USE FOR ONE EXCHANGE |
|---|---|
| Beef (USDA good or choice grades): flank steak, tenderloin, round steak, rump steak, sirloin steak, chipped beef* | 1 oz. |
| Pork: fresh, canned, cured, and boiled ham*; Canadian bacon*; tenderloin | 1 oz. |
| Veal: all cuts except veal cutlet | 1 oz. |
| Poultry: meat without skin of chicken, turkey, Cornish hen | 1 oz. |
| Fish: | |
| Any fresh or frozen (no breaded coating) | 1 oz. |
| Crab, lobster, clams, shrimp (5-6 med.), scallops (8) | 2 oz. |
| Canned water-packed tuna* | ¼ cup |
| Oysters | 6 med. |
| Sardines, drained | 2 med. |
| Herring, uncreamed or smoked | 1 oz. |
| Wild game: venison, rabbit, squirrel, pheasant, duck, goose (without skin) | 1 oz. |
| Cheese (containing less than 55 calories per ounce)* and grated Parmesan | 1 oz. |
| Cottage cheese | ¼ cup |
| Other: | |
| 95% fat-free luncheon meat* | 1 oz. |
| Egg whites | 3 whites |
| Egg substitute with less than 55 calories per ¼ cup | ¼ cup |

*High in salt content.

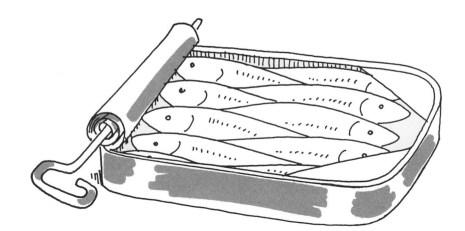

# MEDIUM-FAT MEAT

One exchange contains:
Protein . . . . . . . . . . . . . . . . . . . .7 grams
Fat . . . . . . . . . . . . . . . . . . . . . .5 grams
Calories . . . . . . . . . . . . . . . . . . . . .75

| FOOD ITEM | AMOUNT TO USE FOR ONE EXCHANGE |
|---|---|
| Beef (most beef products): roasts (rib, chuck, rump), steak (cubed, porterhouse, T-bone), meatloaf | 1 oz. |
| Pork (most lean products): chops, loin roast, Boston butt, cutlets | 1 oz. |
| Lamb (most lamb products): chops, leg, roast | 1 oz. |
| Veal: cutlet | 1 oz. |
| Poultry: chicken (with skin), domestic duck or goose (well-drained of fat), ground turkey | 1 oz. |
| Fish: | |
| Tuna* (canned in oil and drained) | ¼ cup |
| Salmon* (canned) | ¼ cup |
| Organ meats: liver, kidney, sweetbreads (high in cholesterol) | 1 oz. |
| Cheese: Mozzarella, Ricotta, farmer, diet cheeses (56-80 calories per oz.) | 1 oz. |
| Eggs (high in cholesterol—limit to 4 per week) | 1 |
| Other: | |
| 86% fat-free luncheon meat* | 1 oz. |
| Egg substitute with 56-90 calories per ¼ cup | ¼ cup |
| Tofu (2½" x 2¾" x 1") | 4 oz. |

*High in salt content.

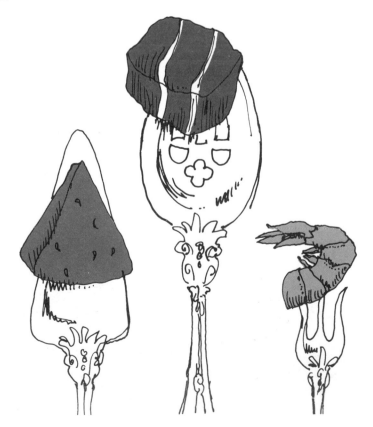

## HIGH-FAT MEAT

One exchange contains:
Protein....................7 grams
Fat ......................8 grams
Calories .....................100

Limit meat from the "high-fat" group to three times per week.

| FOOD ITEM | AMOUNT TO USE FOR ONE EXCHANGE |
|---|---|
| Beef (most USDA prime cuts): ribs, corned beef | 1 oz. |
| Lamb: patties (ground lamb) | 1 oz. |
| Pork: spareribs, ground pork, pork sausage | 1 oz. |
| Fish: any fried product | 1 oz. |
| Cheese*: all regular cheeses, such as American, Cheddar, Swiss, Monterey | 1 oz. |
| Cold cuts* (4½" x ⅛" slices) | 1 oz. |
| Frankfurter* (turkey or chicken) | 1 small (10 per lb.) |
| Frankfurter* (beef, pork, or combination) | 1 (also count as 1 fat exchange) |
| Sausage*: bratwurst, knockwurst, Polish, Italian | 1 oz. |
| Peanut butter (contains unsaturated fat) | 1 T. |

*High in salt content.

## MEAT ALTERNATIVES

If these foods are used as a substitute for meat (as in a vegetarian diet), the carbohydrate content needs to be accounted for as indicated below.

| FOOD ITEM / AMOUNT TO USE | EXCHANGE VALUE |
|---|---|
| Beans† (cooked): | |
| Butter, 1 cup | 1 lean meat and 2 starch/bread |
| Lima, ⅔ cup | 1 lean meat and 1 starch/bread |
| Pinto, ½ cup | 1 lean meat and 2 starch/bread |
| Red, 1 cup | 1 lean meat and 2 starch/bread |
| Soy, ⅓ cup | 1 lean meat and ½ starch/bread |
| White, 1 cup | 1 lean meat and 1 starch/bread |
| Garbanzo beans or chickpeas,† canned, 3½ oz. | 1 lean meat and 2 starch/bread |
| Lentils,† cooked, ⅔ cup | 1 lean meat and 1 starch/bread |
| Peas,† cooked: | |
| Black-eyed, ⅔ cup | ½ lean meat and 1 starch/bread |
| Split, 1 cup | 1 lean meat, 2 starch/bread and 1 vegetable |
| Nuts and seeds: | |
| Peanuts, ¼ cup (25 nuts) | 1 medium-fat meat, 2 fat and 1 vegetable |
| Pumpkin seeds, 1 oz. | 1 high-fat meat, 1 fat and 1 vegetable |
| Sesame seeds, 1 oz. (3 T.) | 1 medium-fat meat and 2 fat |
| Soybean nuts, 1 oz. (¼ cup) | 2 lean meat and ½ vegetable |
| Squash seeds, 1 oz. (3 T.) | 1 high-fat meat, 1 fat and 1 vegetable |
| Sunflower or safflower seeds, 1 oz. (3 T.) | 1 high-fat meat, 1 fat and 1 vegetable |
| Wheat germ, toasted, ¼ cup | 1 lean meat and 1 starch/bread |

†Three or more grams fiber per serving.

# FIGURE 9A: ESTIMATION OF MEAT PORTION SIZE
## (actual size)

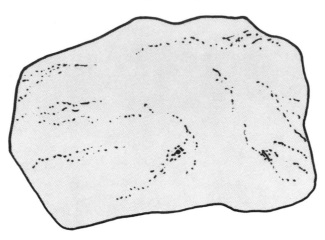

This thick

One slice this size = 1 meat exchange (1 oz. cooked)

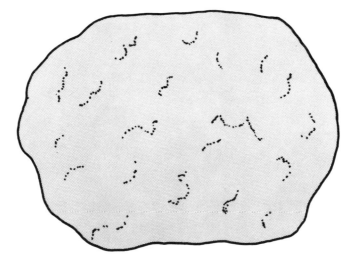

This thick

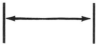

Hamburger (lean)
One patty this size = 3 meat exchanges (3 oz. cooked)

# FIGURE 9B: ESTIMATION OF MEAT PORTION SIZE
## (actual size)

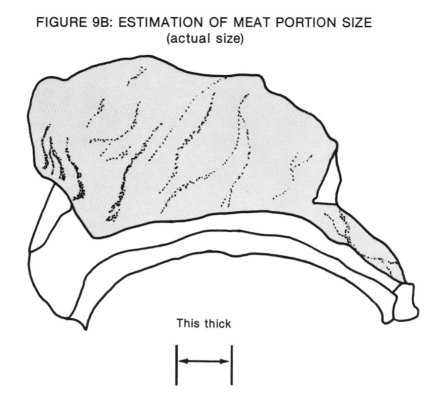

This thick

Two chops this size (fat removed) = 3 meat exchanges (3 oz. cooked)

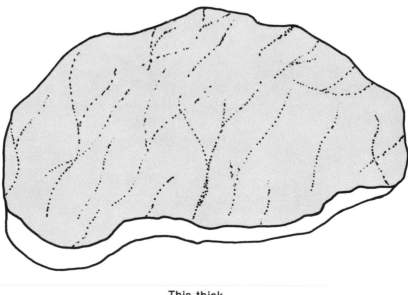

This thick

Lean roast meat
Two slices this size = 3 meat exchanges (3 oz. cooked)

# LIST 3: VEGETABLE EXCHANGES

One exchange contains:

Carbohydrate . . . . . . . . . . . . . .5 grams
Protein . . . . . . . . . . . . . . . . . . . .2 grams
Fiber . . . . . . . . . . . . . . . . .2 to 3 grams
Calories . . . . . . . . . . . . . . . . . . . . . .25

One-half cup cooked or one cup raw of the following equals one exchange:

| | | |
|---|---|---|
| Artichoke (½ med.) | Greens: | Sauerkraut* |
| Asparagus | Chard | Spinach, cooked |
| Bamboo shoots | Collards | String beans (green or |
| Bean sprouts | Dandelion | yellow) |
| Beets | Kale | Summer squash |
| Broccoli | Mustard | Tomato |
| Brussels sprouts | Turnip | Tomato juice* |
| Cabbage, cooked | Kohlrabi | Tomato paste, 2 T. |
| Carrots | Leeks | Tomato sauce, 2 T. |
| Cauliflower | Mushrooms, cooked | Turnips |
| Eggplant | Okra | Vegetable juice cocktail* |
| Green pepper | Onions | Water chestnuts |
| Greens: | Pea pods | Zucchini, cooked |
|   Beet | Rutabaga | |

The following raw vegetables may be used as desired:

| | | |
|---|---|---|
| Cabbage | Escarole | Radishes |
| Celery | Green onion | Romaine |
| Chinese cabbage | Lettuce | Spinach |
| Cucumber | Mushrooms | Watercress |
| Endive | Parsley | Zucchini |

*High in salt content.

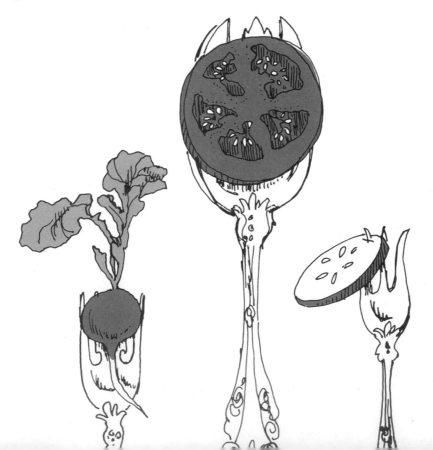

# LIST 4: FRUIT EXCHANGES

One exchange contains:
Carbohydrate . . . . . . . . . . . . .15 grams
Fiber . . . . . . . . . . . . . . . . . . . . .2 grams
Calories . . . . . . . . . . . . . . . . . . . . . .60

Use fresh, dried, cooked, canned or frozen fruit as long as no sugar has been added. Be sure the can or package says "water-packed," "unsweetened" or "no sugar added."

| FOOD ITEM | AMOUNT TO USE FOR ONE EXCHANGE | FOOD ITEM | AMOUNT TO USE FOR ONE EXCHANGE |
|---|---|---|---|
| Apple, 2" across | 1 | Mango | ½ small |
| Apple, dried (4 rings)[†] | ½ cup | Melon: | |
| Apple juice | ½ cup |   Cantaloupe, 5" across | ⅓ |
| Applesauce | ½ cup |   Cantaloupe cubes | 1 cup |
| Apricots, canned | ½ cup |   Honeydew, 7" dia. | ⅛ |
|   dried[†] | 7 halves |   Honeydew cubes | 1 cup |
|   fresh | 4 med. |   Watermelon cubes | 1¼ cups |
| Banana | ½ or 4" length | Nectar: | |
| Berries: | |   Apricot | ⅓ cup |
|   Blackberries, raw[†] | ¾ cup |   Peach | ⅓ cup |
|   Blueberries, raw[†] | ¾ cup |   Pear | ⅓ cup |
|   Raspberries, raw[†] | 1 cup | Nectarine[†] | 1 med. |
|   Strawberries, raw, whole[†] | 1¼ cups | Orange, 2½" across | 1 |
| Cherries, fresh | 12 large | Orange juice, unsweetened | ½ cup |
|   canned | ½ cup | Orange sections | ½ cup |
| Cranberry juice cocktail | ⅓ cup | Papaya | 1 cup |
| Cranberry juice, low-calorie | 1¼ cup | Peaches, canned, halves | 2 med. halves |
| Currants, dried | 1 T. |   canned, sliced | ½ cup |
|   fresh | ⅔ cup |   fresh | 1 med. |
| Dates | 2½ med. | Pears, canned | 2 halves or ½ cup |
| Figs, dried[†] | 1½ |   fresh | 1 small or ½ large |
|   fresh | 2 | Persimmon | 2 |
| Fruit cocktail, canned | ½ cup | Pineapple, canned, chunks | ⅓ cup |
| Grapefruit | ½ med. |   canned, sliced | 2 small or 1 large slice |
| Grapefruit juice, unsweetened | ½ cup |   fresh | ¾ cup |
| Grapefruit sections, canned | ¾ cup | Pineapple juice | ½ cup |
| Grape juice | ⅓ cup | Plums, canned | 2 med. |
| Grapes | 15 small |   fresh | 2 med. |
| Guava | 1 small | Pomegranate[†] | ½ |
| Kiwi | 1 large | Prune juice | ⅓ cup |
| Kumquats, fresh | 5 med. | Prunes, dried[†] | 3 med. |
| Lemon juice | 1 cup | Raisins | 2 T. (level) |
| Mandarin orange | ¾ cup | Tangerine, 2½" across | 2 |

[†]Three or more grams fiber per serving.

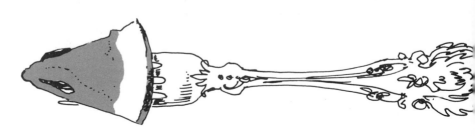

# LIST 5: MILK EXCHANGES

One exchange contains:

|  | Skim &<br>Very Low Fat | Low-Fat | Whole |
|---|---|---|---|
| Carbohydrate (grams) | 12 | 12 | 12 |
| Protein (grams) | 8 | 8 | 8 |
| Fat (grams) | 0 | 5 | 8 |
| Calories | 90 | 120 | 150 |

| FOOD ITEM | AMOUNT TO USE FOR ONE EXCHANGE |
|---|---|
| **Skim and Very Low Fat Milk:** | |
| Buttermilk (from skim milk) | 1 cup |
| Skim, ½% and 1% milk | 1 cup |
| Evaporated skim milk | ½ cup |
| Nonfat dry milk powder | ⅓ cup |
| Plain nonfat yogurt | 8 oz. |
| **Low-Fat Milk:** | |
| 2% milk | 1 cup |
| Plain low-fat yogurt | 8 oz. |
| **Whole Milk:** | |
| Whole milk | 1 cup |
| Evaporated whole milk | ½ cup |
| Whole plain yogurt | 8 oz. |

# LIST 6: FAT EXCHANGES

One exchange contains:

Fat ........................ 5 grams
Calories ........................ 45

| FOOD ITEM | AMOUNT TO USE FOR ONE EXCHANGE |
|---|---|
| **Polyunsaturated Fats** | |
| Avocado, 4" dia. | ⅛ |
| Margarine, soft, tub or stick (made from polyunsaturated oil) | 1 t. |
| diet* | 1 T. |
| Mayonnaise, regular | 1 t. |
| diet* | 1 T. |
| Nuts: | |
| Almonds, dry roasted | 6 |
| Cashews, dry roasted | 1 T. |
| Peanuts: | |
| Spanish | 20 small |
| Virginia | 10 whole |
| Pecans | 2 whole |
| Walnuts | 2 whole |
| Other | 1 T. |
| Oil: corn, cottonseed, safflower, soybean, sunflower, olive | 1 t. |
| Olives* | 10 small or 5 large |
| Salad dressing: | |
| Mayonnaise-type | 2 t. |
| Mayonnaise-type, reduced calorie | 1 T. |
| **Polyunsaturated Fats (continued)** | |
| Salad dressing* (all types) | 1 T. |
| reduced calorie* | 2 T. |
| Seeds: | |
| Pine nuts, sunflower (without shells) | 1 T. |
| Pumpkin | 2 t. |
| **Saturated Fats** | |
| Bacon,* crisp | 1 strip |
| Butter | 1 t. |
| Chitterlings, boiled | ½ cup |
| Coconut | 2 T. |
| Coffee whitener, liquid | 2 T. |
| powder | 4 T. |
| Cream, light (20%) | 2 T. |
| heavy (40%) | 1 T. |
| Cream cheese | 1 T. |
| Lard | 1 t. |
| Salt pork,* 1" cube | 1 |
| Sour cream | 2 T. |

*High in salt content.

# FREE FOODS

These foods may be eaten in any quantity except for those items with an amount listed. Limit those foods to two to three servings per day.

---

**Liquids**
Bouillon* or broth without fat
Bouillon, low-sodium
Carbonated beverages, sugar-free
Carbonated water
Club soda
Cocoa powder, unsweetened (1 T.)
Coffee/Tea
Drink mixes, sugar-free
Tonic water, sugar-free
Water
Nonstick pan spray

**Fruit**
Cranberries, unsweetened (½ cup)
Rhubarb, unsweetened (½ cup)

**Sweet Substitutes**
Candy, hard, sugar-free
Gelatin, sugar-free
Gum, sugar-free
Jam/Jelly, sugar-free (2 t.)
Pancake syrup, sugar-free (1 to 2 T.)
Sugar substitutes (saccharin, aspartame)
Whipped topping (2 T.)

**Condiments**
Barbeque sauce (1 T.)
Cocktail sauce (1 T.)
Catsup (1 T.)
Fat-free butter flavoring
Flavoring extracts
Herbs
Horseradish
Lemon
Lime
Mustard
Pickles,* dill, unsweetened
Salad dressing, low-calorie (2 T.)
Soy sauce*
Soy sauce, low-sodium ("lite")
Spices
Taco sauce (1 T.)
Vinegar
Wine, used in cooking (¼ cup)
Worcestershire sauce

**Dietetic Foods**
Read the label carefully. If the product, together with other "free foods" in that meal, does not total more than 20 calories, it can be used without calculating it into the day's total calories.

---

*High in salt content.

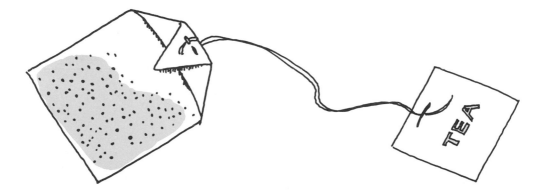

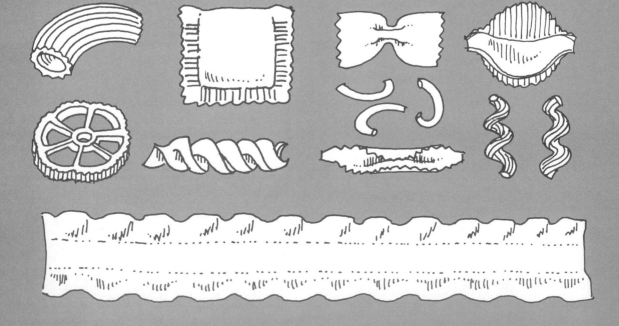

# Chapter 15: 1,200-, 1,500- and 1,800-Calorie Meal Plans

## Selecting a Weight Goal and Meal Plan

Return to chapter 1, table 2, and, with your physician, select your desirable body weight based on height and age. Calculate how many pounds overweight you are. Show your doctor the various meal plans in this monograph and select the one that is most suitable for you. A sensible rate of weight loss should not exceed 10 pounds per month. To accomplish this, it is recommended that the three weight-reduction meal plans be chosen as follows:

(1) 1,200 calories per day: Obese, inactive women under 200 pounds
(2) 1,500 calories per day: Obese, active women and inactive men below 200 pounds
(3) 1,800 calories per day: Obese men and women between 200 and 250 pounds; certain obese, active men below 200 pounds

People whose weight exceeds 250 pounds may need slightly higher caloric intakes, but the final decision must be individualized and decided by one's doctor.

The three meal plans are balanced and nutritious. At the top of each plan is stated the number of grams of protein, fat and carbohydrate. As indicated in the parentheses, the total daily calories are in the range of 50% carbohydrate, 33% fat and 17% protein. The proportions follow the guidelines for good nutrition outlined in chapter 6. The total number of exchanges allowed each day is also listed at the top of each menu plan. These are distributed throughout the day for the three meals and nighttime snack.

Each diet lists the number and type of food exchanges that are allowed for each meal on the left-hand side. On the right are sample menus that follow the plan. As an example, let's look at supper for the 1,200-calorie menu. It allows:

    1 starch/bread exchange (List 1)
    2 meat exchanges (List 2)
    1 vegetable exchange (List 3)
    1 fruit exchange (List 4)
    1 fat exchange (List 6)

For starch/bread exchanges, look at list 1. The menu calls for one exchange. Everything on the list in the amounts given equals one exchange. The sample menu suggests one small baked potato; if potato is desired, also allowed is ½ cup of mashed or ⅓ cup of potato flakes. One-third cup of sweet potato also is possible. If one prefers 10 French fries or ¼ cup of hash browns, this involves frying and extra fat. The fat exchange allowed for this meal will have to be used for this

purpose. One can also select from any of the other possibilities, such as one dinner roll, ½ cup corn or three gingersnaps.

There are two meat exchanges on the supper menu. Since a 1,200-calorie diet has little room for dietary fat, it is best to use the lean meat list as much as possible. Look at the lean meat exchange in list 2. Again, each item in the amounts given is equal to one exchange. If only one kind of meat will be eaten, two times as much (two exchanges) is allowed. That means one could eat 2 ounces of lean cuts of beef, pork or veal, or 2 ounces of fish or wild game, or 6 ounces of seafood, like crab, lobster or shrimp as examples. If more than one type of meat is being served, such as in a buffet-like setting, one could select one exchange of two different meats: for example, 1 ounce each of turkey and pork.

If meat alternatives are chosen, fat and starch/bread content have to be watched. Many of them could provide two meat exchanges, but the starch/bread and fat exchanges in them would be too high for this specific supper meal plan. If only one of the two meat exchanges were a meat alternative, however, one could use ⅔ cup lima beans or 1 cup of white beans (one lean meat and one starch/bread), and that would also use up the one starch/bread allowance. The remaining exchange of meat could be added as the true lean variety. Higher calorie meal plans can accommodate meat alternatives better because of the greater number of exchanges allowed.

One vegetable exchange can be eaten at supper on this 1,200-calorie diet. Look at list 3. One-half cup of cooked or 1 cup of raw vegetables meet the allowance. Note that these vegetables can be combined with several raw vegetables of any amount that do not need to be counted and which are at the bottom of the vegetable exchange list.

Most everyone enjoys fruit during their meals. The supper menu calls for one fruit exchange. Look at list 4. All the fruit in this table in the amounts given equals one exchange. Any single item may be chosen. Remember, many processed fruits that are dried, cooked, canned or frozen may contain sugar. Read the label and be certain they are "water-packed," "unsweetened," or have "no sugar added."

The supper meal plan also includes one fat exchange. List 6 contains the foods high in fat. The amounts given equal one exchange. At supper most individuals would use 1 teaspoon of margarine or butter and place it on their one starch/bread exchange (a slice of bread or baked potato). Or they may have used the fat exchange up by frying their potatoes or meat. Others may use that fat exchange as mayonnaise or salad dressing, etc. It is important to be careful with foods containing fat. Small amounts may be very high in calories (nine calories per gram), and it is easy to make mistakes that are costly with this type of food more than any other.

Milk should be mentioned. Look at list 5. One can see that skim or very low fat milk is only 90 calories per one exchange or 1 cup. Low-fat and whole milk are 120 and 150 calories per cup, respectively, because of their greater fat content. Because of the relatively lower caloric intake of all these meal plans, skim milk is recommended. In addition, it reduces the amount of saturated fat in the diet.

## Some Do's and Don'ts on the Exchange Diet System

- If you or your chapter has a question about the exchange system and your meal plan, consult a *registered* dietitian in a local clinic or hospital. Take your monograph with you. Your chapter may wish to organize a group session with the dietitian.
- Do not use this new edition of the TOPS nutrition monograph along with the older, first edition published in 1980. Since 1988 the American Dietetic Association and the American Diabetes Association have revised the exchange lists. The fruit exchange, for example, is totally different.
- Don't skip meals and save the exchanges for a later time. There is one exception. Those who wish to drink their skim milk at a different meal may do so. Remember, those who eat the fewest meals per day are generally the least successful in weight control.
- Don't crisscross exchanges. In other words, don't substitute a fruit exchange for a starch/bread or a starch/bread for a meat exchange even though the calories of each portion may be the same. This will disturb the balanced nutrition and proper amounts of carbohydrate, protein and fat in your meal plan. If you wish to make any changes, consult a registered dietitian.
- It is recommended that a single, simple multiple vitamin tablet be taken daily by those following 1,200- or 1,500-calorie meal plans. Check the label to ensure that all the vitamins provide between 100 to 150% of the RDA. Calcium supplements should be taken only if advised by a physician.

## Rates of Weight Loss

Amounts of weight lost each month will vary a great deal from one individual to the next. Age, medical condition, physical activity and degree of obesity are some of the factors that explain these differences. Very overweight people tend to lose the most weight initially (10 or more pounds per month) because of greater excesses of body fluids as well as body fat which are both lost on restricted calorie meal plans. Moderately obese and mildly obese people may lose only 5 to 10 pounds or 2 to 5 pounds per month, respectively. They are closer to their weight goals at the beginning and have less weight to lose, so their rates of weight loss will be less.

It should be emphasized that as obese individuals lose more and more weight and begin to approach their goals, the amount of weight lost each month also will become progressively less. This occurs for the same reasons that less obese lose fewer pounds per month than very obese subjects.

For those of you who cannot lose weight or actually gain weight on an appropriate meal plan, it is time to review it with a dietitian after keeping a food diary. This will help you determine where changes need to be made.

## Weight Plateaus

The most common cause of failing to lose weight after weeks or months of successful weight reduction is the failure to be consistent and conscientious about the meal plan. Weight plateaus usually reflect this problem. On the other hand, very heavy TOPS members who begin on an 1,800-calorie per day program and who pass below the 200-pound level may need to switch to a 1,500-calorie per day diet. This may restore better rates of weight loss. For similar reasons, individuals who begin on a 1,500-calorie diet and who are within 10 to 20 pounds of their weight goal may need to lower their intake to 1,200 calories if a plateau is reached for which there is no other explanation.

All changes in diets should be approved by a physician and should be reviewed with a registered dietitian before starting them.

# 1,200-CALORIE EXCHANGE DIET

Carbohydrate ........140 grams (46%)
Protein ..............65 grams (21%)
Fat .................45 grams (33%)

    4 starch/bread exchanges
    5 meat exchanges
    2 vegetable exchanges
    3 fruit exchanges
    2 milk exchanges
    3 fat exchanges

| EXCHANGES | SAMPLE MENU |
|---|---|

**Breakfast**

| | |
|---|---|
| List 5: 1 milk exchange | 1 cup skim milk (1 milk) |
| List 4: 1 fruit exchange | ½ cup orange juice (1 fruit) |
| List 1: 1 starch/bread exchange | 1 slice whole wheat toast (1 starch/bread) |
| List 2: 1 meat exchange | 1 oz. low-fat cheese (1 meat) |
| List 6: 1 fat exchange | 1 t. margarine (1 fat) |
| Free choice | Coffee or tea, ice water |

**Lunch**

| | |
|---|---|
| List 2: 2 meat exchanges | 2 oz. lean roast beef (2 meat) |
| List 1: 1 starch/bread exchange | 2 slices diet whole wheat bread (1 starch/bread) |
| List 3: 1 vegetable exchange | 1 cup raw carrots (1 vegetable) |
| List 4: 1 fruit exchange | 1¼ cups fresh strawberries (1 fruit) |
| List 6: 1 fat exchange | 1 t. margarine (1 fat) |
| Free choice | Coffee or tea, ice water, mustard |

**Supper**

| | |
|---|---|
| List 2: 2 meat exchanges | 2 oz. baked chicken (2 meat) |
| List 1: 1 starch/bread exchange | 1 small baked potato (1 starch/bread) |
| List 6: 1 fat exchange | 1 t. margarine (1 fat) |
| List 3: 1 vegetable exchange | ½ cup green beans (1 vegetable) |
| List 4: 1 fruit exchange | 1 small fresh apple, 2½" dia. (1 fruit) |
| Free choice | Coffee or tea, ice water, lettuce, 1 T. low-calorie salad dressing |

**Snacks**

| | |
|---|---|
| List 1: 1 starch/bread exchange | 3 cups popcorn, air-popped (starch/bread) |
| List 5: 1 milk exchange | 1 cup skim milk (1 milk) |
| Free choices | Ice water, diet soda |

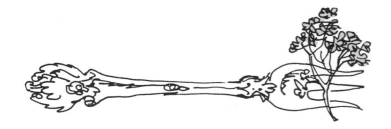

# 1,500-CALORIE EXCHANGE DIET

Carbohydrate ........194 grams (51%)
Protein ...............77 grams (20%)
Fat .................48 grams (29%)

6 starch/bread exchanges
5 meat exchanges
4 vegetable exchanges
4 fruit exchanges
2 milk exchanges
3 fat exchanges

| EXCHANGES | SAMPLE MENU |
|---|---|
| **Breakfast** | **Breakfast** |
| List 4: 1 fruit exchange | 1¼ cups fresh strawberries, blended with yogurt (1 fruit) |
| List 1: 1 starch/bread exchange | ½ bagel (1 starch/bread) |
| List 2: 1 meat exchange | 1 oz. low-fat cheese (1 meat) |
| List 6: 1 fat exchange | 1 t. margarine (1 fat) |
| List 5: 1 milk exchange | 8 oz. plain nonfat yogurt (1 milk) |
| Free choices | Tea, artificial sweetener, ice water |
| **Lunch** | **Lunch** |
| List 2: 2 meat exchanges | 2 oz. low-fat Swiss cheese* (2 meat) |
| List 1: 2 starch/bread exchanges | 1 pita bread (2 starch/bread) |
| List 6: 1 fat exchange | ⅛ avocado* (1 fat) |
| List 3: 2 vegetable exchanges | 1 cup sliced tomato* (1 vegetable) |
| | 1 cup raw carrots (1 vegetable) |
| List 4: 1 fruit exchange | 2 T. raisins (1 fruit) |
| Free choices | ½ cup alfalfa sprouts* and ½ cup celery,* 1 T. low-calorie salad dressing,* tea, ice water |
| | *ingredients for filling pita bread |
| **Supper** | **Supper** |
| List 2: 2 meat exchanges | 2 oz. roast beef (2 meat) |
| List 1: 2 starch/bread exchanges | ½ cup mashed potatoes (1 starch/bread) |
| | 1 dinner roll (1 starch/bread) |
| List 3: 2 vegetable exchanges | 1 cup pea pods (2 vegetable) |
| List 6: 1 fat exchange | 1 t. margarine (1 fat) |
| List 4: 1 fruit exchange | 1 small baked apple (1 fruit) |
| Free choices | Coffee, ice water, bouillon, lettuce, 1 T. low-calorie salad dressing |
| **Snacks** | **Snacks** |
| List 4: 1 fruit exchange | 1 small orange (1 fruit) |
| List 1: 1 starch/bread exchange | 3 cups popcorn, air-popped (1 starch/bread) |
| List 5: 1 milk exchange | 1 cup skim milk (1 milk) |
| Free choices | Ice water, diet soda, raw celery |

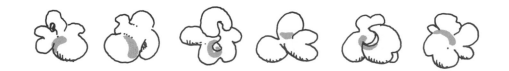

# 1,800-CALORIE EXCHANGE DIET

Carbohydrate ........225 grams (50%)
Protein ..............90 grams (20%)
Fat .................60 grams (30%)

8 starch/bread exchanges
6 meat exchanges
4 vegetable exchanges
4 fruit exchanges
2 milk exchanges
4 fat exchanges

| EXCHANGES | SAMPLE MENU |
|---|---|

**Breakfast**

**Breakfast**

List 4: 1 fruit exchange .......................... ½ cup orange juice (1 fruit)
List 1: 1 starch/bread exchange ................. ½ English muffin (1 starch/bread)
List 2: 1 meat exchange ......................... 1 oz. low-fat cheese (1 meat)
List 6: 1 fat exchange .......................... 1 t. margarine (1 fat)
List 5: 1 milk exchange ......................... 1 cup skim milk (1 milk)
Free choices ................................... Coffee, 1 t. diet jelly, water, artificial sweetener

**Lunch**

**Lunch**

List 2: 2 meat exchanges ........................ ½ cup water-packed tuna (2 meat)
List 1: 2 starch/bread exchanges ................. 2 slices whole wheat bread (2 starch/bread)
List 6: 1 fat exchange .......................... 2 t. mayonnaise-type salad dressing, mixed with tuna (1 fat)
List 3: 2 vegetable exchanges ................... 2 cups raw vegetables (mix of carrots, broccoli, green pepper, cauliflower and tomato) (2 vegetable)
List 4: 1 fruit exchange .......................... 15 small green grapes (1 fruit)
Free choices ................................... Ice water, tea, 1 T. low-calorie salad dressing, lettuce

**Supper**

**Supper**

List 2: 3 meat exchanges ........................ 3 oz. roast chicken (3 meat)
List 1: 3 starch/bread exchanges ................. 1 medium (6 oz.) baked potato (2 starch/bread) 1 dinner roll (1 starch/bread)
List 3: 2 vegetable exchanges ................... 1 cup green beans (2 vegetable)
List 6: 2 fat exchanges .......................... 2 t. margarine (2 fat)
List 4: 1 fruit exchange .......................... ½ cup water-packed peaches (1 fruit)
Free choices ................................... Coffee, ice water, raw cabbage, 1 T. low-calorie salad dressing

**Snacks**

**Snacks**

List 4: 1 fruit exchange .......................... ½ grapefruit (1 fruit)
List 5: 1 milk exchange .......................... 1 cup skim milk (1 milk)
List 1: 2 starch/bread exchanges ................. 1½ oz. pretzels (2 starch/bread)
Free choices ................................... Ice water, diet soda

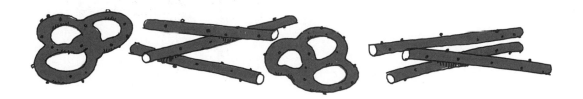

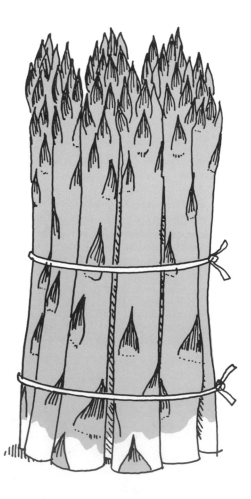

# Chapter 16: 28-Day Menu Plans for Taking Off Pounds Sensibly

This chapter is designed to show how a variety of foods can be worked into the 1,200-, 1,500- and 1,800-calorie per day exchange systems for weight loss over a four-week period. It is not intended to be an easy way out for someone who does not want to take the time to learn the exchange system and their meal plans.

Please read this chapter *after* you have an understanding of chapters 14 and 15!

Look at the organization of each day's meal plan from left to right. The type and number of food exchanges for each meal are listed for the 1,200-, 1,500- and 1,800-calorie meal plans in the first four columns. Next, the specific foods and their amounts for each meal are placed under the 1,200-calorie meal plan and correspond to the number of exchanges allowed for those meals. To the right of the 1,200-calorie meal plan column are the 1,500- and 1,800-calorie diet columns.

As an example, the day 1 menu plans can be reviewed. For breakfast, the same number of exchanges and same amounts of food are eaten on all three meal plans. For lunch, the same amount of food is consumed on the 1,500- and 1,800-calorie diets. The 1,200-calorie plan has one less starch/ bread and vegetable exchange. For the evening meal, the one fruit allowance is the only similarity for the three different calorie levels.

The exchange distribution for the three meals is slightly different for days 15 to 28 than it is for days 1 to 14. If you wish to stay with the distribution you have been following in days 1 to 14, you can repeat those days again. Or if you are not taking insulin, switching to the new distribution will not affect your rate of weight loss. If you are taking insulin and are on the 1,500- or 1,800-calorie diets, subtract one starch/bread exchange from breakfast and add it to the evening meal. You will then have the same distribution for starch/bread exchanges as during days 1 to 14 and your blood sugar should not be affected.

As you will see, the plans make full use of free vegetables and other low-calorie seasonings, foods and beverages.

A word of caution: Look at the beginning of chapter 15 once more. Select the right diet for you based on weight, sex and physical activity. Stick to that meal plan throughout the 28 days. Do not jump back and forth from one calorie level to another.

Since you have several days of menus ahead of time, it will be convenient to shop for the foods well in advance of preparing them. This can be done on a weekly basis. The entire family will enjoy these meals. For the member who has a weight problem, the quantities must be carefully measured. Too much of the foods on these meal plans can also cause weight gain.

Good luck! Up to 5 to 10 pounds can be lost in four weeks on the appropriate plan if there are no errors and no overeating.

Author's Note: Mary Hoettels, R.D., M.S., planned the 1,500- and 1,800-calorie menus and Joan Pleuss, R.D., M.S., planned the 1,200-calorie menus for the 28-day meal plans in chapter 16. This represented a great deal of effort for which we are all grateful.

# DAY 1

| EXCHANGES | | | | MENU | | |
|---|---|---|---|---|---|---|
| TYPE | CALORIE LEVEL | | | | CALORIE LEVEL | |
| | 1,200 | 1,500 | 1,800 | 1,200 | 1,500 | 1,800 |

**Breakfast**

| | | | | | | |
|---|---|---|---|---|---|---|
| Fruit | 1 | 1 | 1 | Grapefruit half, or grapefruit juice, ½ cup | same | same |
| Starch | 1 | 1 | 1 | English muffin, ½ | same | same |
| Meat | 1 | 1 | 1 | Poached egg, 1 med. | same | same |
| Fat | 1 | 1 | 1 | Crisp bacon, 1 slice | same | same |
| Milk | 1 | 1 | 1 | Skim milk, 1 cup | same | same |

**Noon Meal**

| | | | | | | |
|---|---|---|---|---|---|---|
| Meat | 2 | 2 | 2 | Water-packed tuna, ½ cup* | same | same |
| Starch | 1 | 2 | 2 | Whole wheat bread, thin sliced, 2 slices* | Whole wheat bread, regular, 2 slices* | same |
| Fat | 1 | 1 | 1 | Diet mayonnaise, 1 T.* | same | same |
| Vegetable | 1 | 2 | 2 | Carrot sticks, ½ cup | same + tomato juice, ½ cup | same |
| | | | | Green pepper strips, ½ cup | same | same |
| Fruit | 1 | 1 | 1 | Apple, 1 small | same | same |

*Tuna Sandwich Spread: Combine tuna, 1 T. each diced onion and celery, diet mayonnaise, 2 T. plain nonfat yogurt; spread between bread. (For 1,500 and 1,800 calorie levels, double the amount of onion and celery, if desired.)

**Evening Meal**

| | | | | | | |
|---|---|---|---|---|---|---|
| Meat | 2 | 2 | 3 | Roast beef, 2 oz. | same | 3 oz. |
| Starch | 1 | 2 | 3 | Mashed potatoes, ½ cup | same | 1 cup |
| | | | | none | Green peas, ½ cup | same |
| Fat | 1 | 1 | 2 | Diet margarine, 1 T. | same | same + reduced-calorie salad dressing, 2 T. |
| Vegetable | 1 | 2 | 2 | Vegetable Salad, 1 serving* + calorie-free salad dressing | 2 servings | same |
| Fruit | 1 | 1 | 1 | Honeydew melon, ⅛ | same | same |

*Vegetable Salad: For 1 serving, combine ½ med. tomato, chopped; ¼ cup sliced mushrooms; ¼ cup alfalfa sprouts. Arrange on 1 to 2 cups salad greens.

**Snack**

| | | | | | | |
|---|---|---|---|---|---|---|
| Starch | 1 | 1 | 2 | Sugar-free vanilla pudding, ½ cup | same | 1 cup |
| Fruit | 0 | 1 | 1 | none | Fresh cherries, 12* | same |
| Milk | 1 | 1 | 1 | Skim milk, 1 cup | same | same |

*Pit cherries; arrange on pudding. Garnish with 1 T. low-calorie topping, if desired.

# DAY 2

| | EXCHANGES | | | MENU | | |
|---|---|---|---|---|---|---|
| TYPE | CALORIE LEVEL | | | CALORIE LEVEL | | |
| | 1,200 | 1,500 | 1,800 | 1,200 | 1,500 | 1,800 |

**Breakfast**

| | | | | | | |
|---|---|---|---|---|---|---|
| Fruit | 1 | 1 | 1 | Seedless grapes, 15, or grape juice, ⅓ cup | same | same |
| Starch | 1 | 1 | 1 | Whole wheat bread, 1 slice | same | same |
| Meat | 1 | 1 | 1 | Cheddar cheese, 1-oz. cube | same | same |
| Fat | 1 | 1 | 1 | Diet margarine, 1 T. | same | same |
| Milk | 1 | 1 | 1 | Skim milk, 1 cup | same | same |

Use low-fat, low-cholesterol cheese, if desired.

**Noon Meal**

| | | | | | | |
|---|---|---|---|---|---|---|
| Meat | 2 | 2 | 2 | Roast turkey, white meat, cubed, 2 oz.* | same | same |
| Starch | 1 | 2 | 2 | Enriched macaroni, ½ cup cooked* | 1 cup* | same |
| Fat | 1 | 1 | 1 | Diet mayonnaise, 1 T.* | same | same |
| Vegetable | 1 | 2 | 2 | Garden Vegetable Salad** | Double ingredients** | same |
| Fruit | 1 | 1 | 1 | Mandarin orange sections, ¾ cup | same | same |

*Turkey Salad: Combine turkey, macaroni, diet mayonnaise, 2 T. plain nonfat yogurt, ½ t. sage; chill. Serve on 1 cup spinach leaves.

**Garden Vegetable Salad: Combine ¼ cup each chopped tomatoes, green onion, green pepper, broccoli flowerets. (For 1,500 and 1,800 calorie levels, use ½ cup each of vegetables.) Add calorie-free salad dressing.

**Evening Meal**

| | | | | | | |
|---|---|---|---|---|---|---|
| Meat | 2 | 2 | 3 | Speedy Baked Fish, 2 oz. cooked* | same | 3 oz.* |
| Starch | 1 | 2 | 3 | Steamed red potatoes, ½ cup | same | 1 cup |
| | | | | none | Whole wheat roll, 1 | same |
| Fat | 1 | 1 | 2 | Diet margarine, 1 T. | same | 2 T. |
| Vegetable | 1 | 2 | 2 | Steamed green beans, ½ cup | 1 cup | same |
| Fruit | 1 | 1 | 1 | Fresh peach, 1 large, or canned peaches, 2 halves | same | same |

*Speedy Baked Fish: Use 1 lb. frozen fish fillets; place in baking pan. Add 2 cups fat-free chicken broth; ½ t. dill; 2 cups sliced mushrooms, if desired; dash of white pepper. Bake at 425° for 15 to 20 minutes or microwave on high for 8 to 10 minutes until fish flakes.

**Snack**

| | | | | | | |
|---|---|---|---|---|---|---|
| Starch | 1 | 1 | 2 | Flaked bran cereal with raisins, ½ cup | same | 1 cup |
| Fruit | 0 | 1 | 1 | none | Banana, 9″, ½ | same |
| Milk | 1 | 1 | 1 | Skim milk, 1 cup | same | same |

# DAY 3

| EXCHANGES | | | | MENU | | |
|---|---|---|---|---|---|---|
| TYPE | CALORIE LEVEL | | | | CALORIE LEVEL | |
| | 1,200 | 1,500 | 1,800 | 1,200 | 1,500 | 1,800 |

### Breakfast

| | | | | | | |
|---|---|---|---|---|---|---|
| Fruit | 1 | 1 | 1 | Raisins, 2 T.* | same | same |
| Starch | 1 | 1 | 1 | Oatmeal toast, 1 slice* | same | same |
| Meat | 1 | 1 | 1 | Ricotta cheese, ¼ cup* | same | same |
| Fat | 1 | 1 | 1 | Walnuts, chopped, 1 T.* | same | same |
| Milk | 1 | 1 | 1 | Skim milk, 1 cup | same | same |

*Mock Danish: Combine ricotta cheese, raisins, cinnamon, walnuts. Spread on toast. Broil 1 to 2 minutes, if desired.

### Noon Meal

| | | | | | | |
|---|---|---|---|---|---|---|
| Meat | 2 | 2 | 2 | Thin-sliced turkey ham, 2 oz. | same | same |
| Starch | 1 | 2 | 2 | Rye bread, thin sliced, 2 slices | Rye bread, regular, 2 slices | same |
| Fat | 1 | 1 | 1 | Diet mayonnaise, 1 T. | same | same |
| Vegetable | 1 | 2 | 2 | Cherry tomatoes, 3 | 6 | same |
| | | | | Carrot sticks, ¼ cup | 1 cup | same |
| Fruit | 1 | 1 | 1 | Grapefruit sections, ¾ cup | same | same |

1 to 2 t. mustard may be used on sandwich.

### Evening Meal

| | | | | | | |
|---|---|---|---|---|---|---|
| Meat | 2 | 2 | 3 | BBQ chicken legs, 2 legs* | same | 3 legs* |
| Starch | 1 | 2 | 3 | none | Baked beans, ¼ cup | ½ cup |
| | | | | Baking powder biscuit, 2″ dia., 1 | same | same |
| Fat | 1 | 1 | 2 | omit | omit | Diet margarine, 1 T. |
| Vegetable | 1 | 2 | 2 | Steamed broccoli spears, ½ cup | 1 cup | same |
| Fruit | 1 | 1 | 1 | Watermelon, 1¼ cups | same | same |

*Baste chicken legs with regular or salt-free seasoned vegetable juice.

### Snack

| | | | | | | |
|---|---|---|---|---|---|---|
| Starch | 1 | 1 | 2 | Graham crackers, 2½″ squares, 3 | same | 6 |
| Fruit | 0 | 1 | 1 | none | Fresh plums, 2, or canned plums, ½ cup | same |
| Milk | 1 | 1 | 1 | Skim milk, 1 cup | same | same |

Note: Where "omit" is indicated, extra exchange listed is derived from another food item in menu.

# DAY 4

| TYPE | CALORIE LEVEL 1,200 | CALORIE LEVEL 1,500 | CALORIE LEVEL 1,800 | 1,200 | 1,500 | 1,800 |
|------|---------------------|---------------------|---------------------|-------|-------|-------|
| | **EXCHANGES** | | | **MENU** | | |

**Breakfast**

| TYPE | 1,200 | 1,500 | 1,800 | 1,200 | 1,500 | 1,800 |
|------|-------|-------|-------|-------|-------|-------|
| Fruit | 1 | 1 | 1 | Fresh pear, 1 small, or canned pears, 2 halves | same | same |
| Starch | 1 | 1 | 1 | Rye toast, regular, 1 slice, or 2 thin slices | same | same |
| Meat | 1 | 1 | 1 | Swiss cheese, 1-oz. cube | same | same |
| Fat | 1 | 1 | 1 | Diet margarine, 1 T. | same | same |
| Milk | 1 | 1 | 1 | Skim milk, 1 cup | same | same |

**Noon Meal**

| TYPE | 1,200 | 1,500 | 1,800 | 1,200 | 1,500 | 1,800 |
|------|-------|-------|-------|-------|-------|-------|
| Meat | 2 | 2 | 2 | Old-fashioned peanut butter, 2 T. | same | same |
| Starch | 1 | 2 | 2 | Saltine-type crackers, 6 | same + chicken noodle soup, 1 cup | same |
| Fat | 1 | 1 | 1 | Diet mayonnaise, 1 T. | same | same |
| Vegetable | 1 | 2 | 2 | Tomato Salad* | same + carrot and celery sticks, ½ cup each | same |
| Fruit | 1 | 1 | 1 | Tangerines, 2, or orange, 1 med. | same | same |

*Tomato Salad: Slice 1 med. tomato. Arrange on bed of lettuce. Sprinkle with fresh or dried basil. Use calorie-free salad dressing, if desired.

**Evening Meal**

| TYPE | 1,200 | 1,500 | 1,800 | 1,200 | 1,500 | 1,800 |
|------|-------|-------|-------|-------|-------|-------|
| Meat | 2 | 2 | 3 | Meatball, 2 oz. | same | same + Parmesan cheese, 2 T. |
| Starch | 1 | 2 | 3 | Spaghetti noodles, ½ cup | 1 cup | same + Italian bread, 1 slice |
| Fat | 1 | 1 | 2 | omit | omit | Diet margarine, 1 T. |
| Vegetable | 1 | 2 | 2 | Lettuce with raspberry vinegar (free) | same | same |
| | | | | Basic Italian sauce (no meat), ½ cup | same | same |
| | | | | none | Italian green beans, ½ cup | same |
| Fruit | 1 | 1 | 1 | Cantaloupe, 5″ dia., ⅓, or frozen melon balls, 1 cup | same | same |

**Snack**

| TYPE | 1,200 | 1,500 | 1,800 | 1,200 | 1,500 | 1,800 |
|------|-------|-------|-------|-------|-------|-------|
| Starch | 1 | 1 | 2 | Holland rusk, 2 | same | 4 |
| Fruit | 0 | 1 | 1 | none | Fresh or canned apricots, 4 | same |
| Milk | 1 | 1 | 1 | Skim milk, 1 cup | same | same |

Note: Where "omit" is indicated, extra exchange listed is derived from another food item in menu.

# DAY 5

| EXCHANGES | | | | MENU | | |
|---|---|---|---|---|---|---|
| TYPE | CALORIE LEVEL | | | | CALORIE LEVEL | |
| | 1,200 | 1,500 | 1,800 | 1,200 | 1,500 | 1,800 |

### Breakfast

| | | | | | | |
|---|---|---|---|---|---|---|
| Fruit | 1 | 1 | 1 | Mango, ½ small, or orange juice, ½ cup | same | same |
| Starch | 1 | 1 | 1 | Soft tortilla, 6″ dia., 1 | same | same |
| Meat | 1 | 1 | 1 | Julienned cooked chicken, 1 oz. | same | same |
| Fat | 1 | 1 | 1 | Taco salad dressing, 1 T. | same | same |
| Milk | 1 | 1 | 1 | Skim milk, 1 cup | same | same |

Free: You may add ¼ cup chopped fresh tomato, 2 T. each chopped green pepper and onion, 1 T. salsa.

### Noon Meal

| | | | | | | |
|---|---|---|---|---|---|---|
| Meat | 2 | 2 | 2 | Turkey frankfurter, 2 | same | same |
| Starch | 1 | 2 | 2 | Bun, 1 small (1 oz.)§ | 2 | same |
| Fat | 1 | 1 | 1 | Walnuts, 1 T.* | same | same |
| Vegetable | 1 | 2 | 2 | Fruited Carrot Salad* | same + extra vegetables listed in recipe* | same |
| Fruit | 1 | 1 | 1 | Raisins, 1 T.* | same | same |
| | | | | Crushed pineapple, 3 T.* | same | same |

§Lower calorie buns are commercially available.

*Fruited Carrot Salad: Combine 1 cup shredded carrot, walnuts, raisins, and crushed pineapple with 2 T. plain nonfat yogurt. (For 1,500 and 1,800 calorie levels, add 1 cup broccoli flowerets.) Chill. Serve on bed of lettuce.

1 T. catsup or mustard may be used on frankfurter.

### Evening Meal

| | | | | | | |
|---|---|---|---|---|---|---|
| Meat | 2 | 2 | 3 | Boiled medium shrimp, 4 oz. | same | 6 oz. |
| Starch | 1 | 2 | 3 | Confetti Rice, 1 serving* | 2 servings | same + dinner roll, 1 |
| Fat | 1 | 1 | 2 | Reduced-calorie salad dressing, 2 T.** | same | same + diet margarine, 1 T. |
| Vegetable | 1 | 2 | 2 | none | Asparagus spears, 6 to 8 | same |
| | | | | Vegetable Salad** | same | same |
| Fruit | 1 | 1 | 1 | Bing cherries, 12, or canned cherries, ½ cup | same | same |

*Confetti Rice: For 1 serving, steam 2 T. rice with ¼ cup water plus 1 T. each diced green and red pepper.

**Vegetable Salad: Combine 1 cup assorted vegetables of choice and serve on lettuce leaf-lined bowl.

### Snack

| | | | | | | |
|---|---|---|---|---|---|---|
| Starch | 1 | 1 | 2 | Animal crackers, 10 | same | 20 |
| Fruit | 0 | 1 | 1 | none | Blueberries, ¾ cup | same |
| Milk | 1 | 1 | 1 | Skim milk, 1 cup | same | same |

# DAY 6

| EXCHANGES | | | | MENU | |
|---|---|---|---|---|---|
| TYPE | CALORIE LEVEL | | | | CALORIE LEVEL | |
| | 1,200 | 1,500 | 1,800 | 1,200 | 1,500 | 1,800 |

**Breakfast**

| Fruit | 1 | 1 | 1 | Orange, 1 med., or orange juice, ½ cup | same | same |
|---|---|---|---|---|---|---|
| Starch | 1 | 1 | 1 | Raisin toast, 1 slice | same | same |
| Meat | 1 | 1 | 1 | Old-fashioned peanut butter, 1 T. | same | same |
| Fat | 1 | 1 | 1 | omit | omit | omit |
| Milk | 1 | 1 | 1 | Skim milk, 1 cup | same | same |

**Noon Meal**

| Meat | 2 | 2 | 2 | Canned salmon, ½ cup* | same | same |
|---|---|---|---|---|---|---|
| Starch | 1 | 2 | 2 | Ry Krisp, 3 crackers | 6 crackers | same |
| Fat | 1 | 1 | 1 | Diet mayonnaise, 1 T.* | same | same |
| Vegetable | 1 | 2 | 2 | ¼ cup each chopped green pepper, tomato, onion, wax beans* | ½ cup each* | same |
| Fruit | 1 | 1 | 1 | Seedless grapes, 15 | same | same |

*Salmon Salad: Combine salmon, vegetables, diet mayonnaise, 2 T. plain nonfat yogurt, 1 t. dill. Chill. Serve on bed of salad greens.

**Evening Meal**

| Meat | 2 | 2 | 3 | Roast pork, 2 oz. | same | 3 oz. |
|---|---|---|---|---|---|---|
| Starch | 1 | 2 | 3 | Baked potato, 1 small (3 oz.) | same | same |
| | | | | none | Rye bread, 1 slice | 2 slices |
| Fat | 1 | 1 | 2 | Diet margarine, 1 T. | same | 2 T. |
| Vegetable | 1 | 2 | 2 | Steamed cabbage wedge with caraway seed, ½ cup | 1 cup | same |
| Fruit | 1 | 1 | 1 | Baked apple, 1* | same | same |

*Core 1 small apple. Sprinkle with cinnamon or apple pie spice. Bake at 350° for 30 minutes or microwave on high for 2 to 4 minutes until soft.

**Snack**

| Starch | 1 | 1 | 2 | Raspberry sherbet, ¼ cup | same | ½ cup |
|---|---|---|---|---|---|---|
| Fruit | 0 | 1 | 1 | none | Fresh or frozen raspberries, 1 cup* | same |
| Milk | 1 | 1 | 1 | Skim milk, 1 cup | same | same |

*For 1,500 and 1,800 calorie levels, top berries with sherbet. If fresh or frozen unsweetened berries are unavailable, use ½ cup frozen variety with sugar.

Note: Where "omit" is indicated, extra exchange listed is derived from another food item in menu.

# DAY 7

| EXCHANGES | | | | MENU | | |
|---|---|---|---|---|---|---|
| TYPE | CALORIE LEVEL | | | CALORIE LEVEL | | |
| | 1,200 | 1,500 | 1,800 | 1,200 | 1,500 | 1,800 |

### Breakfast

| | | | | | | |
|---|---|---|---|---|---|---|
| Fruit | 1 | 1 | 1 | Raisins, 2 T.* | same | same |
| Starch | 1 | 1 | 1 | Wheat germ, ¼ cup* | same | same |
| Meat | 1 | 1 | 1 | omit | omit | omit |
| Fat | 1 | 1 | 1 | Walnuts, chopped, 1 T.* | same | same |
| Milk | 1 | 1 | 1 | Skim milk, 1 cup | same | same |

*Top wheat germ cereal with raisins and nuts; add enough milk to moisten. Let stand a few minutes before serving.

### Noon Meal

| | | | | | | |
|---|---|---|---|---|---|---|
| Meat | 2 | 2 | 2 | 1 to 2% cottage cheese, ½ cup | same | same |
| Starch | 1 | 2 | 2 | Saltine-type crackers, regular or salt-free, 6 | same + tomato soup, 1 cup (commercial variety diluted with water) | same |
| Fat | 1 | 1 | 1 | Diet margarine, 1 T. | same | same |
| Vegetable | 1 | 2 | 2 | ¼ cup each cauliflower, green pepper, carrots, zucchini | ½ cup each | same |
| Fruit | 1 | 1 | 1 | Fresh peach, 1 large, or canned peaches, 2 halves | same | same |

### Evening Meal

| | | | | | | |
|---|---|---|---|---|---|---|
| Meat | 2 | 2 | 3 | Broiled whitefish with lemon, 2 oz. cooked | same | 3 oz. |
| Starch | 1 | 2 | 3 | Spinach noodles, ½ cup | same | same |
| | | | | none | Whole wheat bread, 1 slice | 2 slices |
| Fat | 1 | 1 | 2 | Diet margarine, 1 T. | same | 2 T. |
| Vegetable | 1 | 2 | 2 | Steamed wax beans with red pepper strips, ½ cup | 1 cup | same |
| Fruit | 1 | 1 | 1 | Broiled grapefruit half* | same | same |

*Top grapefruit with 1 to 2 t. no-sugar strawberry jelly before broiling.

### Snack

| | | | | | | |
|---|---|---|---|---|---|---|
| Starch | 1 | 1 | 2 | Crisp flat bread, 2 crackers | same | 4 crackers |
| Fruit | 0 | 1 | 1 | none | Fresh plums, 2, or prunes, 3 regular or 5 snack size | same |
| Milk | 1 | 1 | 1 | Skim milk, 1 cup | same | same |

Note: Where "omit" is indicated, extra exchange listed is derived from another food item in menu.

# DAY 8

| EXCHANGES | | | | MENU | | |
|---|---|---|---|---|---|---|
| TYPE | CALORIE LEVEL | | | | CALORIE LEVEL | |
| | 1,200 | 1,500 | 1,800 | 1,200 | 1,500 | 1,800 |

### Breakfast

| | | | | | | |
|---|---|---|---|---|---|---|
| Fruit | 1 | 1 | 1 | Fresh fruit cup, ¾ cup, or no-sugar frozen fruit, ½ cup | same | same |
| Starch | 1 | 1 | 1 | Popover, 1 small | same | same |
| Meat | 1 | 1 | 1 | Fat-free scrambled egg* | same | same |
| Fat | 1 | 1 | 1 | omit | omit | omit |
| Milk | 1 | 1 | 1 | Skim milk, 1 cup | same | same |

*Use 1 med. egg or ¼ cup egg substitute.

### Noon Meal

| | | | | | | |
|---|---|---|---|---|---|---|
| Meat | 2 | 2 | 2 | Thin-sliced cold roast turkey, 2 oz. | same | same |
| Starch | 1 | 2 | 2 | Bran bread, thin sliced, 2 slices | Bran bread, regular, 2 slices | same |
| Fat | 1 | 1 | 1 | Diet mayonnaise, 1 T. | same | same |
| Vegetable | 1 | 2 | 2 | Homemade Vegetable Soup, 1 serving* | 2 servings* | same |
| Fruit | 1 | 1 | 1 | Fresh apricots, 4, or canned apricots, 4 halves | same | same |

*Homemade Vegetable Soup: To 1 cup fat-free broth, add ¼ cup each sliced mushrooms, sliced zucchini, shredded cabbage, shredded carrot. Simmer until tender. Float parsley sprig for garnish. Makes 1 serving.

### Evening Meal

| | | | | | | |
|---|---|---|---|---|---|---|
| Meat | 2 | 2 | 3 | Shredded Cheddar cheese, ½ oz.* | same | 1 oz.* |
| | | | | Ground beef or turkey, 1½ oz.* | same | 2 oz.* |
| Starch | 1 | 2 | 3 | Soft tortilla, 6″ dia., 1* | same | 2* |
| | | | | none | Refried beans, ⅓ cup | same |
| Fat | 1 | 1 | 2 | omit | omit | Avocado, ⅛ |
| Vegetable | 1 | 2 | 2 | ½ cup chopped tomato, ¼ cup diced green pepper, 2 T. chopped onion, ½ cup shredded lettuce* | same + raw carrots, 1 cup | same |
| Fruit | 1 | 1 | 1 | Kiwi, 1 large, sliced, or mandarin orange sections, ¾ cup | same | same |

*Tortillas: Brown meat in nonstick pan. Drain. Season with chili powder and/or taco seasoning to taste. Place on tortilla; add vegetables; top with cheese.

### Snack

| | | | | | | |
|---|---|---|---|---|---|---|
| Starch | 1 | 1 | 2 | High-fiber (12 grams per serving) cereal, ½ cup | same | 1 cup |
| Fruit | 0 | 1 | 1 | none | Banana, 9″, ½, sliced | same |
| Milk | 1 | 1 | 1 | Skim milk, 1 cup | same | same |

Note: Where "omit" is indicated, extra exchange listed is derived from another food item in menu.

# DAY 9

| EXCHANGES | | | | MENU | | |
|---|---|---|---|---|---|---|
| TYPE | CALORIE LEVEL | | | | CALORIE LEVEL | |
| | 1,200 | 1,500 | 1,800 | 1,200 | 1,500 | 1,800 |

**Breakfast**

| | 1,200 | 1,500 | 1,800 | 1,200 | 1,500 | 1,800 |
|---|---|---|---|---|---|---|
| Fruit | 1 | 1 | 1 | Grapefruit half, or grapefruit juice, ½ cup | same | same |
| Starch | 1 | 1 | 1 | Whole wheat toast, thin sliced, 2 slices | same | same |
| Meat | 1 | 1 | 1 | Poached egg, 1 med., or fat-free scrambled egg using ¼ cup egg substitute | same | same |
| Fat | 1 | 1 | 1 | Diet margarine, 1 T. | same | same |
| Milk | 1 | 1 | 1 | Skim milk, 1 cup | same | same |

**Noon Meal**

| | 1,200 | 1,500 | 1,800 | 1,200 | 1,500 | 1,800 |
|---|---|---|---|---|---|---|
| Meat | 2 | 2 | 2 | Thin-sliced cold roast beef, 2 oz. | same | same |
| Starch | 1 | 2 | 2 | Rye bread, thin sliced, 2 slices | Dark pumpernickel, 2 slices | same |
| Fat | 1 | 1 | 1 | Diet margarine or mayonnaise, 1 T. | same | same |
| Vegetable | 1 | 2 | 2 | Tomato, 1 med., sliced, on lettuce leaves | same + ½ cup each carrot and green pepper strips | same |
| Fruit | 1 | 1 | 1 | Pear, 1 small, or canned pears, 2 halves | same | same |

**Evening Meal**

| | 1,200 | 1,500 | 1,800 | 1,200 | 1,500 | 1,800 |
|---|---|---|---|---|---|---|
| Meat | 2 | 2 | 3 | Roast turkey breast, 2 oz. | same | 3 oz. |
| Starch | 1 | 2 | 3 | Bread dressing, ¼ cup | same | ½ cup |
| | | | | none | Mashed potatoes, ½ cup | same |
| Fat | 1 | 1 | 2 | Diet margarine, 1 T. | same | 2 T. |
| Vegetable | 1 | 2 | 2 | Brussels sprouts, ½ cup | 1 cup | same |
| Fruit | 1 | 1 | 1 | Fruited Gelatin Mold, 1 cup* | same | same |

*Use sugar-free gelatin and juice-packed unsweetened canned fruit. Follow package directions.

**Snack**

| | 1,200 | 1,500 | 1,800 | 1,200 | 1,500 | 1,800 |
|---|---|---|---|---|---|---|
| Starch | 1 | 1 | 2 | Graham crackers, 2½" squares, 3 | same | 6 |
| Fruit | 0 | 1 | 1 | none | Raisins, 2 T. | same |
| Milk | 1 | 1 | 1 | Skim milk, 1 cup | same | same |

MADE BY CHICKENS

# DAY 10

| EXCHANGES | | | | MENU | | |
|---|---|---|---|---|---|---|
| TYPE | CALORIE LEVEL | | | | CALORIE LEVEL | |
| | 1,200 | 1,500 | 1,800 | 1,200 | 1,500 | 1,800 |

### Breakfast

| | | | | | | |
|---|---|---|---|---|---|---|
| Fruit | 1 | 1 | 1 | Fresh or frozen blueberries, ¾ cup,* or orange juice, ½ cup | same | same |
| Starch | 1 | 1 | 1 | Pancakes, 4″ dia., 2 | same | same |
| Meat | 1 | 1 | 1 | Broiled ham, 1 oz. | same | same |
| Fat | 1 | 1 | 1 | omit | omit | omit |
| Milk | 1 | 1 | 1 | Skim milk, 1 cup | same | same |

*Use berries over pancakes or eat separately and use 1 to 2 T. sugar-free syrup.

### Noon Meal

| | | | | | | |
|---|---|---|---|---|---|---|
| Meat | 2 | 2 | 2 | Sliced cold chicken, 2 oz. | same | same |
| Starch | 1 | 2 | 2 | Whole wheat bread, thin sliced, 2 slices | Whole wheat bread, regular, 2 slices | same |
| Fat | 1 | 1 | 1 | Diet mayonnaise or margarine, 1 T. | same | same |
| Vegetable | 1 | 2 | 2 | Vegetable juice cocktail, regular or salt-free, 6 oz. | same + carrot sticks, 1 cup | same |
| Fruit | 1 | 1 | 1 | Tangerines, 2, or orange, 1 med. | same | same |

### Evening Meal

| | | | | | | |
|---|---|---|---|---|---|---|
| Meat | 2 | 2 | 3 | Roast beef (top round), 2 oz. | same | 3 oz. |
| Starch | 1 | 2 | 3 | Baked potato, 1 small (3 oz.) | same | same |
| | | | | none | Dinner roll, 1 (1 oz.) | 2 rolls |
| Fat | 1 | 1 | 2 | Diet margarine, 1 T. | same | 2 T. |
| Vegetable | 1 | 2 | 2 | Steamed wax/green bean mix, ½ cup | 1 cup | same |
| Fruit | 1 | 1 | 1 | Cantaloupe, 5″ dia., ⅓, or melon cubes, 1 cup | same | same |

### Snack

| | | | | | | |
|---|---|---|---|---|---|---|
| Starch | 1 | 1 | 2 | Pineapple sherbet, ¼ cup | same | ½ cup |
| Fruit | 0 | 1 | 1 | none | Canned pineapple chunks, ⅓ cup* | same |
| Milk | 1 | 1 | 1 | Skim milk, 1 cup | same | same |

*For 1,500 and 1,800 calorie levels, top sherbet with fruit for fruited sundae.

Note: Where "omit" is indicated, extra exchange listed is derived from another food item in menu.

# DAY 11

| EXCHANGES | | | | MENU | | |
|---|---|---|---|---|---|---|
| TYPE | CALORIE LEVEL | | | CALORIE LEVEL | | |
| | 1,200 | 1,500 | 1,800 | 1,200 | 1,500 | 1,800 |

### Breakfast

| | | | | | | |
|---|---|---|---|---|---|---|
| Fruit | 1 | 1 | 1 | Fresh peach, 1, or canned peach slices, ½ cup* | same | same |
| Starch | 1 | 1 | 1 | Raisin toast, 1 slice | same | same |
| Meat | 1 | 1 | 1 | 1 to 2% cottage cheese, ¼ cup | same | same |
| Fat | 1 | 1 | 1 | Diet margarine, 1 T. | same | same |
| Milk | 1 | 1 | 1 | Skim milk, 1 cup | same | same |

*Top cottage cheese with peaches; sprinkle lightly with cinnamon.

### Noon Meal

| | | | | | | |
|---|---|---|---|---|---|---|
| Meat | 2 | 2 | 2 | Thin-sliced ham, 4% fat, 2 oz. | same | same |
| Starch | 1 | 2 | 2 | Whole wheat bread, thin sliced, 2 slices | Whole wheat bread, regular, 2 slices | same |
| Fat | 1 | 1 | 1 | Diet mayonnaise, 1 T.* | same | same |
| Vegetable | 1 | 2 | 2 | Vegetable Slaw* | Double ingredients* | same |
| Fruit | 1 | 1 | 1 | Orange, 1 med. | same | same |

*Vegetable Slaw: Combine ½ cup shredded cabbage, ¼ cup shredded carrots, ¼ cup green pepper, 1 t. dill seed, diet mayonnaise, 2 T. plain nonfat yogurt. Mix and chill. (For 1,500 and 1,800 calorie levels, double ingredients, except mayonnaise.)

### Evening Meal

| | | | | | | |
|---|---|---|---|---|---|---|
| Meat | 2 | 2 | 3 | Sage baked chicken, 1 thigh (2 oz.) | same | 1 leg and 1 thigh (3 oz.) |
| Starch | 1 | 2 | 3 | Biscuit, 2″ dia., 1 | same | 2 |
| | | | | none | Peas, ½ cup | same |
| Fat | 1 | 1 | 2 | omit | omit | omit |
| Vegetable | 1 | 2 | 2 | Steamed cauliflower, ½ cup | 1 cup | same |
| Fruit | 1 | 1 | 1 | Baked apple, 1* | same | same |

*Core 1 small apple. Fill with 1 t. raisins; add dash of cinnamon. Place in small baking dish with 1 T. orange juice. Bake at 350° for 30 minutes or until soft.

### Snack

| | | | | | | |
|---|---|---|---|---|---|---|
| Starch | 1 | 1 | 2 | Rice cakes, 2 | same | same + 3 graham crackers |
| Fruit | 0 | 1 | 1 | none | Banana, 9″, ½ | same |
| Milk | 1 | 1 | 1 | Skim milk, 1 cup | same | same |

Try 1 to 2 t. low-sugar jam or jelly on rice cakes.

Note: Where "omit" is indicated, extra exchange listed is derived from another food item in menu.

# DAY 12

| TYPE | CALORIE LEVEL 1,200 | CALORIE LEVEL 1,500 | CALORIE LEVEL 1,800 | 1,200 | CALORIE LEVEL 1,500 | 1,800 |
|------|------|------|------|------|------|------|
| **EXCHANGES** | | | | **MENU** | | |

## EXCHANGES / MENU

| TYPE | 1,200 | 1,500 | 1,800 | 1,200 | 1,500 | 1,800 |
|------|-------|-------|-------|-------|-------|-------|
| **Breakfast** | | | | | | |
| Fruit | 1 | 1 | 1 | Fresh or frozen raspberries, 1 cup, or strawberries, sliced, 1¼ cups* | same | same |
| Starch | 1 | 1 | 1 | Commercial frozen waffle, 4½" dia., 1 | same | same |
| Meat | 1 | 1 | 1 | Broiled sausage link, 1 oz. | same | same |
| Fat | 1 | 1 | 1 | Diet margarine, 1 T. | same | same |
| Milk | 1 | 1 | 1 | Skim milk, 1 cup | same | same |

*Use fruit over heated waffle or eat separately and use 1 to 2 T. no-sugar syrup.

| TYPE | 1,200 | 1,500 | 1,800 | 1,200 | 1,500 | 1,800 |
|------|-------|-------|-------|-------|-------|-------|
| **Noon Meal** | | | | | | |
| Meat | 2 | 2 | 2 | Cooked small shrimp, 4 oz.* | same | same |
| Starch | 1 | 2 | 2 | Plain toasted bagel, ½ | Toasted bagel, split, whole | same |
| Fat | 1 | 1 | 1 | Diet mayonnaise, 1 T.* | same | same |
| Vegetable | 1 | 2 | 2 | Tomato, 1 med.* | same + carrot sticks, 1 cup | same |
| Fruit | 1 | 1 | 1 | Seedless red and/or green grapes, 15 | same | same |

*Shrimp-Stuffed Tomato: Combine shrimp, diet mayonnaise, 2 T. plain nonfat yogurt, 1 T. peas, 2 T. each chopped green onion and red pepper. Split tomato almost through into 5 to 6 wedges and arrange on lettuce leaf. Stuff with shrimp mixture.

| TYPE | 1,200 | 1,500 | 1,800 | 1,200 | 1,500 | 1,800 |
|------|-------|-------|-------|-------|-------|-------|
| **Evening Meal** | | | | | | |
| Meat | 2 | 2 | 3 | Cube steak, 2 oz.* | same | 3 oz. |
| Starch | 1 | 2 | 3 | Parslied rice, ⅓ cup cooked** | ⅔ cup | same + dinner roll, 1 |
| Fat | 1 | 1 | 2 | Diet margarine, 1 T. | same | 2 T. |
| Vegetable | 1 | 2 | 2 | Vegetable Combo, 1 serving*** | 2 servings | same |
| Fruit | 1 | 1 | 1 | Orange sections, ½ cup | same | same |

*Use 3 t. of diet margarine allowance to brown cube steak; then use small amount fat-free broth to finish cooking. Season with pepper.

**For parslied rice, use chicken broth in place of water. Add chopped fresh parsley to taste.

***Vegetable Combo: For 1 serving, simmer until tender: ½ cup summer-type squash slices (crookneck or zucchini), ¼ cup chopped tomato, ¼ onion (cut in wedges).

| TYPE | 1,200 | 1,500 | 1,800 | 1,200 | 1,500 | 1,800 |
|------|-------|-------|-------|-------|-------|-------|
| **Snack** | | | | | | |
| Starch | 1 | 1 | 2 | Air-popped popcorn, 3 cups | same | 6 cups |
| Fruit | 0 | 1 | 1 | none | Apple, 1 small | same |
| Milk | 1 | 1 | 1 | Skim milk, 1 cup | same | same |

# DAY 13

| EXCHANGES | | | | MENU | | |
|---|---|---|---|---|---|---|
| TYPE | CALORIE LEVEL | | | | CALORIE LEVEL | |
| | 1,200 | 1,500 | 1,800 | 1,200 | 1,500 | 1,800 |

### Breakfast

| TYPE | 1,200 | 1,500 | 1,800 | 1,200 | 1,500 | 1,800 |
|---|---|---|---|---|---|---|
| Fruit | 1 | 1 | 1 | Fresh fruit cup, ¾ cup, or cranberry juice, ⅓ cup | same | same |
| Starch | 1 | 1 | 1 | Nut bread, ½″ slice, 1 | same | same |
| Meat | 1 | 1 | 1 | Canadian bacon, 1 oz. | same | same |
| Fat | 1 | 1 | 1 | omit | omit | omit |
| Milk | 1 | 1 | 1 | Skim milk, 1 cup | same | same |

### Noon Meal

| TYPE | 1,200 | 1,500 | 1,800 | 1,200 | 1,500 | 1,800 |
|---|---|---|---|---|---|---|
| Meat | 2 | 2 | 2 | Thin-sliced cold turkey, 2 oz. | same | same |
| Starch | 1 | 2 | 2 | Rye bread, thin sliced, 2 slices | Caraway rye, regular, 2 slices | same |
| Fat | 1 | 1 | 1 | Diet mayonnaise, 1 T. | same | same |
| Vegetable | 1 | 2 | 2 | Marinated Vegetables* | Use ½ cup each of vegetables listed in recipe + ¼ cup very low calorie Italian salad dressing* | same |
| Fruit | 1 | 1 | 1 | Grapefruit sections, ¾ cup | same | same |

*Marinated Vegetables: Several hours before serving, combine ¼ cup each: sliced mushrooms, bean sprouts, cauliflowerets, green beans, and 2 T. very low calorie Italian dressing (4 to 6 calories per T.). (For 1,500 and 1,800 calorie levels, use ½ cup each of vegetables and ¼ cup dressing.) Serve on 2 to 3 lettuce leaves.

### Evening Meal

| TYPE | 1,200 | 1,500 | 1,800 | 1,200 | 1,500 | 1,800 |
|---|---|---|---|---|---|---|
| Meat | 2 | 2 | 3 | Scalloped Potatoes and Ham, 1 cup* | same | 1½ cups |
| Starch | 1 | 2 | 3 | omit | Dinner roll, 1 (1 oz.) | same + croutons, ½ cup |
| Fat | 1 | 1 | 2 | Reduced-calorie French dressing, 2 T. | same | same + margarine, 1 t. |
| Vegetable | 1 | 2 | 2 | Lettuce (free) | same + broccoli, ½ cup | same |
| Fruit | 1 | 1 | 1 | Watermelon, 1¼ cups | same | same |

*For recipe, see chapter 24.

### Snack

| TYPE | 1,200 | 1,500 | 1,800 | 1,200 | 1,500 | 1,800 |
|---|---|---|---|---|---|---|
| Starch | 1 | 1 | 2 | Flat or crisp bread, 2 crackers | same | 4 crackers |
| Fruit | 0 | 1 | 1 | none | Raisins, 2 T. | same |
| Milk | 1 | 1 | 1 | Skim milk, 1 cup | same | same |

Note: Where "omit" is indicated, extra exchange listed is derived from another food item in menu.

# DAY 14

| | EXCHANGES | | | MENU | | |
|---|---|---|---|---|---|---|
| TYPE | CALORIE LEVEL | | | CALORIE LEVEL | | |
| | 1,200 | 1,500 | 1,800 | 1,200 | 1,500 | 1,800 |

### Breakfast

| | | | | | | |
|---|---|---|---|---|---|---|
| Fruit | 1 | 1 | 1 | Applesauce, ½ cup | same | same |
| Starch | 1 | 1 | 1 | Whole wheat bread, 1 slice* | same | same |
| Meat | 1 | 1 | 1 | Egg, 1 med., or egg substitute, ¼ cup* | same | same |
| Fat | 1 | 1 | 1 | Diet margarine, 1 T* | same | same |
| Milk | 1 | 1 | 1 | Skim milk, 1 cup | same | same |

*French toast: Beat egg with 1 T. of allotted skim milk; flavor with 1 t. vanilla extract and dash of cinnamon. Dip both sides of bread into egg; then allow to absorb egg. Brown with diet margarine in nonstick pan. Serve applesauce over French toast or serve separately and use 1 to 2 T. sugar-free syrup on French toast.

### Noon Meal

| | | | | | | |
|---|---|---|---|---|---|---|
| Meat | 2 | 2 | 2 | Low-fat Cheddar cheese, 2 oz.* | same | same |
| Starch | 1 | 2 | 2 | Baked potato, ½ large (3 oz.)* | 1 large (6 oz.)* | same |
| Fat | 1 | 1 | 1 | Diet mayonnaise, 1 T.* | same | same |
| Vegetable | 1 | 2 | 2 | Cooked broccoli, chopped, ½ cup* | 1 cup* | same |
| Fruit | 1 | 1 | 1 | Orange, 1 med. | same | same |

*Stuffed Potato: Scoop out potato, leaving ½" shell. Mix potato with chopped, cooked broccoli, diet mayonnaise, 2 T. plain nonfat yogurt, Cheddar cheese (cubed). Stuff into shell and place under broiler until lightly browned.

### Evening Meal

| | | | | | | |
|---|---|---|---|---|---|---|
| Meat | 2 | 2 | 3 | Broiled pork chop, 2 oz. | same | 3 oz. |
| Starch | 1 | 2 | 3 | Boiled potato, 1 small (3 oz.) | same | same |
| | | | | none | Corn-on-the-cob, 6" ear, 1 ear | 2 ears |
| Fat | 1 | 1 | 2 | Diet margarine, 1 T. | same | 2 T. |
| Vegetable | 1 | 2 | 2 | Cooked tomatoes (seasoned with green onions, celery), ½ cup | 1 cup | same |
| Fruit | 1 | 1 | 1 | Fruited Gelatin Mold, 1 cup* | same | same |

*Use sugar-free gelatin and juice-packed unsweetened canned fruit. Follow package directions. Top with 2 T. whipped topping.

### Snack

| | | | | | | |
|---|---|---|---|---|---|---|
| Starch | 1 | 1 | 2 | Graham crackers, 2½" squares, 3 | same | 6 |
| Fruit | 0 | 1 | 1 | none | Apple, 1 small | same |
| Milk | 1 | 1 | 1 | Skim milk, 1 cup | same | same |

# DAY 15

| EXCHANGES | | | | MENU | | |
|---|---|---|---|---|---|---|
| TYPE | CALORIE LEVEL | | | | CALORIE LEVEL | |
| | 1,200 | 1,500 | 1,800 | 1,200 | 1,500 | 1,800 |

### Breakfast

| | | | | | | |
|---|---|---|---|---|---|---|
| Fruit | 1 | 1 | 1 | Kiwi, 1 large, sliced, or cranberry juice, ⅓ cup | same | same |
| Starch | 1 | 2 | 2 | Toasted whole wheat English muffin, split, half | whole | same |
| Fat | 1 | 1 | 1 | Diet margarine, 1 T. | same | same |
| Milk | 1 | 1 | 1 | Skim milk, 1 cup | same | same |

### Noon Meal

| | | | | | | |
|---|---|---|---|---|---|---|
| Meat | 2 | 2 | 2 | Bean soup, 1 cup | same | same |
| | | | | Low-fat Cheddar cheese, 1 oz. | same | same |
| Starch | 1 | 2 | 2 | omit | Saltine-type crackers, regular or salt-free, 6 | same |
| Fat | 1 | 1 | 1 | Reduced-calorie salad dressing, 2 T. | same | same |
| Vegetable | 1 | 2 | 2 | Tossed green salad | same + carrot sticks, 1 cup | same |
| Fruit | 1 | 1 | 1 | Golden Delicious apple, 1 small | same | same |

### Evening Meal

| | | | | | | |
|---|---|---|---|---|---|---|
| Meat | 3 | 3 | 4 | Broiled beef patty, 3 oz. | same | 4 oz. |
| Starch | 1 | 1 | 2 | Hamburger bun, 1 small (1 oz.) | same | 1 regular size |
| Fat | 1 | 1 | 2 | Diet margarine, 1 T.* | same | 2 T. |
| Vegetable | 1 | 2 | 2 | Vegetable Kabob* | 2 kabobs | same |
| Fruit | 1 | 1 | 1 | Watermelon, 1¼ cups | same | same |

*Kabob for One: Place on skewer: 4 1″ green pepper chunks, 3 small onions, 4 1″ chunks summer squash, 3 cherry tomatoes. Baste with melted diet margarine and dash of oregano. Grill until tender.

### Snack

| | | | | | | |
|---|---|---|---|---|---|---|
| Starch | 1 | 1 | 2 | Frozen yogurt, ⅓ cup | same | ⅔ cup |
| Fruit | 0 | 1 | 1 | none | Mango, ½,* or strawberries, 1¼ cups | same |
| Milk | 1 | 1 | 1 | Skim milk, 1 cup | same | same |

*For 1,500 and 1,800 calorie levels, serve yogurt on mango half.

Note: Where "omit" is indicated, extra exchange listed is derived from another food item in menu.

# DAY 16

| EXCHANGES | | | | MENU | | |
|---|---|---|---|---|---|---|
| TYPE | CALORIE LEVEL | | | CALORIE LEVEL | | |
| | 1,200 | 1,500 | 1,800 | 1,200 | 1,500 | 1,800 |

### Breakfast

| TYPE | 1,200 | 1,500 | 1,800 | 1,200 | 1,500 | 1,800 |
|---|---|---|---|---|---|---|
| Fruit | 1 | 1 | 1 | Seedless raisins, 2 T. | same | same |
| Starch | 1 | 2 | 2 | none | Cooked oatmeal, ½ cup | same |
| | | | | Whole wheat toast, 1 slice | same | same |
| Fat | 1 | 1 | 1 | Diet margarine, 1 T. | same | same |
| Milk | 1 | 1 | 1 | Skim milk, 1 cup | same | same |

### Noon Meal

| TYPE | 1,200 | 1,500 | 1,800 | 1,200 | 1,500 | 1,800 |
|---|---|---|---|---|---|---|
| Meat | 2 | 2 | 2 | Water-packed tuna, ½ cup* | same | same |
| Starch | 1 | 2 | 2 | Pita bread, 6″ dia., ½* | Whole, cut in half* | same |
| Fat | 1 | 1 | 1 | Diet mayonnaise, 1 T.* | same | same |
| Vegetable | 1 | 2 | 2 | Tomato juice, regular or salt-free, 6 oz. | same + carrot sticks, 1 cup | same |
| Fruit | 1 | 1 | 1 | Orange, 1 med., cut in wedges | same | same |

*Tuna-Stuffed Pita: Combine tuna; diet mayonnaise; 2 T. plain nonfat yogurt; ¼ cup each alfalfa or bean sprouts; 2 T. each chopped green onion, tomato, green pepper; dash of white pepper. Stuff pita bread with tuna mixture.

### Evening Meal

| TYPE | 1,200 | 1,500 | 1,800 | 1,200 | 1,500 | 1,800 |
|---|---|---|---|---|---|---|
| Meat | 3 | 3 | 4 | Braised pork chop, 3 oz. | same | 4 oz. |
| Starch | 1 | 1 | 2 | Noodles, ½ cup | same | same + rye bread, 1 slice |
| Fat | 1 | 1 | 2 | Diet margarine, 1 T. | same | 2 T. |
| Vegetable | 1 | 2 | 2 | Asparagus spears, 6 to 8 | 12 to 16 | same |
| Fruit | 1 | 1 | 1 | Applesauce, ½ cup* | same | same |

*Dust applesauce with cinnamon. Garnish with mint.

### Snack

| TYPE | 1,200 | 1,500 | 1,800 | 1,200 | 1,500 | 1,800 |
|---|---|---|---|---|---|---|
| Starch | 1 | 1 | 2 | Graham crackers, 2½″ squares, 3 | same | 6 |
| Fruit | 0 | 1 | 1 | none | Fruit cocktail, ½ cup | same |
| Milk | 1 | 1 | 1 | Skim milk, 1 cup | same | same |

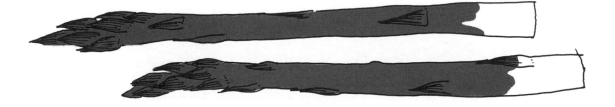

# DAY 17

| EXCHANGES | | | | MENU | | |
|---|---|---|---|---|---|---|
| TYPE | CALORIE LEVEL | | | | CALORIE LEVEL | |
| | 1,200 | 1,500 | 1,800 | 1,200 | 1,500 | 1,800 |
| **Breakfast** | | | | | | |
| Fruit | 1 | 1 | 1 | Ready-to-eat snack prunes, 5, or prune juice, ⅓ cup | same | same |
| Starch | 1 | 2 | 2 | none | Multi-vitamin mineral ready-to-eat cereal, ¾ cup | same |
| | | | | Rye toast, 1 slice | same | same |
| Fat | 1 | 1 | 1 | Diet margarine, 1 T. | same | same |
| Milk | 1 | 1 | 1 | Skim milk, 1 cup | same | same |
| **Noon Meal** | | | | | | |
| Meat | 2 | 2 | 2 | Thin-sliced/shaved chicken, 2 oz. | same | same |
| Starch | 1 | 2 | 2 | Whole wheat roll, 1 small (1 oz.) | 2 | same |
| Fat | 1 | 1 | 1 | Diet margarine, 1 T. | same | same |
| Vegetable | 1 | 2 | 2 | Vegetable juice, regular or salt-free, 6 oz. | same + carrot and green pepper strips, ½ cup each | same |
| Fruit | 1 | 1 | 1 | Fresh pineapple chunks, ¾ cup, or canned pineapple chunks, ⅓ cup | same | same |
| **Evening Meal** | | | | | | |
| Meat | 3 | 3 | 4 | Beef stew (select or good grade chuck roast), 3 oz. | same | 4 oz. |
| Starch | 1 | 1 | 2 | Potato, 1 small (3 oz.) | same | same + whole wheat bread, 1 slice |
| Fat | 1 | 1 | 2 | Reduced-calorie salad dressing, 2 T. | same | same + diet margarine, 1 T. |
| Vegetable | 1 | 2 | 2 | Cooked carrots, ½ cup | same | same |
| | | | | none | Cooked onion, ½ cup | same |
| | | | | Tossed green salad (free) | same | same |
| Fruit | 1 | 1 | 1 | Orange, 1 med. | same | same |
| **Snack** | | | | | | |
| Starch | 1 | 1 | 2 | Rice cakes, 2 | same | 4 |
| Fruit | 0 | 1 | 1 | none | Fruit cocktail, ½ cup | same |
| Milk | 1 | 1 | 1 | Skim milk, 1 cup | same | same |

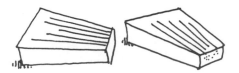
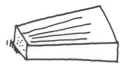

# DAY 18

| | EXCHANGES | | | MENU | | |
|---|---|---|---|---|---|---|
| TYPE | CALORIE LEVEL | | | CALORIE LEVEL | | |
| | 1,200 | 1,500 | 1,800 | 1,200 | 1,500 | 1,800 |

**Breakfast**

| | | | | | | |
|---|---|---|---|---|---|---|
| Fruit | 1 | 1 | 1 | Orange, 1 med., sliced, or orange juice, ½ cup | same | same |
| Starch | 1 | 2 | 2 | none | Toasted oat cereal, ¾ cup | same |
| | | | | Raisin toast, 1 slice | same | same |
| Fat | 1 | 1 | 1 | Diet margarine, 1 T. | same | same |
| Milk | 1 | 1 | 1 | Skim milk, 1 cup | same | same |

**Noon Meal**

| | | | | | | |
|---|---|---|---|---|---|---|
| Meat | 2 | 2 | 2 | Low-fat Swiss cheese (for broiled cheese sandwich), 2 oz. | same | same |
| Starch | 1 | 2 | 2 | Rye bread, thin sliced, 2 slices | Pumpernickel rye, 2 slices | same |
| Fat | 1 | 1 | 1 | Olives, 5 large | same | same |
| Vegetable | 1 | 2 | 2 | Raw broccoli, ½ cup | 1 cup | same |
| | | | | Raw cauliflower ½ cup | 1 cup | same |
| Fruit | 1 | 1 | 1 | Cantaloupe, 5" dia., ⅓, or frozen melon cubes, 1 cup | same | same |

**Evening Meal**

| | | | | | | |
|---|---|---|---|---|---|---|
| Meat | 3 | 3 | 4 | Baked ham studded with cloves and basted with orange juice, 3 oz. | same | 4 oz. |
| Starch | 1 | 1 | 2 | Scalloped potatoes, ½ cup | same | 1 cup |
| Fat | 1 | 1 | 2 | omit | omit | omit |
| Vegetable | 1 | 2 | 2 | Whole baby carrots, ½ cup | 1 cup | same |
| Fruit | 1 | 1 | 1 | Apple, 1 small, or applesauce, ½ cup | same | same |

**Snack**

| | | | | | | |
|---|---|---|---|---|---|---|
| Starch | 1 | 1 | 2 | Graham crackers, 2½" squares, 3 | same | 6 |
| Fruit | 0 | 1 | 1 | none | Fresh pear, 1 small, or canned pears, 2 halves | same |
| Milk | 1 | 1 | 1 | Skim milk, 1 cup | same | same |

Note: Where "omit" is indicated, extra exchange listed is derived from another food item in menu.

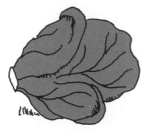

# DAY 19

| EXCHANGES | | | | MENU | | |
|---|---|---|---|---|---|---|
| TYPE | CALORIE LEVEL | | | | CALORIE LEVEL | |
| | 1,200 | 1,500 | 1,800 | 1,200 | 1,500 | 1,800 |

**Breakfast**

| | | | | | | |
|---|---|---|---|---|---|---|
| Fruit | 1 | 1 | 1 | Fresh apricots, 4, or canned apricots, 4 halves | same | same |
| Starch | 1 | 2 | 2 | none | Shredded Wheat Biscuit, 1 large | same |
| | | | | Banana bread, ½″ slice, 1 slice | same | same |
| Fat | 1 | 1 | 1 | omit | omit | omit |
| Milk | 1 | 1 | 1 | Skim milk, 1 cup | same | same |

**Noon Meal**

| | | | | | | |
|---|---|---|---|---|---|---|
| Meat | 2 | 2 | 2 | Thin-sliced/shaved roast beef, 2 oz. | same | same |
| Starch | 1 | 2 | 2 | Whole wheat bread, thin sliced, 2 slices | Whole wheat bread, regular, 2 slices | same |
| Fat | 1 | 1 | 1 | Diet margarine or mayonnaise, 1 T. | same | same |
| Vegetable | 1 | 2 | 2 | Cherry tomatoes, 3 | 6 | same |
| | | | | Carrot sticks, ½ cup | 1 cup | same |
| Fruit | 1 | 1 | 1 | Tangerines, 2, or orange, 1 med. | same | same |

**Evening Meal**

| | | | | | | |
|---|---|---|---|---|---|---|
| Meat | 3 | 3 | 4 | Baked chicken breast, 3 oz. | same | 4 oz. |
| Starch | 1 | 1 | 2 | Spinach noodles, ½ cup | same | 1 cup |
| Fat | 1 | 1 | 2 | Diet margarine, 1 T. | same | 2 T. |
| Vegetable | 1 | 2 | 2 | Steamed cauliflower, ½ cup* | 1 cup | same |
| Fruit | 1 | 1 | 1 | Cherries, 12, or canned cherries, ½ cup | same | same |

*Dust cauliflower with paprika.

**Snack**

| | | | | | | |
|---|---|---|---|---|---|---|
| Starch | 1 | 1 | 2 | Sugar-free vanilla pudding, ½ cup | same | 1 cup |
| Fruit | 0 | 1 | 1 | none | Banana, 9″, ½, sliced* | same |
| Milk | 1 | 1 | 1 | Skim milk, 1 cup | same | same |

*For 1,500 and 1,800 calorie levels, combine banana slices with pudding. Garnish with 1 to 2 T. low-calorie topping.

Note: Where "omit" is indicated, extra exchange listed is derived from another food item in menu.

# DAY 20

| | EXCHANGES | | | MENU | | |
|---|---|---|---|---|---|---|
| TYPE | CALORIE LEVEL | | | | CALORIE LEVEL | |
| | 1,200 | 1,500 | 1,800 | 1,200 | 1,500 | 1,800 |

### Breakfast

| | | | | | | |
|---|---|---|---|---|---|---|
| Fruit | 1 | 1 | 1 | Fresh Fruit Cup* | same | same |
| Starch | 1 | 2 | 2 | none | High-fiber cereal, ½ cup | same |
| | | | | Small plain donut, 1 | same | same |
| Fat | 1 | 1 | 1 | omit | omit | omit |
| Milk | 1 | 1 | 1 | Skim milk, 1 cup | same | same |

*Fresh Fruit Cup: Use ¾ cup strawberries, ⅓ cup blueberries, 1″ segment of banana (sliced).

### Noon Meal

| | | | | | | |
|---|---|---|---|---|---|---|
| Meat | 2 | 2 | 2 | Lean meat, 2 oz.* | same | same |
| Starch | 1 | 2 | 2 | Brown or white rice, ⅓ cup cooked* | ⅔ cup cooked* | same |
| Fat | 1 | 1 | 1 | Cashews, 1 T. | same | same |
| Vegetable | 1 | 2 | 2 | Raw pea pods or shredded cabbage, 1 cup* | 2 cups* | same |
| | | | | Mushrooms, ½ cup* | 1 cup* | same |
| Fruit | 1 | 1 | 1 | Mandarin orange sections, ¾ cup | same | same |

*Stir Fry: Heat wok (or electric fry pan) until several drops of water dance on surface. Add meat, 2 T. beef broth; brown, stirring continuously. Push aside and add vegetables, continuing to stir. Add ½ t. cornstarch, ⅛ t. garlic, ⅛ t. ginger to ½ cup water; stir into meat-vegetable mixture. Cover; simmer until crisp-tender. Serve over rice.

### Evening Meal

| | | | | | | |
|---|---|---|---|---|---|---|
| Meat | 3 | 3 | 4 | Roast turkey, 3 oz. | same | 4 oz. |
| Starch | 1 | 1 | 2 | Baked acorn squash, ½* | same | 2 halves* |
| Fat | 1 | 1 | 2 | Diet margarine, 1 T.* | same | 2 T.* |
| Vegetable | 1 | 2 | 2 | Steamed broccoli, ½ cup | 1 cup | same |
| | | | | Tossed green salad with herbed vinegar | same | same |
| Fruit | 1 | 1 | 1 | Seedless grapes, 15 | same | same |

*Bake squash in oven or microwave until tender. Cut in half. Remove seeds. Dot each half with 1 T. diet margarine and 1 T. low-calorie maple syrup. Add dash of allspice. Serve immediately.

### Snack

| | | | | | | |
|---|---|---|---|---|---|---|
| Starch | 1 | 1 | 2 | Gingersnaps, 3 | same | 6 |
| Fruit | 0 | 1 | 1 | none | Apple, 1 small, or applesauce, ½ cup | same |
| Milk | 1 | 1 | 1 | Skim milk, 1 cup | same | same |

Note: Where "omit" is indicated, extra exchange listed is derived from another food item in menu.

# DAY 21

| | EXCHANGES | | | MENU | | |
|---|---|---|---|---|---|---|
| TYPE | CALORIE LEVEL | | | | CALORIE LEVEL | |
| | 1,200 | 1,500 | 1,800 | 1,200 | 1,500 | 1,800 |
| **Breakfast** | | | | | | |
| Fruit | 1 | 1 | 1 | Fresh or frozen blueberries, ¾ cup | same | same |
| Starch | 1 | 2 | 2 | none | Puffed rice, 1¼ cups | same |
| | | | | Whole wheat toast, 1 slice | same | same |
| Fat | 1 | 1 | 1 | Diet margarine, 1 T. | same | same |
| Milk | 1 | 1 | 1 | Skim milk, 1 cup | same | same |
| **Noon Meal** | | | | | | |
| Meat | 2 | 2 | 2 | Diced chicken, 2 oz.* | same | same |
| Starch | 1 | 2 | 2 | Bread sticks, ⅔ oz. | 1⅓ oz. | same |
| Fat | 1 | 1 | 1 | Diet mayonnaise, 1 T.* | same | same |
| Vegetable | 1 | 2 | 2 | Assorted diced vegetables, 1 cup* | same + vegetable juice cocktail, regular or salt-free, 6 oz. | same |
| Fruit | 1 | 1 | 1 | Seedless green grapes, cluster of 15 | same | same |

*Chicken-Vegetable Salad Plate: Combine chicken, vegetables, diet mayonnaise, 2 T. plain nonfat yogurt, dash of curry (if desired). Chill. Serve on bed of salad greens. Arrange bread sticks and cluster of grapes alongside salad.

For 1,500 and 1,800 calorie levels, serve vegetable juice cocktail hot or on ice.

| | EXCHANGES | | | MENU | | |
|---|---|---|---|---|---|---|
| **Evening Meal** | | | | | | |
| Meat | 3 | 3 | 4 | Lean ground round, 3 oz. cooked (individual meat loaves)* | same | 4 oz. cooked* |
| Starch | 1 | 1 | 2 | Whole kernel corn, ½ cup | same | 1 cup |
| Fat | 1 | 1 | 2 | Diet margarine, 1 T. | same | 2 T. |
| Vegetable | 1 | 2 | 2 | French green beans, ½ cup | 1 cup | same |
| Fruit | 1 | 1 | 1 | Fresh peach, 1 small, or canned peaches, 2 halves | same | same |

*Individual meat loaves: Use lean ground round in your favorite meat loaf recipe. Form 4 oz. raw (5 oz. for 1,800 calorie level) into a round. Bake on rack at 350° for 20 to 30 minutes or until done.

| | EXCHANGES | | | MENU | | |
|---|---|---|---|---|---|---|
| **Snack** | | | | | | |
| Starch | 1 | 1 | 2 | Frozen fruit yogurt, ⅓ cup | same | ⅔ cup |
| Fruit | 0 | 1 | 1 | none | Fresh peach, 1 large, or canned peaches, 2 halves* | same |
| Milk | 1 | 1 | 1 | Skim milk, 1 cup | same | same |

*For 1,500 and 1,800 calorie levels, serve fruit over frozen yogurt.

# DAY 22

| EXCHANGES | | | | MENU | | |
|---|---|---|---|---|---|---|
| TYPE | CALORIE LEVEL | | | | CALORIE LEVEL | |
| | 1,200 | 1,500 | 1,800 | 1,200 | 1,500 | 1,800 |
| **Breakfast** | | | | | | |
| Fruit | 1 | 1 | 1 | Apple, 1 small, chopped* | same | same |
| Starch | 1 | 2 | 2 | none | Grape Nuts cereal, 3 T.* | same |
| | | | | Boston brown bread, ½″, 1 slice | same | same |
| Fat | 1 | 1 | 1 | Diet margarine, 1 T. | same | same |
| Milk | 1 | 1 | 1 | Plain nonfat yogurt, ¾ cup* | same | same |

*Breakfast Yogurt: Combine fruit, yogurt, dash of cinnamon. (For 1,500 and 1,800 calorie levels, add cereal.) For a fast breakfast, make the night before and store in refrigerator.

| | | | | **Noon Meal**<br>**(for Lunch-on-the-Run)** | | |
|---|---|---|---|---|---|---|
| Meat | 2 | 2 | 2 | String cheese, 2 oz. | same | same |
| Starch | 1 | 2 | 2 | English water crackers, 4 | 8 | same |
| Fat | 1 | 1 | 1 | Peanuts, 10 large | same | same |
| Vegetable | 1 | 2 | 2 | Carrot sticks, 1 cup | same + green zucchini sticks, 1 cup | same |
| Fruit | 1 | 1 | 1 | Tangerines, 2, or orange, 1 med. | same | same |

| | | | | **Evening Meal** | | |
|---|---|---|---|---|---|---|
| Meat | 3 | 3 | 4 | Broiled whitefish, 3 oz.* | same | 4 oz.* |
| Starch | 1 | 1 | 2 | Boiled small red potatoes, 3 oz. | same | same + rye bread, 1 slice |
| Fat | 1 | 1 | 2 | Diet margarine, 1 T. | same | 2 T. |
| Vegetable | 1 | 2 | 2 | Steamed broccoli spears, ½ cup | 1 cup | same |
| Fruit | 1 | 1 | 1 | Fresh pineapple, ¾ cup | same | same |

*Brush whitefish with 1 t. of diet margarine allowance and squeeze of lemon.

| | | | | **Snack** | | |
|---|---|---|---|---|---|---|
| Starch | 1 | 1 | 2 | Ry Krisp, 3 crackers | same | 6 crackers |
| Fruit | 0 | 1 | 1 | none | Nectarine, 1½″ dia., 1, or canned pears, 2 halves | same |
| Milk | 1 | 1 | 1 | Skim milk, 1 cup | same | same |

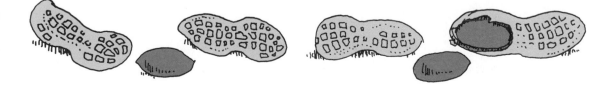

# DAY 23

| | EXCHANGES | | | MENU | | |
|---|---|---|---|---|---|---|
| TYPE | CALORIE LEVEL | | | | CALORIE LEVEL | |
| | 1,200 | 1,500 | 1,800 | 1,200 | 1,500 | 1,800 |

### Breakfast

| | | | | | | |
|---|---|---|---|---|---|---|
| Fruit | 1 | 1 | 1 | Orange, 1 med., or orange juice, ½ cup | same | same |
| Starch | 1 | 2 | 2 | none | Shredded Wheat Squares, ½ cup | same |
| | | | | Raisin toast, 1 slice | same | same |
| Fat | 1 | 1 | 1 | Diet margarine, 1 T. | same | same |
| Milk | 1 | 1 | 1 | Skim milk, 1 cup | same | same |

### Noon Meal

| | | | | | | |
|---|---|---|---|---|---|---|
| Meat | 2 | 2 | 2 | Thin-sliced/shaved roast beef, 2 oz. | same | same |
| Starch | 1 | 2 | 2 | Whole wheat bread, thin sliced, 2 slices | Whole wheat bread, regular, 2 slices | same |
| Fat | 1 | 1 | 1 | Diet mayonnaise, 1 T. | same | same |
| Vegetable | 1 | 2 | 2 | Tomato, 1 med., sliced, on lettuce leaves (free) | same + raw cauliflower, 1 cup | same |
| Fruit | 1 | 1 | 1 | Fresh peach, 1 large, or canned peaches, 2 halves | same | same |

Try fresh cracked pepper with fresh lemon juice on tomato salad.

### Evening Meal

| | | | | | | |
|---|---|---|---|---|---|---|
| Meat | 3 | 3 | 4 | Roast turkey, 3 oz. | same | 4 oz. |
| Starch | 1 | 1 | 2 | Sweet potato slices, ¼ cup | same | ½ cup |
| Fat | 1 | 1 | 2 | Diet margarine, 1 T. | same | same + reduced-calorie salad dressing, 2 T. |
| Vegetable | 1 | 2 | 2 | Steamed spinach, ½ cup | 1 cup | same |
| | | | | Tossed salad greens | same | same |
| Fruit | 1 | 1 | 1 | Fresh fruit cup, ½ cup | same | same |

Cranberry sauce, ¼ to ½ cup (free exchange): To make sauce, cook cranberries with water. When cranberries are tender, cool and add sugar substitute to taste.

### Snack

| | | | | | | |
|---|---|---|---|---|---|---|
| Starch | 1 | 1 | 2 | Toasted English muffin, ½ | same | Whole muffin |
| Fruit | 0 | 1 | 1 | none | Fresh plums, 2, or canned plums, ½ cup | same |
| Milk | 1 | 1 | 1 | Sugar-Free Cocoa* | same | same |

*Sugar-Free Cocoa: Combine ⅓ cup nonfat dry milk, 2 t. unsweetened cocoa. Add ¾ cup hot water. Stir. Add 1 to 2 packets sugar substitute to taste.

# DAY 24

| EXCHANGES | | | | MENU | | |
|---|---|---|---|---|---|---|
| TYPE | CALORIE LEVEL | | | | CALORIE LEVEL | |
| | 1,200 | 1,500 | 1,800 | 1,200 | 1,500 | 1,800 |

### Breakfast

| | | | | | | |
|---|---|---|---|---|---|---|
| Fruit | 1 | 1 | 1 | Fresh pineapple, ¾ cup, or pineapple juice, ½ cup | same | same |
| Starch | 1 | 2 | 2 | none | Cooked oatmeal, ½ cup | same |
| | | | | Blueberry muffin, 2″ dia., 1 | same | same |
| Fat | 1 | 1 | 1 | omit | omit | omit |
| Milk | 1 | 1 | 1 | Skim milk, 1 cup | same | same |

### Noon Meal

| | | | | | | |
|---|---|---|---|---|---|---|
| Meat | 2 | 2 | 2 | Water-packed tuna, ½ cup* | same | same |
| Starch | 1 | 2 | 2 | Ry Krisp, 3 crackers | 6 crackers | same |
| Fat | 1 | 1 | 1 | Diet mayonnaise, 1 T.* | same | same |
| Vegetable | 1 | 2 | 2 | Tomato, 1 med.* | same | same |
| Fruit | 1 | 1 | 1 | Fresh pear, 1 small, or canned pears, 2 halves | same | same |

*Tuna-Stuffed Tomato: Combine tuna, diet mayonnaise, 2 T. nonfat plain yogurt, 1 to 2 T. each diced onion and green pepper. Split tomato almost through into 5 to 6 wedges and arrange on chilled lettuce. Stuff with tuna mixture.

### Evening Meal

| | | | | | | |
|---|---|---|---|---|---|---|
| Meat | 3 | 3 | 4 | Meat loaf, 3 oz. | same | 4 oz. |
| Starch | 1 | 1 | 2 | Baked potato, 1 small (3 oz.) | same | 6 oz. |
| Fat | 1 | 1 | 2 | Diet margarine, 1 T. | same | 2 T. |
| Vegetable | 1 | 2 | 2 | Steamed green beans, ½ cup | 1 cup | same |
| Fruit | 1 | 1 | 1 | Grapefruit half* | same | same |

*Spread grapefruit half with 1 to 2 t. no-sugar strawberry jam. Broil. Garnish with fresh whole strawberry.

### Snack

| | | | | | | |
|---|---|---|---|---|---|---|
| Starch | 1 | 1 | 2 | Bread sticks, ⅔ oz. | same | 1⅓ oz. |
| Fruit | 0 | 1 | 1 | none | Nectarine, 1 med., or apple, 1 small | same |
| Milk | 1 | 1 | 1 | Skim milk, 1 cup | same | same |

Note: Where "omit" is indicated, extra exchange listed is derived from another food item in menu.

# DAY 25

| | EXCHANGES | | | MENU | | |
|---|---|---|---|---|---|---|
| TYPE | CALORIE LEVEL | | | CALORIE LEVEL | | |
| | 1,200 | 1,500 | 1,800 | 1,200 | 1,500 | 1,800 |

**Breakfast**

| | | | | | | |
|---|---|---|---|---|---|---|
| Fruit | 1 | 1 | 1 | Grapefruit half, or pine-apple juice, ½ cup | same | same |
| Starch | 1 | 2 | 2 | none | Cream of wheat, ½ cup | same |
| | | | | Bran muffin, 2″ dia., 1 | same | same |
| Fat | 1 | 1 | 1 | omit | omit | omit |
| Milk | 1 | 1 | 1 | Skim milk, 1 cup | same | same |

**Noon Meal**

| | | | | | | |
|---|---|---|---|---|---|---|
| Meat | 2 | 2 | 2 | 1 to 2% cottage cheese, ½ cup* | same | same |
| Starch | 1 | 2 | 2 | Crisp flat bread, 2 crackers* | 4 crackers* | same |
| Fat | 1 | 1 | 1 | Walnuts, chopped, 1 T.* | same | same |
| Vegetable | 1 | 2 | 2 | Homemade Vegetable Soup, 1 serving** | 2 servings** | same |
| Fruit | 1 | 1 | 1 | Fresh peach, 1 small, sliced or half-sliced* | same | same |
| | | | | Seedless grapes, 7 to 8* | same | same |

*Cottage Cheese Fruit Plate: On lettuce leaf-lined plate, arrange cottage cheese, fruit, crackers. Sprinkle with walnuts. Dust with cinnamon.

**Homemade Vegetable Soup: To 1 cup fat-free chicken or beef broth, add 1 cup assorted chopped vegetables (cabbage, onion, mushrooms, zucchini, spinach). Simmer until tender. Makes 1 serving.

**Evening Meal**

| | | | | | | |
|---|---|---|---|---|---|---|
| Meat | 3 | 3 | 4 | Broiled orange roughie, 3 oz. | same | 4 oz. |
| Starch | 1 | 1 | 2 | Steamed rice, ⅓ cup cooked | same | ⅔ cup cooked |
| Fat | 1 | 1 | 2 | Diet margarine, 1 T. | same | same + reduced-calorie salad dressing, 2 T. |
| Vegetable | 1 | 2 | 2 | Sliced beets, ½ cup | 1 cup | same |
| | | | | Tossed green salad with balsamic vinegar | same | Tossed green salad |
| Fruit | 1 | 1 | 1 | Fruit Gelatin Mold, 1 cup* | same | same |

*Use sugar-free gelatin and juice-packed unsweetened canned fruit. Follow package directions. Garnish with 2 T. whipped topping.

**Snack**

| | | | | | | |
|---|---|---|---|---|---|---|
| Starch | 1 | 1 | 2 | Air-popped popcorn, 3 cups | same | 6 cups |
| Fruit | 0 | 1 | 1 | none | Fresh figs, 2, or dried figs, 1½ | same |
| Milk | 1 | 1 | 1 | Skim milk, 1 cup | same | same |

Note: When "omit" is indicated, extra exchange listed is derived from another food item in menu.

# DAY 26

| | EXCHANGES | | | MENU | | |
|---|---|---|---|---|---|---|
| TYPE | CALORIE LEVEL | | | CALORIE LEVEL | | |
| | 1,200 | 1,500 | 1,800 | 1,200 | 1,500 | 1,800 |

**Breakfast**

| | | | | | | |
|---|---|---|---|---|---|---|
| Fruit | 1 | 1 | 1 | Cantaloupe, 5″ dia., ⅓, or cantaloupe cubes, 1 cup, or grapefruit juice, ½ cup | same | same |
| Starch | 1 | 2 | 2 | Toasted bagel, split, half | whole | same |
| Fat | 1 | 1 | 1 | Cream cheese, 1 T. | same | same |
| Milk | 1 | 1 | 1 | Skim milk, 1 cup | same | same |

**Noon Meal**

| | | | | | | |
|---|---|---|---|---|---|---|
| Meat | 2 | 2 | 2 | Old-fashioned peanut butter, 2 T. | same | same |
| Starch | 1 | 2 | 2 | Rice cakes, 2 | 4 | same |
| Fat | 1 | 1 | 1 | Diet mayonnaise, 1 T.* | same | same |
| Vegetable | 1 | 2 | 2 | Cabbage slaw, 1 cup* | same + carrot sticks, 1 cup | same |
| Fruit | 1 | 1 | 1 | Apple, 1 small | same | same |

*Cabbage Slaw: Combine 1 cup shredded cabbage with diet mayonnaise. Add 1 T. plain nonfat yogurt if creamier texture is desired.

**Evening Meal**

| | | | | | | |
|---|---|---|---|---|---|---|
| Meat | 3 | 3 | 4 | Baked chicken breast, 3 oz. | same | 4 oz. |
| Starch | 1 | 1 | 2 | Baked potato (with chives), 1 small (3 oz.) + 2 T. plain yogurt | same | same + whole wheat roll, 1 |
| Fat | 1 | 1 | 2 | Reduced-calorie salad dressing, 2 T. | same | same + diet margarine, 1 T. |
| Vegetable | 1 | 2 | 2 | Steamed summer squash, ½ cup | 1 cup | same |
| | | | | Tossed salad, 1 cup | same | same |
| Fruit | 1 | 1 | 1 | Grapes, 15 | same | same |

**Snack**

| | | | | | | |
|---|---|---|---|---|---|---|
| Starch | 1 | 1 | 2 | Flaked bran cereal, ½ cup | same | 1 cup |
| Fruit | 0 | 1 | 1 | none | Banana, 9″, ½, sliced | same |
| Milk | 1 | 1 | 1 | Skim milk, 1 cup | same | same |

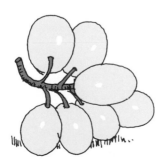

# DAY 27

| | EXCHANGES | | | MENU | | |
|---|---|---|---|---|---|---|
| TYPE | CALORIE LEVEL | | | CALORIE LEVEL | | |
| | 1,200 | 1,500 | 1,800 | 1,200 | 1,500 | 1,800 |

**Breakfast**

| | | | | | | |
|---|---|---|---|---|---|---|
| Fruit | 1 | 1 | 1 | Orange, 1 med., or orange juice, ½ cup | same | same |
| Starch | 1 | 2 | 2 | none | High-fiber cereal, ½ cup | same |
| | | | | Rye toast, 1 slice | same | same |
| Fat | 1 | 1 | 1 | Diet margarine, 1 T. | same | same |
| Milk | 1 | 1 | 1 | Skim milk, 1 cup | same | same |

**Noon Meal**

| | | | | | | |
|---|---|---|---|---|---|---|
| Meat | 2 | 2 | 2 | Cold sliced/shaved roast turkey, 2 oz. | same | same |
| Starch | 1 | 2 | 2 | Whole wheat bread, thin sliced, 2 slices | Whole wheat bread, regular, 2 slices | same |
| Fat | 1 | 1 | 1 | Diet mayonnaise, 1 T. | same | same |
| Vegetable | 1 | 2 | 2 | Cherry tomatoes, 6 | same + carrot sticks, 1 cup | same |
| Fruit | 1 | 1 | 1 | Plums, 2 | same | same |

Try alfalfa sprouts on sandwich.

**Evening Meal**

| | | | | | | |
|---|---|---|---|---|---|---|
| Meat | 3 | 3 | 4 | Lasagna, 3″ x 4″ piece | same | same + ¼ cup 1 to 2% cottage cheese on lettuce leaf liner |
| Starch | 1 | 1 | 2 | omit | omit | Italian garlic toast, 1 oz. slice* |
| Fat | 1 | 1 | 2 | omit | omit | Diet margarine, 1 T.* |
| Vegetable | 1 | 2 | 2 | Italian green beans, ½ cup | 1 cup | same |
| Fruit | 1 | 1 | 1 | Fresh pineapple, ¾ cup, or canned pineapple chunks, ⅓ cup | same | same |

*Garlic toast: Combine melted diet margarine with a dash of garlic powder. Spread on bread. Run under broiler.

**Snack**

| | | | | | | |
|---|---|---|---|---|---|---|
| Starch | 1 | 1 | 2 | Pretzels, regular or salt-free, ¾ oz. | same | 1½ oz. |
| Fruit | 0 | 1 | 1 | none | Raisins, 2 T. | same |
| Milk | 1 | 1 | 1 | Skim milk, 1 cup | same | same |

Note: Where "omit" is indicated, extra exchange listed is derived from another food item in menu.

# DAY 28

| EXCHANGES | | | | MENU | | |
|---|---|---|---|---|---|---|
| TYPE | CALORIE LEVEL | | | | CALORIE LEVEL | |
| | 1,200 | 1,500 | 1,800 | 1,200 | 1,500 | 1,800 |

### Breakfast

| | | | | | | |
|---|---|---|---|---|---|---|
| Fruit | 1 | 1 | 1 | Grapefruit half, or grapefruit juice, ⅓ cup | same | same |
| Starch | 1 | 2 | 2 | Multi-grain bread, 1 slice | 2 slices | same |
| Fat | 1 | 1 | 1 | Diet margarine, 1 T. | same | same |
| Milk | 1 | 1 | 1 | Skim milk, 1 cup | same | same |

Try no-sugar jam or jelly.

### Noon Meal

| | | | | | | |
|---|---|---|---|---|---|---|
| Meat | 2 | 2 | 2 | Thin-sliced/shaved ham, 2 oz. | same | same |
| Starch | 1 | 2 | 2 | Rye bread, 2 slices | Caraway rye, 2 slices | same |
| Fat | 1 | 1 | 1 | Diet margarine or mayonnaise, 1 T. | same | same |
| Vegetable | 1 | 2 | 2 | Green pepper strips, ½ cup | 1 cup | same |
| | | | | Tomato slices, ½ cup | 1 cup | same |
| Fruit | 1 | 1 | 1 | Apple, 1 small, or applesauce, ½ cup | same | same |

1 or 2 t. mustard may be used on sandwich.

### Evening Meal

| | | | | | | |
|---|---|---|---|---|---|---|
| Meat | 3 | 3 | 4 | Roast Cornish game hen, 3 oz. | same | 4 oz. |
| Starch | 1 | 1 | 2 | Bread dressing, ¼ cup | same | ½ cup |
| Fat | 1 | 1 | 2 | omit | omit | omit |
| Vegetable | 1 | 2 | 2 | Brussels sprouts, ½ cup | 1 cup | same |
| Fruit | 1 | 1 | 1 | Fresh pear, 1 small, or canned pears, 2 halves | same | same |

### Snack

| | | | | | | |
|---|---|---|---|---|---|---|
| Starch | 1 | 1 | 2 | Air-popped popcorn, 3 cups | same | 6 cups |
| Fruit | 0 | 1 | 1 | none | Dried apricot halves, 7 | same |
| Milk | 1 | 1 | 1 | Skim milk, 1 cup | same | same |

Note: Where "omit" is indicated, extra exchange listed is derived from another food item in menu.

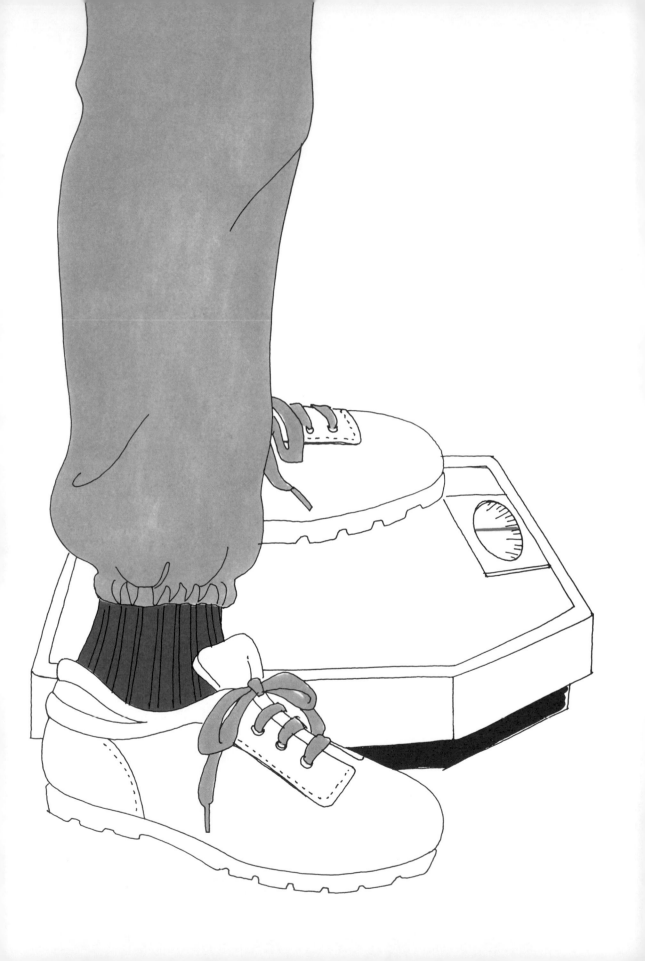

# PART SIX:
# Keeping Off Pounds Sensibly

Chapter 17: How To Prevent Backsliding


Chapter 18: Weight-Maintenance Meal Plans

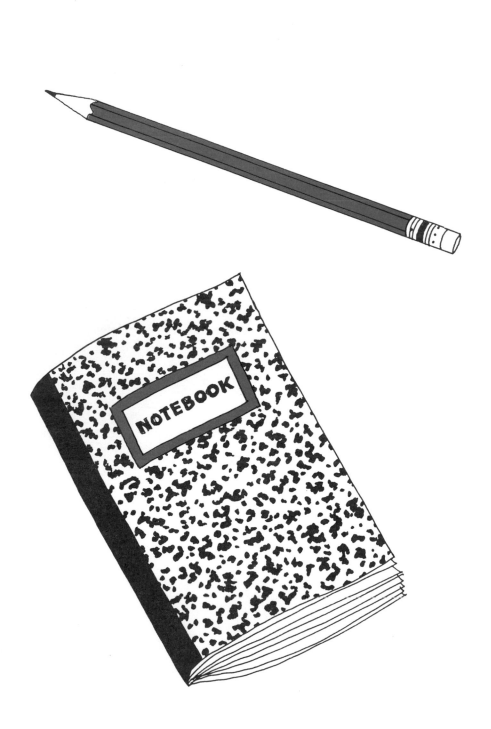

# Chapter 17: How To Prevent Backsliding

After you reach a weight goal, it is easy to drop your guard, slip back into bad habits and regain lost weight. For whatever reason, reduced overweight people have a greater tendency to gain weight—much more so than an individual who has never been obese before. KEEPING OFF POUNDS SENSIBLY requires a great deal of motivation and perseverance. A planned, objective approach is just as important as the one you took to lose weight in the first place. In fact, the two approaches are quite similar, if not identical.

## Continue Follow-Up Care with Health Professionals

Before beginning a weight-maintenance program, it is essential that you revisit your physician for another health checkup for reasons outlined in chapter 10. At this point your new meal plan can be selected and reviewed with a registered dietitian. More than one visit is frequently necessary. You may wish to have your physician's input on the degree of exercising you can perform now that you have lost weight. Laboratory tests, an electrocardiogram and chest x-ray may be repeated. All other aspects of health care maintenance can be reviewed at this time and at regular intervals thereafter. Your doctor may wish you to see other health professionals for special problems that were described previously in chapter 10.

## Continue Your Exercise Program

Reaching your weight goal should not be a signal to stop exercising. If it is not continued with equal or even greater intensity, weight gain will result. Review chapter 11 once more. Remember, for those of you who are able and who have the approval of your physician, rigorous exercise for at least 20 minutes three times per week is a good rule to follow. It not only will sustain your physical fitness and health, it will help hold down your appetite. Idleness and physical inactivity promote overeating to a much greater extent than does exercise. Seek new kinds of physical activity if you can. Always select the kinds of exercise that are the most enjoyable and appropriate for you.

## Anticipate Problems with Bad Eating Habits

Bad eating habits and an ill-advised lifestyle brought on your personal problem with obesity. Obviously, you made some corrections in order to lose weight and achieve your goal. Now it is time to increase the total number of calories in your meal plan for weight maintenance. During this transition to more food intake, there may be a false sense of security that you can be less strict about meal planning. However, just one extra starch/bread exchange per day can cause weight gains of as much as 1 pound each month; within six months, 6 pounds; within one year, 12 pounds. Your KOPS status will be long gone. See how easy it is to regain! You can do the same thing with extra fruits, meats, dairy products and especially with too many calorie-dense desserts and hidden fat calories found in many fast foods and convenience foods.

Don't relax your guard. Read chapters 12 and 13 again. Know what strategies are necessary to avoid going back to bad eating habits. Review what foods to avoid to make health and a good body weight possible.

## Keeping Records

Now more than ever a logbook should be kept. Take the time to record dates, types and duration of exercise, resting and maximum pulse rates. Show evidence in your book of meal planning. Keep track of the types and amounts of food eaten each day with proof that the correct number of food exchanges were consumed at each meal. Place your weekly weights and monthly body measurements in there, too. This logbook will serve three purposes. It will remind you that you have a weight problem that needs daily attention. It will tell you when the weight-maintaining program is going well and when it is not. It will provide a record for your physician and dietitian should problems arise and trouble-shooting is necessary.

## The Eventual Goal

An eventual goal is simple to state but difficult to achieve. You have learned what lifestyle is necessary to maintain your desirable weight. Your eventual goal is to become so well adapted to this new way of life that it becomes automatic and the rule rather than the exception. Start off in the right way so that you can reach this ultimate objective.

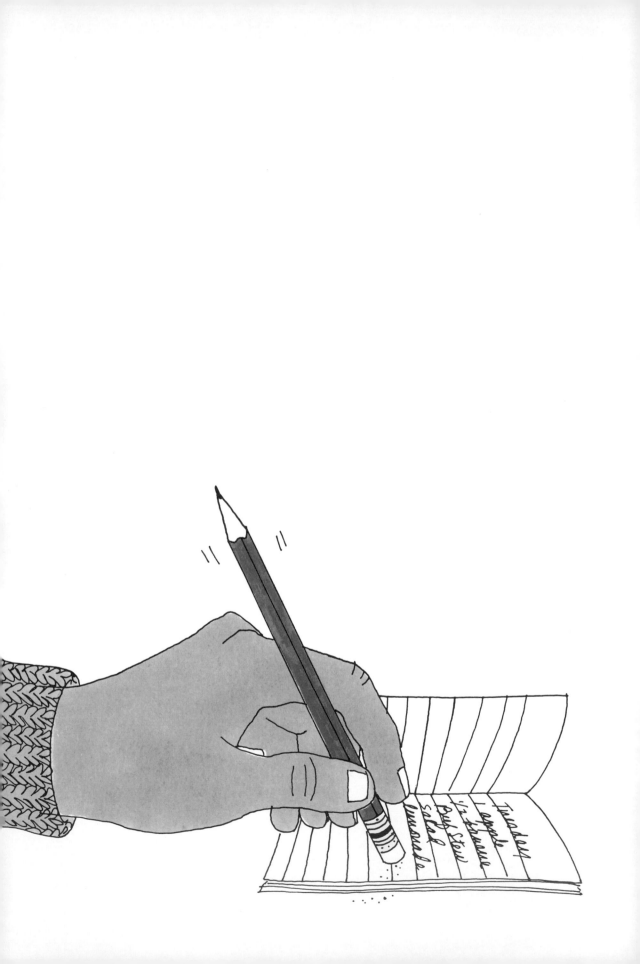

# Chapter 18: Weight-Maintenance Meal Plans

## Using the Exchange System of Meal Planning For Weight Maintenance

In chapter 15, 1,200-, 1,500- and 1,800-calorie meal plans were described for weight loss. The specific plan that was selected should be discontinued as soon as the weight goal is reached; otherwise, weight loss may continue below the desirable value selected by you and your physician.

In the present chapter, additional meal plans ranging from 2,000 to 3,000 calories per day are listed. Each meal plan is defined in the same way as was done in chapter 15. The grams of carbohydrate, protein and fat as well as the total number of exchanges are listed at the very top. The number of exchanges for each meal and snack appear in the left-hand column. Sample menus appear in the right-hand column. The reader will have to refer back to chapter 14 for the correct food portions within each of the six exchange lists.

Table 11 defines the average number of calories of food needed each day to maintain a given desirable weight level. Each daily requirement is to the nearest 100 calories. If your desirable weight is not the same as values in the table, select the one that is closest to your own. If your desirable weight is 152 pounds, choose the meal plan for 150 pounds (2,000 calories per day). If your desirable weight is 158, the 160 pounds maintenance

diet is selected (2,200 calories per day). If your desirable weight is halfway between 150 and 160 (155 pounds), the daily calorie intake also would be halfway between 2,000 and 2,200 or 2,100 calories. The range of calories above or below this average takes into account variations in physical activity. Very inactive individuals, including those with physical or medical handicaps, frequently require less than average calories (low range). Very physically active adults are often in the higher ranges. In fact, some individuals, like athletes, may exceed the upper ranges for weight maintenance and will require even more calories.

Meal plans to maintain weight below 150 pounds are mostly for women and some men with small frames. Weights at or above 150 pounds are selected mostly for men and some taller women with large frames.

## Adjusting Your Meal Plan

Table 12 lists in the left-hand column all the meal plans that are in this chapter as well as in chapter 15. Some of you may choose one that is slightly below or above one of these diets (middle column). To make adjustments upward or downward, it is best to subtract or add a single starch/bread exchange. This exchange list is in chapter 14.

For example, if a 1,900-calorie diet is selected, it

### TABLE 11: CALORIES REQUIRED FOR DESIRABLE WEIGHT MAINTENANCE

| DESIRABLE WEIGHT (pounds) | AVERAGE LEVEL (calories/day) | RANGE (calories/day) |
|---|---|---|
| 100 | 1,400 | 1,200-1,600 |
| 110 | 1,500 | 1,300-1,700 |
| 120 | 1,600 | 1,400-1,900 |
| 130 | 1,800 | 1,500-2,000 |
| 140 | 1,900 | 1,600-2,200 |
| 150 | 2,000 | 1,700-2,300 |
| 160 | 2,200 | 1,900-2,500 |
| 170 | 2,300 | 2,000-2,700 |
| 180 | 2,400 | 2,100-2,800 |
| 190 | 2,600 | 2,200-3,000 |
| 200 | 2,700 | 2,300-3,100 |
| 210 | 2,900 | 2,400-3,300 |
| 220 | 3,000 | 2,500-3,400 |

NOTES: Average daily caloric requirements are calculated to the nearest 100 calories for adults with average physical activity. The range of calories reflects differences in physical activity (very inactive to very active).

Author's Note: Joan Pleuss, R.D., M.S., formulated the 2,000- to 3,000-calorie exchange lists in chapter 18. We appreciate her efforts.

126

is not described in the monograph. An 1,800-calorie plan is given in chapter 15. Simply add one starch/bread exchange to one of the three meals on the 1,800-calorie diet. This will add 80 more calories and will bring you close enough to the 1,900-calorie level you desire. Other examples of adjustments are given in the right-hand column of table 12. These adjustments also may become useful when changes are needed to maintain your desired weight.

## Selecting the Meal Plan That Is Right for You

*For Adults with Average to Above Average Physical Activity*

This would include adults who participate in some form of exercise program. The frequency and duration of exercise determine whether it is average or above average exertion. For example, it could be a woman who began at 160 pounds and who easily achieved her weight goal of 130 pounds within six months. Or it could be a man who dropped his weight from 220 to a desirable level of 180 pounds in seven months. Table 11 indicates that for average adults, weight-maintenance meal plans would be 1,800 calories for the woman (130 pounds) and 2,400 calories for the man (180 pounds). However, this may not be enough calories

for the very physically active person. The following approach is recommended:

- Select the meal plan for the average situation and stay on that plan for four weeks.
- If weight remains at the same level after four weeks, stay with this plan.
- If additional weight is lost, add 100 calories to the meal plan per pound lost during this four-week period. For example, if the very active woman lost 2 pounds the first month, she would add 200 calories to her 1,800-calorie diet and follow the 2,000-calorie meal plan. If the man lost 3 pounds during the first month, he would add 300 calories and follow the 2,700-calorie meal plan (see table 12). Further adjustments can be made after additional four-week periods.
- If slight amounts of weight are gained initially, this would be most unusual for the very active person but not unusual for people of average physical activity. Subtract 100 calories per pound gained in the initial four-week period. If 2 pounds are gained, subtract 200 calories, etc. Follow this new, slightly lower level for another four weeks. Readjust again, if necessary, on a month-to-month basis.

*For the Very Inactive*

These are individuals who have limited abilities

## TABLE 12: ADJUSTING CALORIES FOR MEAL PLANS

| MEAL PLANS IN MONOGRAPH (calories/day) | MEAL PLANS NOT IN MONOGRAPH (calories/day) | STARCH/BREAD EXCHANGE ADJUSTMENT* |
|---|---|---|
| 1,200 | | |
| | 1,300 | 1,200 plus 1 starch/bread |
| | 1,400 | 1,500 minus 1 starch/bread |
| 1,500 | | |
| | 1,600 | 1,500 plus 1 starch/bread |
| | 1,700 | 1,800 minus 1 starch/bread |
| 1,800 | | |
| | 1,900 | 1,800 plus 1 starch/bread |
| 2,000 | | |
| | 2,100 | 2,000 plus 1 starch/bread |
| 2,200 | | |
| | 2,300 | 2,200 plus 1 starch/bread |
| 2,400 | | |
| | 2,500 | 2,400 plus 1 starch/bread |
| 2,600 | | |
| | 2,700 | 2,600 plus 1 starch/bread |
| 2,800 | | |
| | 2,900 | 2,800 plus 1 starch/bread |
| 3,000 | | |
| | >3,000 | Requires assistance from a registered dietitian |

*Addition or subtraction of one starch/bread exchange may be made at breakfast, lunch or supper.

to exercise because of specific medical problems. In many cases it may have been a real struggle to reach a weight goal. Examples might include a woman with crippling arthritis who reduced from 170 to 140 pounds on a 1,200-calorie diet or a man with heart disease who lost weight from 190 to 160 pounds on a 1,500-calorie plan over several months.

Table 11 indicates that in an average situation the 140-pound woman and 160-pound man require weight-maintenance diets of 1,900 and 2,200 calories per day, respectively. For the very inactive this may be too much food, and weight may be gained.

- Begin a meal plan about halfway between the weight-loss diet and the average weight-maintaining diet. For the 140-pound woman coming off a 1,200-calorie diet, a 1,600-calorie plan should be selected. For the 160-pound man, a 1,900-calorie diet is in order.
- Try these below average weight-maintenance diets for at least four weeks.
- After four weeks continue this plan if weight is unchanged. If weight changes, readjust the diet upward or downward by 100 calories per pound gained or lost. If weight remains the same after another four weeks, stay with the new adjustment. If not, adjust for additional four-week periods until weight remains stable.

*For the True Backslider*

There are individuals who never really follow a weight-maintaining meal plan consistently after reaching their weight goal. Within four to eight weeks, gains of 5 to 10 pounds or more indicate significant backsliding. For these backsliders the following approach is recommended:

- Don't allow too much time to pass before doing something positive about the weight gain. It should be aggressively managed within four to eight weeks into the backsliding period.
- Resume your original weight-reduction meal plan until your desirable weight is reached once more.
- Read chapters 9 through 13 in this monograph and decide what factors were responsible for regaining weight.
- See your physician and/or dietitian before beginning a weight-maintenance diet. Keep records and be honest about what you enter into your record book!

**Some Additional Comments about Weight Maintenance**

Table 13 summarizes a suggested strategy for maintaining desirable weight. There are other problems to keep in mind. During the first week or two of the new meal plan there may be slight weight gains even though the diet is being followed very carefully. Don't be discouraged. This frequently indicates slight fluid retention, which may occur when calories are increased from a weight-loss to a weight-maintenance plan. This will end shortly and your weight will stabilize. If weight continues to rise beyond two weeks, re-

## TABLE 13: ADJUSTING MEAL PLANS FOR WEIGHT MAINTENANCE

| | ACTIVITY LEVEL | | |
|---|---|---|---|
| GROUP | Very Active | Average | Very Inactive |
| Initial meal plan* | Average diet | Average diet | Halfway between weight-loss diet and average diet |
| No weight gain after 4 weeks | Continue the same meal plan | | |
| Slight weight loss after 4 weeks | Add 100 calories per pound lost per month | | |
| Slight weight gain after 4 weeks | Subtract 100 calories per pound gained per month | | |
| Major weight gain within 4 weeks | Return to original weight-reduction diet until desirable weight is reached. Review new weight-maintenance diet with physician and/or dietitian before beginning new plan. | | |

*See table 11.

adjustments of the calories downward may be necessary, because this very likely represents fat tissue weight gain, not fluid retention in most cases. If there is confusion about fluid vs. fat gain, see your physician.

Another common problem is seasonal variation in physical activity. If warm weather months include more exercise in contrast to cold weather months, weight gain may be experienced between late fall and spring. If this occurs, there is nothing wrong with adjusting the weight-maintenance diet downward during seasonal periods of reduced physical activity.

Similar adjustments may be necessary whenever exercise comes to an abrupt halt. Examples include injuries or illnesses that require significant periods of convalescence. Anticipate weight gain unless your diet is readjusted to accommodate the reduced calorie need. Your physician should decide what is necessary, since good nutrition is also important during periods of recovery from illness, trauma or surgery.

## Summary

Weight-maintenance meal plans in this chapter are guidelines. Caloric needs vary a great deal from one individual to the next. In fact, caloric needs often vary in the same individual from time to time. For these reasons, careful monitoring of body weight, exercise and health are necessary for weight stability. Individuals must be flexible in adjusting their meal plans when it is appropriate. The initial adjustments should occur only at monthly intervals until the right level is established. This should not take more than two to three months. Thereafter, adjustments should be done relatively infrequently and only when clearly indicated. In this regard, the advice and guidance of your physician and dietitian are very important. The sharing of your progress with fellow TOPS members at chapter meetings is another means of gaining motivation and encouragement.

# 2,000-CALORIE EXCHANGE DIET

Carbohydrate ........255 grams (51%)
Protein ...............95 grams (19%)
Fat .................65 grams (29%)

10 starch/bread exchanges
6 meat exchanges
4 vegetable exchanges
4 fruit exchanges
2 milk exchanges
5 fat exchanges

| EXCHANGES | SAMPLE MENU |
|---|---|

**Breakfast** | **Breakfast**

List 4: 1 fruit exchange..........................½ small banana (1 fruit)
List 1: 2 starch/bread exchanges.................¾ cup rice flakes (1 starch/bread)
1 slice whole wheat toast (1 starch/bread)
List 6: 1 fat exchange...........................1 t. margarine (1 fat)
List 5: 1 milk exchange..........................1 cup skim milk (1 milk)
Free choices...................................Coffee, ice water, artificial sweetener

**Lunch** | **Lunch**

List 2: 2 meat exchanges........................2 oz. cold turkey (2 meat)
List 1: 2 starch/bread exchanges.................1 hard roll (2 starch/bread)
Lists 6 and 1: 1 fat exchange and
1 starch/bread exchange...........6 vanilla wafers (1 fat + 1 starch/bread)
List 6: 1 fat exchange...........................2 t. mayonnaise-type salad dressing (1 fat)
List 3: 1 vegetable exchange.....................1 cup raw carrots (1 vegetable)
List 4: 1 fruit exchange..........................1 small apple (1 fruit)
Free choices...................................Diet soda, 1 cup shredded cabbage

**Supper** | **Supper**

List 2: 4 meat exchanges........................4 oz. lean hamburger (4 meat)
List 1: 3 starch/bread exchanges.................1 cup macaroni (2 starch/bread)
1 dinner roll (1 starch/bread)
List 3: 2 vegetable exchanges....................1 cup stewed tomatoes (2 vegetable)
List 6: 1 fat exchange...........................1 t. margarine (1 fat)
List 4: 1 fruit exchange..........................1 large kiwi (1 fruit)
List 5: 1 milk exchange..........................1 cup skim milk (1 milk)
Free choices...................................Tea, ice water, 1 cup lettuce, 1 T. low-calorie salad dressing

**Snacks** | **Snacks**

List 4: 1 fruit exchange..........................½ cup orange juice (1 fruit)
List 1: 2 starch/bread exchanges.................1½ oz. pretzels (2 starch/bread)
List 6: 1 fat exchange...........................2 T. dip (1 fat)
List 3: 1 vegetable exchange.....................1 cup raw cauliflower (1 vegetable)
Free choices...................................Diet soda

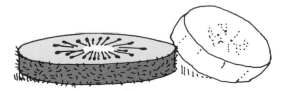
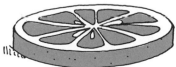

# 2,200-CALORIE EXCHANGE DIET

Carbohydrate ........300 grams (55%)
Protein ..............105 grams (19%)
Fat ..................65 grams (27%)

13 starch/bread exchanges
6 meat exchanges
4 vegetable exchanges
4 fruit exchanges
2 milk exchanges
5 fat exchanges

| EXCHANGES | SAMPLE MENU |
|---|---|

**Breakfast** — **Breakfast**

List 4: 2 fruit exchanges .........................1 banana (2 fruit)
List 1: 3 starch/bread exchanges .................¾ cup dry cereal (1 starch/bread)
2 slices whole wheat toast (2 starch/bread)
List 6: 2 fat exchanges .........................2 t. margarine (2 fat)
List 5: 1 milk exchange..........................1 cup skim milk (1 milk)
Free choices ..................................Coffee, ice water

**Lunch** — **Lunch**

List 2: 2 meat exchanges ........................2 oz. hamburger (2 meat)
List 1: 2 starch/bread exchanges .................1 hamburger bun (2 starch/bread)
Lists 1 + 6: 1 starch/bread exchange and
1 fat exchange ......................10 French fries (1 starch/bread + 1 fat)
List 6: 1 fat exchange ...........................1 T. French dressing (1 fat)
List 3: 1 vegetable exchange ....................1 cup raw vegetables (tomatoes, broccoli, onion, cauliflower) (1 vegetable)
List 4: 1 fruit exchange .........................1 small apple (1 fruit)
Free choices ..................................1 cup lettuce, bouillon, diet soda, ice water

**Supper** — **Supper**

List 2: 4 meat exchanges ........................4 oz. lean roast pork (4 meat)
List 1: 4 starch/bread exchanges .................1 med. (6 oz.) baked potato (2 starch/bread)
½ cup corn (1 starch/bread)
1 dinner roll (1 starch/bread)
List 3: 2 vegetable exchanges ...................1 cup green beans (2 vegetable)
List 6: 1 fat exchange ...........................1 t. margarine (1 fat)
List 4: 1 fruit exchange .........................½ broiled grapefruit (1 fruit)
List 5: 1 milk exchange..........................1 cup skim milk (1 milk)
Free choices ..................................Iced tea, diet gelatin

**Snacks** — **Snacks**

List 3: 1 vegetable exchange ....................1 cup raw carrots (1 vegetable)
List 1: 3 starch/bread exchanges .................½ cup pudding (2 starch/bread)
3 gingersnaps (1 starch/bread)

# 2,400-CALORIE EXCHANGE DIET

Carbohydrate ........300 grams (50%)
Protein ..............120 grams (20%)
Fat .................80 grams (30%)

13 starch/bread exchanges
8 meat exchanges
4 vegetable exchanges
4 fruit exchanges
2 milk exchanges
6 fat exchanges

| EXCHANGES | SAMPLE MENU |
|---|---|

**Breakfast**

**Breakfast**

List 4: 1 fruit exchange ..........................2 T. raisins (1 fruit)
List 1: 3 starch/bread exchanges .................1 bagel (2 starch/bread)
½ cup oatmeal (1 starch/bread)
List 6: 1 fat exchange ..........................1 T. cream cheese (1 fat)
List 5: 1 milk exchange.........................1 cup skim milk (1 milk)
Free choices ..................................Coffee, artificial sweetener

**Lunch**

**Lunch**

List 2: 2 meat exchanges ........................2 oz. cold chicken (2 meat)
List 1: 2 starch/bread exchanges .................2 slices rye bread (2 starch/bread)
Lists 1 + 6: 1 starch/bread exchange and
2 fat exchanges .....................½ cup mayonnaise potato salad
(1 starch/bread + 2 fat)
List 3: 1 vegetable exchange ....................1 cup sliced tomato (1 vegetable)
List 4: 1 fruit exchange ..........................1 small apple (1 fruit)
Free choices ..................................Ice water, dill pickle

**Supper**

**Supper**

List 2: 6 meat exchanges ........................6 oz. broiled cod (6 meat)
List 1: 3 starch/bread exchanges .................2 slices rye bread (2 starch/bread)
½ cup boiled potatoes (1 starch/bread)
Lists 1 + 6: 1 starch/bread exchange and
1 fat exchange .....................½ cup ice milk (1 starch/bread + 1 fat)
List 3: 2 vegetable exchanges ...................1 cup cooked broccoli (2 vegetable)
List 6: 2 fat exchanges ..........................2 t. margarine (2 fat)
List 4: 1 fruit exchange..........................½ cup canned unsweetened peaches (1 fruit)
List 5: 1 milk ................................1 cup skim milk (1 milk)
Free choices ..................................Lemon, coffee

**Snacks**

**Snacks**

List 4: 1 fruit exchange..........................15 small grapes (1 fruit)
List 1: 3 starch/bread exchanges .................9 squares graham crackers (3 starch/bread)
List 3: 1 vegetable exchange ....................4 oz. tomato juice (1 vegetable)

# 2,600-CALORIE EXCHANGE DIET

Carbohydrate . . . . . . . .330 grams (51%)
Protein . . . . . . . . . . . . . .120 grams (18%)
Fat . . . . . . . . . . . . . . . . .90 grams (31%)

14 starch/bread exchanges
8 meat exchanges
4 vegetable exchanges
5 fruit exchanges
2 milk exchanges
7 fat exchanges

| EXCHANGES | SAMPLE MENU |
|---|---|

**Breakfast**

**Breakfast**

List 4: 2 fruit exchanges . . . . . . . . . . . . . . . . . . . . . . . . .8 oz. orange juice (2 fruit)
List 1: 4 starch/bread exchanges . . . . . . . . . . . . . . . . .1½ cups rice flakes (2 starch/bread)
2 slices whole wheat toast (2 starch/bread)
List 6: 1 fat exchange . . . . . . . . . . . . . . . . . . . . . . . . . .1 t. margarine (1 fat)
List 5: 1 milk exchange . . . . . . . . . . . . . . . . . . . . . . . . .1 cup skim milk (1 milk)

**Lunch**

**Lunch**

List 3: 2 meat exchanges . . . . . . . . . . . . . . . . . . . . . . . .2 oz. turkey (2 meat)
List 1: 4 starch/bread exchanges . . . . . . . . . . . . . . . . .2 slices rye bread (2 starch/bread)
1 cup vegetable soup (1 starch/bread)
6 saltines (1 starch/bread)
List 3: 1 vegetable exchange . . . . . . . . . . . . . . . . . . . .1 cup raw tomatoes (1 vegetable)
List 4: 2 fruit exchanges . . . . . . . . . . . . . . . . . . . . . . . .⅔ cup canned unsweetened pineapple (2 fruit)
List 6: 1 fat exchange . . . . . . . . . . . . . . . . . . . . . . . . . .1 t. margarine (1 fat)
Free choices . . . . . . . . . . . . . . . . . . . . . . . . . . . . . . . . .1 cup celery, club soda

**Supper**

**Supper**

List 3: 6 meat exchanges . . . . . . . . . . . . . . . . . . . . . . . .6 oz. broiled sirloin steak (6 meat)
List 1: 4 starch/bread exchanges . . . . . . . . . . . . . . . . .1 large (9 oz.) baked potato (3 starch/bread)
1 dinner roll (1 starch/bread)
List 3: 3 vegetable exchanges . . . . . . . . . . . . . . . . . . .4 oz. tomato juice (1 vegetable)
1 cup asparagus (2 vegetable)
List 6: 4 fat exchanges . . . . . . . . . . . . . . . . . . . . . . . . .2 T. sour cream (1 fat)
2 t. margarine (2 fat)
1 T. French dressing (1 fat)
List 4: 1 fruit exchange . . . . . . . . . . . . . . . . . . . . . . . . .1 cup cantaloupe (1 fruit)
List 5: 1 milk exchange . . . . . . . . . . . . . . . . . . . . . . . . .1 cup skim milk (1 milk)
Free choices . . . . . . . . . . . . . . . . . . . . . . . . . . . . . . . . .Coffee, 1 cup lettuce

**Snacks**

**Snacks**

List 1: 1 starch/bread exchange . . . . . . . . . . . . . . . . . .½ cup sugar-free pudding (1 starch/bread)
Lists 6 + 1: 1 fat exchange and
1 starch/bread exchange . . . . . . . . . . . . . .6 vanilla wafers (1 starch/bread + 1 fat)

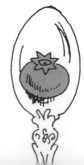

# 2,800-CALORIE EXCHANGE DIET

Carbohydrate ........370 grams (53%)
Protein ..............135 grams (19%)
Fat ................90 grams (28%)

15 starch/bread exchanges
8 meat exchanges
4 vegetable exchanges
6 fruit exchanges
3 milk exchanges
7 fat exchanges

| EXCHANGES | SAMPLE MENU |
|---|---|

**Breakfast**

**Breakfast**

List 4: 2 fruit exchanges .........................1 banana (2 fruit)
List 1: 4 starch/bread exchanges ................1½ cups oat flakes (2 starch/bread)
1 English muffin (2 starch/bread)
List 6: 2 fat exchanges .........................2 t. margarine (2 fat)
List 5: 1 milk exchange.........................1 cup skim milk (1 milk)
Free choices ..................................Coffee, water, 1 t. diet jelly

**Lunch**

**Lunch**

List 2: 2 meat exchanges .......................2 oz. broiled beef patty (2 meat)
List 1: 2 starch/bread exchanges ................1 hamburger bun (2 starch/bread)
Lists 1 + 6: 2 starch/bread exchanges and
2 fat exchanges .....................8 oz. cream of mushroom soup
(1 starch/bread + 1 fat)
10 French fries (1 starch/bread + 1 fat)
List 6: 1 fat exchange ..........................1 T. French dressing (1 fat)
List 3: 1 vegetable exchange ....................2 cups tossed salad with lemon consisting of
1 cup lettuce (free), with 1 cup total of raw broc-
coli, cauliflower, green pepper, tomato (1 vegetable)
List 4: 2 fruit exchanges .........................1 med. apple (2 fruit)
List 5: 1 milk exchange.........................1 cup skim milk (1 milk)
Free choices ..................................Water

**Supper**

**Supper**

List 2: 6 meat exchanges .......................1 baked whole chicken breast (6 meat)
List 1: 4 starch/bread exchanges ................1 cup rice (3 starch/bread)
1 slice rye bread (1 starch/bread)
List 3: 3 vegetable exchanges ...................1 cup cooked broccoli (2 vegetable)
1 cup raw tomato (1 vegetable)
List 6: 2 fat exchanges .........................2 t. margarine (2 fat)
List 4: 1 fruit exchange .........................2 tangerines (1 fruit)
List 5: 1 milk exchange.........................1 cup skim milk (1 milk)
Free choices ..................................Iced tea, water

**Snacks**

**Snacks**

List 1: 3 starch/bread exchanges ................6 bread sticks, 7¾" (3 starch/bread)
List 4: 1 fruit exchange .........................15 small grapes (1 fruit)
Free choices ..................................Water, diet soda, 1 cup raw celery

# 3,000-CALORIE EXCHANGE DIET

Carbohydrate ........390 grams (52%)
Protein .............135 grams (18%)
Fat ................100 grams (30%)

16 starch/bread exchanges
8 meat exchanges
4 vegetable exchanges
6 fruit exchanges
3 milk exchanges
9 fat exchanges

| EXCHANGES | SAMPLE MENU |
|---|---|

**Breakfast** | **Breakfast**

List 4: 2 fruit exchanges ........................4 oz. orange juice (1 fruit)
⅓ cantaloupe (1 fruit)
List 1: 4 starch/bread exchanges .................1 cup raisin bran (2 starch/bread)
2 slices toast (2 starch/bread)
List 6: 2 fat exchanges .........................2 t. margarine (2 fat)
List 5: 1 milk exchange.........................1 cup skim milk (1 milk)
Free choices .................................Artificial sweetener, coffee, water

**Lunch** | **Lunch**

List 2: 2 meat exchanges .......................1 oz. turkey (1 meat)
1 oz. cheese (1 meat)
List 1: 3 starch/bread exchanges .................2 slices rye bread (2 starch/bread)
1 cup vegetable soup (1 starch/bread)
Lists 1 + 6: 1 starch/bread exchange and
1 fat exchange ......................10 French fries (1 starch/bread + 1 fat)
List 6: 2 fat exchanges .........................1 t. margarine (1 fat)
1 T. French dressing (1 fat)
List 4: 1 fruit exchange .........................1 small apple (1 fruit)
List 3: 1 vegetable exchange ....................½ cup raw tomato and ½ cup bean sprouts
(1 vegetable)
List 5: 1 milk exchange.........................1 cup skim milk (1 milk)
Free choices .................................Tea, water, 1 cup lettuce

**Supper** | **Supper**

List 2: 6 meat exchanges .......................6 oz. broiled haddock (6 meat)
List 1: 3 starch/bread exchanges .................1 med. (6 oz.) baked potato (2 starch/bread)
1 dinner roll (1 starch/bread)
Lists 1 + 6: 1 starch/bread exchange and
1 fat exchange ......................2 small cookies (1 starch/bread + 1 fat)
List 3: 3 vegetable exchanges ....................½ cup broccoli (1 vegetable)
4 oz. tomato juice (1 vegetable)
½ cup sauteed mushrooms (1 vegetable)
List 6: 3 fat exchanges .........................2 T. sour cream (1 fat)
2 t. margarine (2 fat)
List 4: 1 fruit exchange .........................¾ cup fresh pineapple (1 fruit)
List 5: 1 milk exchange.........................1 cup skim milk (1 milk)
Free choices .................................Coffee, water

**Snacks** | **Snacks**

List 1: 4 starch/bread exchanges .................1 cinnamon raisin bagel (2 starch/bread)
½ cup sherbet (2 starch/bread)
List 4: 2 fruit exchanges ........................1 banana (2 fruit)
Free choices .................................Diet soda, water

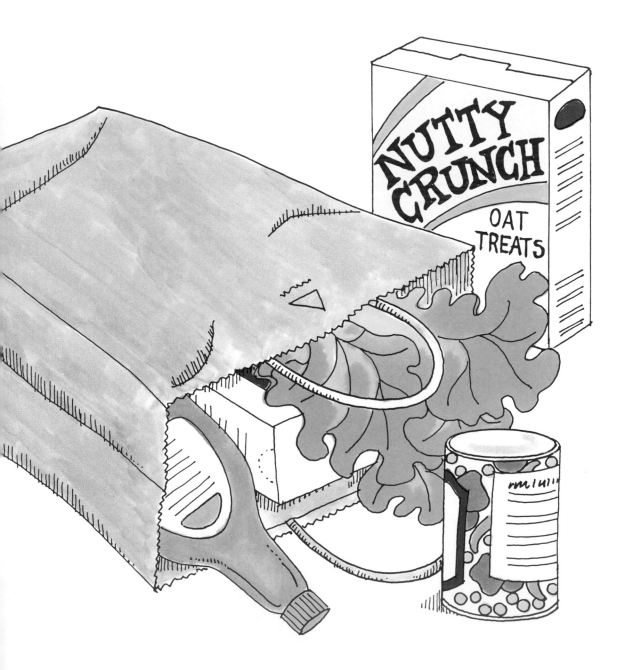

# PART SEVEN:
## Helpful Hints

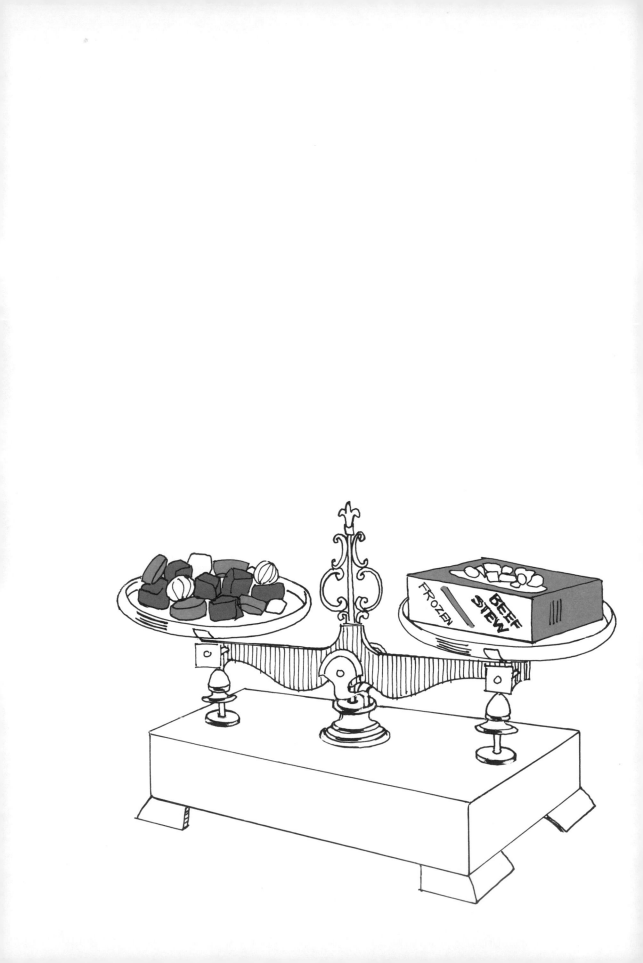

# Chapter 19: Converting Recipes and Food Labels on Processed Foods to Exchanges

Often there are recipes and convenience foods that some families really enjoy. If one of the family members is following a meal plan, he or she may wish to convert some of these favorite dishes into exchange list equivalents to work the food content into a diet.

## Recipes

(1) Write down the amounts of all ingredients in your recipe. In some instances you may have to convert English to metric weights and vice-versa (see table 10).
(2) Convert the amounts to total number of exchanges from the lists in chapter 14.
(3) Add the number of exchanges from each list.
(4) Divide by the serving size. (For example, if there are six equal serving sizes, divide the total number of exchanges by six.) You may omit fractions of exchanges that are less than one-half exchange. Anything above one-half can be rounded off to the next highest number.
(5) You may also want to have the information in calories. Multiply the number of exchanges in each serving by the number of calories per ex-

change (shown at the top of each exchange list in chapter 14 and in table 15).

An example of how to do this is shown in table 14. It is a recipe for beef stew. All the above steps were followed to calculate the exchanges and calories.

To practice your ability to convert recipes, you might look at the various kinds found in chapter 24. Compare your exchange list analysis with what is already given for each recipe.

## Processed Foods

Converting processed foods to exchange lists is more difficult, because the amounts of each ingredient are not given. Moreover, some food labels do not have sufficient information to estimate exchanges.

A satisfactory food label lists:

(1) All ingredients in order of amounts
(2) Serving size
(3) Calories per serving size
(4) Grams of carbohydrate, protein and fat per

## TABLE 14: CONVERTING A BEEF STEW RECIPE (6 SERVINGS) TO EXCHANGES

| INGREDIENTS | TOTAL EXCHANGES | EXCHANGES PER SERVING (divide by 6 servings) | CALORIES PER SERVING |
|---|---|---|---|
| 1½ pounds (24 oz.) of medium-fat stew meat | 18 medium-fat meat* | 18 divided by 6 = 3 medium-fat meat | 225 calories |
| 1 tablespoon flour | ½ starch/bread | negligible | —— |
| 1 tablespoon vegetable oil (for browning) | 3 fat | 3 divided by 6 = ½ fat | 22 calories |
| ½ cup sliced onion | ½ vegetable | negligible | —— |
| 6 small carrots | 6 vegetable | 6 divided by 6 = 1 vegetable | 25 calories |
| 6 small potatoes | 6 starch/bread | 6 divided by 6 = 1 starch/bread | 80 calories |
| TOTAL | | 3 medium-fat meat, 1 vegetable, 1 starch/bread and ½ fat | 352 calories |

*Weights of meat for exchanges are always estimated after cooking. Cooked meat is three-fourths the weight of raw meat (¾ of 24 ounces = 18 ounces).

Author's Note: The input of Joan Pleuss, R.D., M.S., and Mary Hoettels, R.D., M.S., in chapter 19 is greatly appreciated.

serving size. Some also break down the carbo-hydrate into grams of complex (starch) and simple (sugar, corn syrup, etc.) carbohydrate.

In addition, a good food label provides the amount of sodium and food fiber.

If the food label is unsatisfactory, do not use the item in your meal plan. A great many processed foods are high in calories, fat and/or sugar content. If more information is needed about a product, the manufacturer can be contacted by mail. In addition to standard information, the content of the product may also be expressed in food exchanges and can be obtained on request. Ask for both. Major companies also may have toll-free telephone numbers for consumers seeking this kind of information.

Another alternative is to locate a registered dietitian in a local clinic, hospital or medical center and ask for help. They can usually assist you. Books that convert convenience foods to exchange lists are also available for purchase, if necessary.[1]

## An Example of Food Label Conversion

Below is a description of a frozen beef pepper steak dinner. One section of the tray contains the beef pepper steak in tomato sauce. Another section contains a vegetable medley and a third section contains rice.

*Step 1:* List all ingredients on the food label and determine what exchange list they best represent.

| Main Ingredients | Exchange List |
|---|---|
| Water | Free |
| Tomatoes | Vegetable |
| Green pepper | Vegetable |
| Onion | Vegetable |
| Water chestnut | Vegetable |
| Broccoli | Vegetable |
| Carrots | Vegetable |
| Modified food starch | Starch/bread |
| Rice | Starch/bread |
| Butter | Fat |
| Beef | Medium-fat meat |
| Salt | Free |
| Natural flavoring | Free |
| Vegetable oil | Fat |

*Step 2:* List the serving size. In this case it is one 12-ounce serving.

*Step 3:* List nutritional analysis data. This frozen dinner has the following breakdown.

38 grams of carbohydrate

20 grams of protein

11 grams of fat

Total calories = 330

*Step 4:* Begin with the carbohydrate analysis.

There are 38 grams of carbohydrate (starch) in this dinner. Looking at the ingredients, the primary sources of starch are rice, tomatoes, green pepper, broccoli, and carrots. The modified food starch additive and onion are probably negligible.

## TABLE 15: COMPOSITION AND CALORIES IN VARIOUS EXCHANGES

| EXCHANGE | CARBOHYDRATES (grams) | PROTEIN (grams) | FAT (grams) | CALORIES |
|---|---|---|---|---|
| Starch/Bread | 15 | 3 | trace | 80 |
| Meat | | | | |
|   Lean | 0 | 7 | 3 | 55 |
|   Medium-Fat | 0 | 7 | 5 | 75 |
|   High-Fat | 0 | 7 | 8 | 100 |
| Vegetable | 5 | 2 | 0 | 25 |
| Fruit | 15 | 0 | 0 | 60 |
| Milk | | | | |
|   Skim | 12 | 8 | trace | 90 |
|   Low-Fat | 12 | 8 | 5 | 120 |
|   Whole | 12 | 8 | 8 | 150 |
| Fat | 0 | 0 | 5 | 45 |

[1]A. Monk and M. Franz, *Convenience Food Facts: Help for the Healthy Meal Planner*, 2nd ed., 1987 (Wellness and Nutrition Library, Diabetes Center, Inc., P.O. Box 739, Wayazata MN).

There are 15 grams of carbohydrate in each starch/bread exchange. The number of these exchanges in the dinner are 38 grams divided by 15 grams or 2½ starch exchanges.

At this point a sensible estimate is that two starch/bread exchanges are coming from rice and tomato sauce, and the remaining starch is derived from the vegetables. Look at table 15. One can see that each starch/bread exchange contains 15 grams of carbohydrate, 3 grams of protein, and trace fat. Multiply this by 2 to arrive at the total amounts of carbohydrate and protein from starch/bread in the dinner.

Next, look at table 15 for the breakdown of vegetable exchanges. One exchange contains 5 grams of carbohydrate and 2 grams of protein. Estimate that 1½ exchanges are contained in the dinner.

The complex carbohydrate as starch/bread and vegetable, then, is as follows:

| 2 starch/bread | 30 grams carbohydrate | 6 grams protein |
| 1½ vegetable | 7.5 grams carbohydrate | 3 grams protein |
| Total | 38 grams carbohydrate | 9 grams protein |

*Step 5:* Subtract all carbohydrate (starch/bread and vegetable exchanges) from the total dinner breakdown.

| | Carbohydrate | Protein | Fat |
|---|---|---|---|
| Total Dinner | 38 g | 20 g | 11 g |
| Carbohydrate | 38 g | 9 g | 0 g |
| | 0 g | 11 g | 11 g |

The bottom line represents the remaining protein and fat in the dinner.

*Step 6:* Calculate the meat exchanges in the ingredients. The protein in the dinner is derived mostly from beef. The relative amounts of hydrolyzed plant protein are probably negligible. The beef is usually a medium-fat meat in commercial products. We will assume that most of the protein is medium-fat meat.

Each medium-fat meat exchange contains 7 grams of protein and 5 grams of fat. Since there are 11 grams of protein left in the dinner after accounting for carbohydrate, there are approximately 1½ medium-fat meat exchanges, which we will round off to two exchanges.

*Step 7:* Subtract two protein (medium-fat meat) from the remaining dinner breakdown.

| | Protein | Fat |
|---|---|---|
| Remaining Dinner | 11 g | 11 g |
| − 2 Medium-Fat Meat | 14 g | 10 g |
| | 0 g | 1 g |

We were left with 1 gram of fat to express as fat exchanges.

*Step 8:* Summarize your analysis.

| Exchange | Carbohydrate | Protein | Fat |
|---|---|---|---|
| 2 Starch/Bread | 30 g | 6 g | 0 g |
| 1½ Vegetable | 8 g | 3 g | 0 g |
| 2 Medium-Fat Meat | 0 g | 14 g | 10 g |
| Total | 38 g | 23 g | 10 g |

*Step 9:* Check your analysis against the food label. In the left column we have placed our analysis. In the right column we have placed the label analysis. Remember that 1 gram of protein or carbohydrate equals four calories. One gram of fat equals nine calories.

| | Our Analysis | Food Label |
|---|---|---|
| Carbohydrate | 38 g (152 calories) | 38 g (152 calories) |
| Protein | 23 g (92 calories) | 20 g (80 calories) |
| Fat | 10 g (90 calories) | 11 g (99 calories) |
| Total | 334 calories | 331 calories |

By rounding off the medium-fat meat exchanges upward, we have gained four extra calories in our analysis as compared with the food label. This overestimate is less than 10% of total calories and is allowable. If your estimate exceeds 10% or 30 to 40 calories indicated on the food label, you should go over the above comparisons and seek errors!

**Working the Recipe or Processed Food Into a Meal Plan**

The two examples given in this chapter provide the necessary information to determine if they are suitable for your meal plan. For example, if you are on a 1,200-, 1,500- or 1,800-calorie meal plan, look at the exchange lists for dinner, since the recipe and frozen food are both dinner items.

Table 16 compares the exchanges and total calories among them. From the standpoint of total calories, both the recipe and the frozen dinner fall within the calories allowed for the three meal plan suppers. However, when the distribution of exchanges is considered, some shifting needs to be made. Let's consider the recipe first.

If you are following the *1,200*-calorie plan, you will need to add one fruit and one-half fat exchange. Since the beef stew provides one more meat than is allowed, you can either omit the meat exchange at breakfast or if you have already eaten breakfast, weigh out 1 ounce of meat from the one-sixth portion of the recipe and add it to your family's portion.

If you are following the *1,500*-calorie plan, you need to add one starch/bread, one vegetable, one fruit and one-half fat exchange. Since the beef stew provides one more meat than is allowed, you can either omit the meat exchange at breakfast or if you have already eaten breakfast, weigh out 1 ounce of meat from the one-sixth portion of the recipe and add it to your family's portion.

If you are following the *1,800*-calorie plan, you need to add two starch/bread, one vegetable, one fruit and 1½ fat exchanges.

If you are eating the frozen dinner:
• for the 1,200-calorie plan, add one fruit and one fat exchange. Omit a starch/bread exchange at snack. The extra half vegetable exchange is negligible;
• for the 1,500-calorie plan, add one-half vegetable, one fruit and one fat exchange;
• for the 1,800-calorie plan, add one starch/bread, one meat, one-half vegetable, one fruit and two fat exchanges.

## Summary

Do not use processed foods unless the food label is adequate and an estimate of various exchanges and total calories can be made.

Recipes and processed foods must be analyzed for the total number of exchanges and calories before they can be worked into a given meal on the various plans described in this monograph.

The food item should not exceed a given meal in calories or various exchanges. If the food item does not meet the total requirements of a meal, add more food exchanges until the correct number is achieved.

## TABLE 16:
## COMPARISON OF RECIPE AND FROZEN DINNER EXCHANGES WITH THOSE ALLOWED FOR SUPPER ON 1,200-, 1,500-, AND 1,800-CALORIE MEAL PLANS

| TYPE OF EXCHANGE | EXCHANGES | | EXCHANGES ALLOWED | | |
|---|---|---|---|---|---|
| | Recipe | Frozen Dinner | Supper (1,200 Plan) | Supper (1,500 Plan) | Supper (1,800 Plan) |
| Starch/Bread | 1 | 2 | 1 | 2 | 3 |
| Meat* | 3 | 2 | 2 | 2 | 3 |
| Vegetable | 1 | 1½ | 1 | 2 | 2 |
| Fruit | 0 | 0 | 1 | 1 | 1 |
| Milk | 0 | 0 | 0 | 0 | 0 |
| Fat | ½ | 0 | 1 | 1 | 2 |
| Calories | 352 | 334 | 360 | 465 | 665 |

*Meat exchanges are medium-fat meat.

# Chapter 20: Food Preparation for Good Health

Throughout this monograph TOPS members are encouraged to reduce consumption of fat, cholesterol, sodium (salt) and sugar. Guidelines also suggest food fiber intake is increased by using more whole grain products, fruits and vegetables.

Favorite recipes that you enjoy often can be part of a healthy eating plan. Simple changes, such as using fat-free cooking methods and substituting or reducing an ingredient, will produce lighter fare that tastes good. Many of these suggestions reenforce what foods to avoid and what foods to consume (see chapter 13).

Try these cooking techniques:

(1) Roast, broil, oven-bake or microwave instead of frying or pan frying. Be sure cuts of meat are on a rack during the cooking process to allow the fat to drip away. Remove skin from all poultry before cooking. Trim visible fat from red meat.
(2) Brown meats for chili, spaghetti sauce or stews in a nonstick pan; remove from pan with a slotted spoon and place in a colander. Press out fat with back of spoon. Catch the fat with a pie plate and discard.
(3) Chill soups, stews, sauces and broths prior to serving; remove the hardened fat from the top.
(4) Use nonstick cookware. Try paper liners for cupcakes and muffins.
(5) Cut and serve SMALLER PORTIONS.

*Analyze the recipe and determine if the ingredient could be reduced, eliminated or substituted with a more acceptable ingredient.*

INGREDIENT REDUCTION:

• Fat can be reduced by one-fourth to one-third in baked goods, gravies, sauces and desserts. Use 1 to 2 T. of oil or fat for each cup of flour. Compensate by using a moist low-fat ingredient, such as buttermilk, yogurt or applesauce.
• Sugar can be reduced by one-fourth to one-third in desserts and baked goods. Try to use no more than ¼ cup sweetener (granulated or brown sugar, honey, molasses, maple syrup) per cup of flour used. Enhance sweetness with vanilla extract, cinnamon, other spices or lemon. Dried fruit can add sweetness naturally.
• Reduce the amount of nuts, coconut or chips (such as chocolate) by half. The flavor will be there with less fat.
• Reduce the amount of animal protein (such as meat, cheese, eggs or poultry) in entrees and casseroles. Three ounces of lean cooked meat, poultry or fish (without the bone or skin) per person is adequate. If you do not have a scale, a portion of the size of a deck of playing cards is about three ounces.

INGREDIENT ELIMINATION:

• Skip the frosting on a cake; serve plain or with a dusting of powdered sugar.
• Skip the gravy and sauces.
• Eliminate salt in all recipes except yeast breads. The leavenings in baked goods add plenty of sodium.
• Cook vegetables and rice in fat-free broth for flavor without salt.

INGREDIENT SUBSTITUTION:

See next page for suggestions.

We hope these suggestions will help you enjoy family favorites all year long.

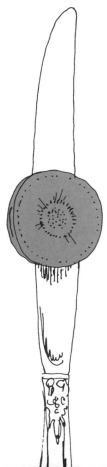

Author's Note: Mary Hoettels, R.D., M.S., greatly aided the author in the preparation of chapter 20.

INGREDIENT SUBSTITUTION:

**To reduce fat and cholesterol try:**

| INGREDIENT | QUANTITY | SUBSTITUTION |
|---|---|---|
| •Shortening | ½ cup | ⅓ cup vegetable oil |
| •Whole milk, 2% milk | 1 cup | 1 cup skim milk |
| •Regular evaporated milk, light or heavy cream | 1 cup | 1 cup evaporated skim milk |
| •Sour cream | 1 cup | 1 cup plain nonfat yogurt OR 1 cup blenderized cottage cheese |
| •Cheese | 1 ounce | 1 ounce low-fat cheese with 5 grams or less of fat per ounce |
| •Ground beef | 1 pound | ½ pound of lean ground round OR ground turkey |
| •Creamed cottage cheese | ½ cup | ½ cup 1% or 2% cottage cheese |
| •Salad dressing or mayonnaise | 1 T. | 1 T. calorie-reduced salad dressing or mayonnaise |
| •Condensed soup | 1 can | 1 cup white sauce using 2 T. margarine, 2 T. flour, 1 cup skim milk, dash white pepper plus ¼ cup cooked mushrooms or celery |
| •Bacon | 2 strips (1 oz.) | 1 ounce Canadian bacon |
| •Whole egg | 1 | 2 egg whites or ¼ cup egg substitute |
| •Baking chocolate | 1 ounce | 3 T. unsweetened baking cocoa |
| •Double pie crust | | Single pie crust |

**To reduce sugar content:**

| INGREDIENT | QUANTITY | SUBSTITUTION |
|---|---|---|
| •Fruit-flavored gelatin | 1 box | Sugar-free gelatin or plain juice |
| •Jam/jelly | 1 T. | 1 T. low-sugar jam/jelly |
| •Frozen or canned sweetened fruit | 1 cup | 1 cup unsweetened frozen or canned fruit |
| •Maple syrup | ¼ cup | Sugar-reduced syrup |

**To increase fiber content:**

| INGREDIENT | QUANTITY | SUBSTITUTION |
|---|---|---|
| •All-purpose flour | 1 cup | 1 cup whole wheat flour OR ½ cup whole wheat and all-purpose flour OR ¾ cup flour plus ¼ cup wheat germ or bran |
| •White rice | 1 cup | 1 cup brown rice |

*Hint:* Add fiber to soups and stews with beans. Add a cup for delicious fiber.

# Chapter 21: Low-Calorie Sugar and Fat Substitutes and Seasoning

## Calorie-Containing Sugar Substitutes

### Sorbitol, Xylitol and Mannitol

These sweeteners are true carbohydrate, and some, like sorbitol, are found naturally in many fruits. They are alcohol sugars and contain four calories per gram like any other sugar. Unlike table sugar or sucrose, they do not promote tooth decay. They also are not absorbed as rapidly from the intestinal tract and do not cause as rapid a rise in blood sugar as do table sugar or other natural sugars, such as glucose or fructose. For this reason they are often used to sweeten candy and other desserts for use by diabetic individuals.

Many "sugarless," "sugar-free" and "diabetic" items like chewing gums and candy actually contain sorbitol, xylitol or mannitol. This type of food labeling is confusing. Although table sugar (sucrose) is not the sweetener, a carbohydrate is used, and the calories may be less, the same or even higher. It is important to read labels and determine what sweetener is being used and how many calories actually are present. Heavy consumption of these carbohydrates can cause very uncomfortable intestinal gas with bloating and diarrhea.

### Aspartame (NutraSweet®)

This sweetener is composed of certain amino acids and contains four calories per gram. However, it is so intensely sweeter than table sugar that small amounts with few calories can be used to achieve the same degree of sweetness as table sugar.

Aspartame has enjoyed great popularity in recent years and is a frequent ingredient in many low-calorie soft drinks, gelatin and pudding desserts, and other food items. To date, aspartame cannot be used in foods that must be baked or heated in any other way. However, some industries are attempting to modify aspartame so that it will not break down during heating.

Although there has been some concern about possible side effects of aspartame, the FDA has found no evidence to support any risks involved in its use. In patients with phenylketonuria, a rare inherited disorder of amino acid metabolism, aspartame should not be consumed, because the phenylalanine (an amino acid) in it may aggravate this disease.

### Acesulfame-K

This is another low-calorie sweetener that has been approved by the FDA very recently. It has sweetening properties that are 200-fold greater than table sugar. It is also stable at high temperatures so that eventually it may be approved for several different uses by the food industry. In Europe, for example, it has enjoyed wide acceptance. Because it appears to enhance sweetness of other products like aspartame, acesulfame-K and aspartame are already being added in combination to some low-calorie beverages and desserts produced in other countries.

## Calorie-Free Sugar Substitutes

### Saccharin

This is the only calorie-free sweetener available in the United States currently. Although animal toxicity studies forced the FDA to ban saccharin, Congress has lifted the ban five times between 1977 and 1987 on the basis of consumer pressure and the lack of evidence for human toxicity.

Saccharin continues to be used as a sweetener in beverages and certain dessert items, although its popularity has been displaced recently by other sweeteners such as aspartame.

### Cyclamate

Cyclamate is another type of no-calorie sweetener that was banned by the FDA in 1967 based on animal and human studies. In recent years the results of those studies have been challenged by newer investigations supporting its safety and efficacy. Petitions have been filed to reconsider its use as an artificial sweetener. However, this controversy is not likely to be resolved in the near future, if at all.

## Table Top Sweeteners

There are several table top sweeteners in use today. Some are in liquid form; others are granulated or powdered. Some are completely calorie free, because saccharin is the only important ingredient.

Others contain low-calorie sweeteners like aspartame or are mixtures of sugar or corn syrup derivatives and other no- or low-calorie sweeteners. Table 17 provides a partial list of products representative of different sweetening agents.

## Polydextrose: A Low-Calorie Bulking Agent

The FDA has approved polydextrose, a low-calorie bulking agent, for use in a number of candies, toppings, frozen desserts, puddings, gelatins and bakery goods.

Polydextrose contains only one calorie per gram

and can be substituted for sugars and fat that normally provide bulk and moisture-containing properties to food. Up to 50% reductions of calories are possible. Food products using this additive are expanding and provide another means of reducing calories in processed foods.

## Fat Substitutes

Everyone realizes that fat is the most calorie-dense food (nine calories per gram). Fake fat or low-fat substitutes that are similar in form to animal or vegetable fats would greatly reduce calories in one's meal plan. Several are being developed by the food industry with an eye on weight-conscious adults.

Two products are being reviewed by the FDA at present, but only one has been approved as of the writing of this monograph. That product, Sim-

plesse, is made by NutraSweet, a division of Monsanto Co. in St. Louis. Simplesse is derived from a process that converts natural protein into microscopic spheres that have the smoothness and texture of cream. Simplesse cannot be heated without destroying its physical properties. Its use will be confined mostly to foods resembling dairy products, salad dressings and other toppings. It is estimated that Simplesse products will have half the calories of comparable foods containing fat.

Olestra is being developed by Proctor & Gamble in Cincinnati. It is chemically synthesized from sucrose (table sugar) and food oils and is a type of sucrose polyester. These compounds have the consistency and taste of vegetable oils but are not absorbed by the intestinal tract. They have no caloric value. Initial research indicates that Olestra is quite palatable in desserts and other foods that require a cream or oil base. Olestra does not

## TABLE 17: LOW-CALORIE SWEETENERS AND TABLE SUGAR EQUIVALENCIES

Find the amount of table sugar to be replaced in the top row. Locate the amount of your sweetener that is equal in sweetness in the columns directly below that amount of table sugar.

| | 1 tsp. | ¼ cup | ½ cup | 1 cup |
|---|---|---|---|---|
| SUGAR (granulated sucrose) | 1 tsp. (16 calories) | ¼ cup (192 calories) | ½ cup (385 calories) | 1 cup (770 calories) |
| EQUAL (powdered aspartame) | ½ packet (2 calories) | 6 packets (24 calories) | 12 packets (48 calories) | 24 packets (96 calories) |
| SPRINKLE SWEET (granulated saccharin) | 1 tsp. (2 calories) | ¼ cup (24 calories) | ½ cup (48 calories) | 1 cup (96 calories) |
| SUGAR TWIN (granulated saccharin) | 1 tsp. (1½ calories) | ¼ cup (18 calories) | ½ cup (36 calories) | 1 cup (72 calories) |
| SWEET 'N LOW (granulated saccharin) | Special spoon (2 calories) | 1 tsp. (17 calories) | 2 tsp. (34 calories) | 4 tsp. (68 calories) |
| SWEET 'N LOW (liquid saccharin) | 10 drops (0 calories) | _____ | 1 tbsp. (0 calories) | 2 tbsp. (0 calories) |
| SWEET ONE (powdered acesulfame-K) | ½ packet (2 calories) | 6 packets (24 calories) | 12 packets (48 calories) | 24 packets (96 calories) |
| SWEET-10 (liquid saccharin) | 10 drops (2 calories) | _____ | 1 tbsp. (48 calories) | 2 tbsp. (96 calories) |

break down during baking or frying and can be used in place of oils, margarine and butter in a variety of bakery goods, like cookies, as well as in frozen desserts, salad dressings, etc.

These kinds of fat substitutes have obvious appeal to people with weight problems. Fat, which contains nine calories per gram, may be replaced either with no-calorie Olestra or very low calorie Simplesse. Hidden fat calorie problems will be controlled better with dietetic foods containing these substitutes. It probably will have a beneficial effect on blood cholesterol as well.

### Substituting Spices for Salt

In chapter 13 it was recommended that the use of salt in cooking or at the table be reduced. This does not mean you have to sacrifice flavor, because there are many ways to improve flavor with no salt spices. In a relatively short time you can become an expert in the use of a variety of spices to improve the taste of food on your meal plan.

Table 18 provides an extensive list of what spices can be used to enhance flavor and what kinds are appropriate for specific meats and vegetables.

### Summary

Over the last 10 years many new low-calorie products have entered the food market. Individuals who must control their weight have a variety of low-calorie sweeteners they can use. Processed foods and beverages that use these sweeteners reduce the calorie content of many favorite items. Now fat substitutes are becoming available.

Adults are encouraged to use the products to aid in weight reduction or weight control. However, low-calorie does not mean calorie-free. Read

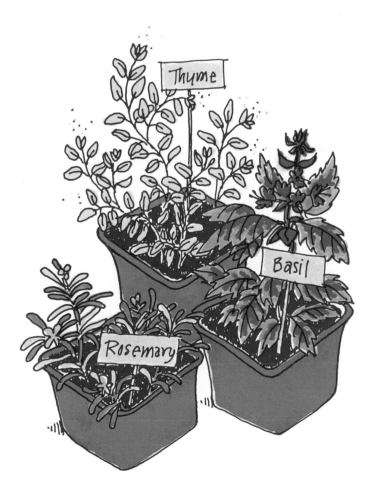

labels on containers carefully. Decide what advantage they have over regular foods and how many calories you are actually saving. Dietetic foods also must be worked into a meal plan.

*Note:* The FDA does not recommend the use of food products containing sugar substitutes by growing children or pregnant women.

## TABLE 18: THE MAGIC OF SPICES ON A LOW-SODIUM DIET

Use in small amounts to enhance flavor:

| | | | |
|---|---|---|---|
| Allspice | Curry | Nutmeg | Red pepper |
| Basil | Dill | Onion | Black pepper |
| Bay leaf | Garlic | Onion juice | Pimento |
| Caraway | Garlic juice | Onion powder | Poultry seasoning |
| Chili powder | Garlic powder | Oregano | Sage |
| Chives | Ginger | Paprika | Vinegar |
| Cinnamon | Lemon juice | Parsley | |
| Cloves | Dry mustard | Green pepper | |

Add-a-spice to meats:
Beef: dry mustard, nutmeg, onion, sage, thyme, pepper, bay leaf
Lamb: garlic, curry, broiled pineapple rings
Veal: bay leaf, ginger, curry
Chicken: paprika, thyme, sage, parsley, cranberry sauce
Fish: dry mustard, paprika, curry, bay leaf, lemon juice
Eggs: pepper, green pepper, dry mustard, paprika, curry

Add-a-spice to vegetables:
Asparagus: lemon juice, caraway
Green beans: lemon juice, nutmeg, dill seed, onion
Broccoli: lemon juice, oregano
Cabbage: mustard, dill seed, caraway seed
Cauliflower: nutmeg
Corn: green pepper, tomatoes, pimento, parsley, chives
Peas: fresh mushrooms, onion, green pepper
Potatoes: parsley, chopped green pepper, chives, onions
Squash: ginger, mace, onions, basil, oregano
Tomatoes: basil, oregano, marjoram, onions
Sweet potatoes: cinnamon, nutmeg

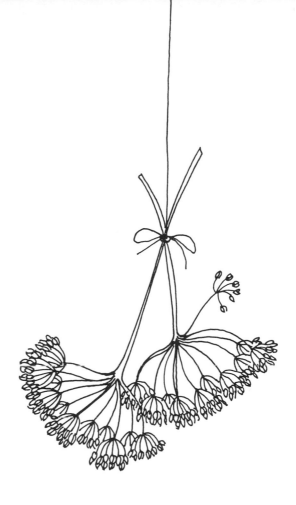

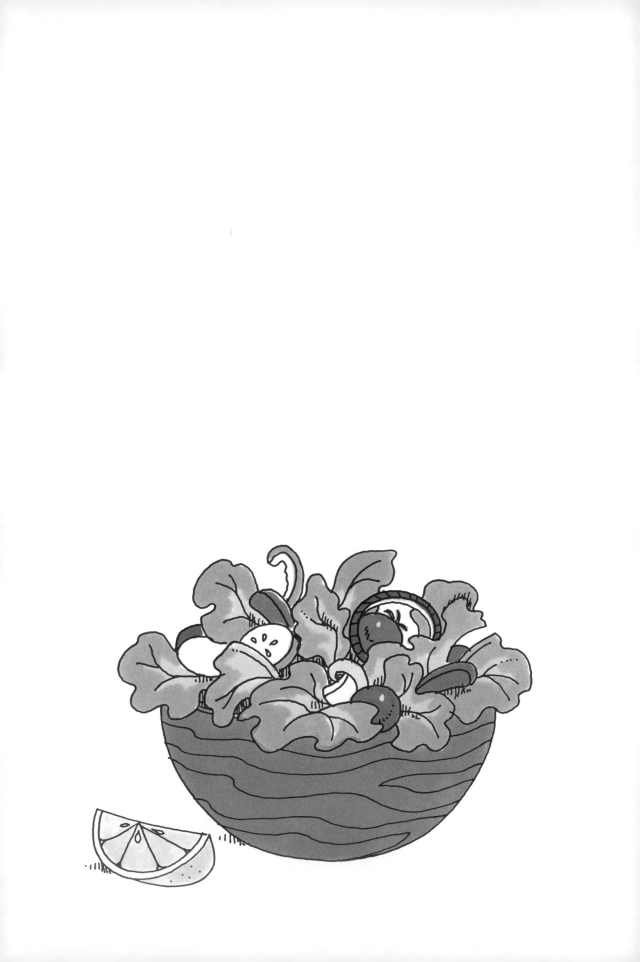

# PART EIGHT:
# Additional Exchange Lists

Chapter 22: Fast Food Restaurants

Chapter 23: Convenience Foods

Chapter 24: Recipes

Chapter 25: Alcoholic Beverages

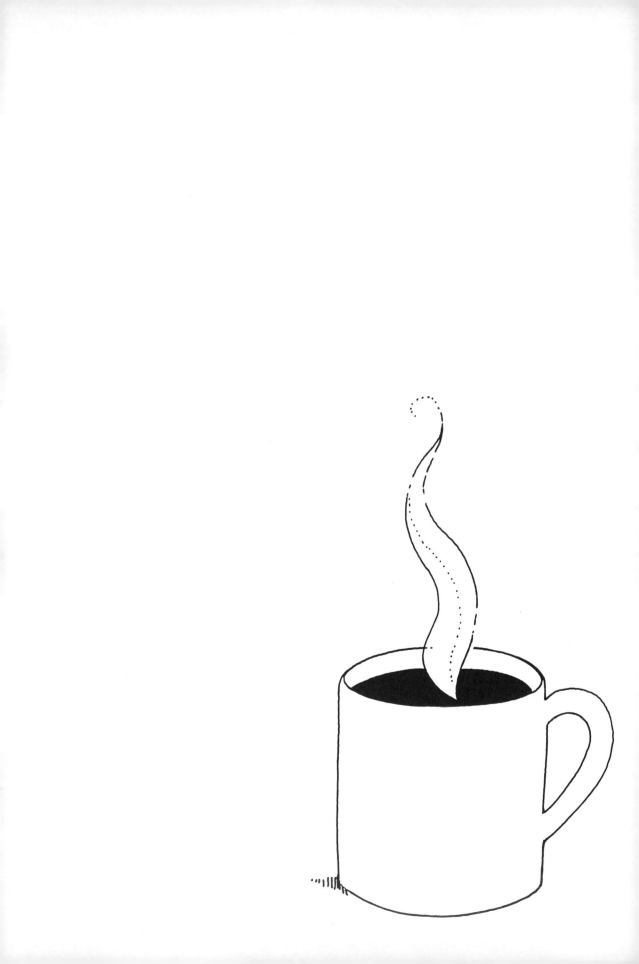

# Chapter 22: Fast Food Restaurants

Eating at fast food outlets can also be eating right when you plan ahead. The effects of fast foods on your meal plan depend on the following:

(1) How often fast foods are eaten
(2) What is selected from available menu items
(3) What you eat the rest of the day

Visits to fast food restaurants that are no more than one or two times per week will have a small impact on the overall nutritional quality and quantity of your meal plan over the course of a week. The concentration of calories and nutrients will vary depending upon the menu items selected. Although fast food meals can supply a significant source of protein, they can also be a concentrated source of fats (especially saturated forms), cholesterol, sugars and sodium, and a poor source of fiber and vitamin A when a salad is not available. The recommended goal of limiting the number of calories and the percentage of calories from fat can still be reached if you select the fast foods carefully and adjust fat exchanges during the rest of the day if necessary. Calories, Sugar and Fat: It's All in the Selection!

Look at a typical fast food meal:

Large ¼-pound meat patty cheeseburger with condiments and vegetables:

| Calories | Carbo-hydrate | Protein | Fat | Sodium | Chol | % Fat |
|---|---|---|---|---|---|---|
| 569 | 38 g | 28 g | 33 g | 1,107 mg | 88 mg | 53 |

Regular order of French fries:

| Calories | Carbo-hydrate | Protein | Fat | Sodium | Chol | % Fat |
|---|---|---|---|---|---|---|
| 237 | 29 g | 3 g | 12 g | 124 mg | 13 mg | 46 |

Regular (10 oz.) vanilla shake:

| Calories | Carbo-hydrate | Protein | Fat | Sodium | Chol | % Fat |
|---|---|---|---|---|---|---|
| 314 | 50 g | 10 g | 8 g | 232 mg | 133 mg | 23 |

TOTALS:

| Calories | Carbo-hydrate | Protein | Fat | Sodium | Chol | % Fat |
|---|---|---|---|---|---|---|
| 1,120 | 117 g | 41 g | 53 g | 1,463 mg | 234 mg | 43 |

Depending upon the calorie level of your meal plan, this could be up to 92% of your allowed daily intake. Note the high sodium and cholesterol values. The percentage of calories from fat is 43%. This is the same as eating 4 tablespoons of solid shortening. The shake also contributes 3 tablespoons of sugar.

A better choice would be a regular hamburger (single meat patty, plain), ½ pint of 2% milk, and a small salad (2 cups of iceberg lettuce, 1 tablespoon of green pepper, ¼ cup of sliced tomatoes, 2 radishes, 4 cucumber slices, ¼ medium size carrot, with lemon juice or vinegar).

Regular hamburger, single meat patty, plain:

| Calories | Carbo-hydrate | Protein | Fat | Sodium | Chol | % Fat |
|---|---|---|---|---|---|---|
| 275 | 30 g | 12 g | 12 g | 387 mg | 36 mg | 39 |

½ pint of 2% milk:

| Calories | Carbo-hydrate | Protein | Fat | Sodium | Chol | % Fat |
|---|---|---|---|---|---|---|
| 121 | 11 g | 8 g | 5 g | 122 mg | 18 mg | 37 |

Small salad:

| Calories | Carbo-hydrate | Protein | Fat | Sodium | Chol | % Fat |
|---|---|---|---|---|---|---|
| 50 | 10 g | 4 g | 0 | 17 mg | 0 | 0 |

TOTALS:

| Calories | Carbo-hydrate | Protein | Fat | Sodium | Chol | % Fat |
|---|---|---|---|---|---|---|
| 446 | 51 g | 24 g | 17 g | 526 mg | 54 mg | 34 |

With 34% of calories from fat, this meal contains only 4 teaspoons of hidden fat as compared with 12 teaspoons as noted previously and is sugar free. Most important of all, the total calories of only 446 is more appropriate for a weight-reduction meal plan.

## Salads: A Quick Avenue to Hidden Calories

Salad bars and prepackaged salads are becoming increasingly popular. Depending upon your choice, a salad can range from about 60 to 1,500 calories!

Salad dressing can contribute many calories. A typical ladle holds a 2-ounce portion of salad dressing. When regular salad dressing is used, this amount is about 300 calories. Calorie-reduced salad dressing is about 150 calories. To control the amount of salad dressing, place 1 to 2 teaspoons of regular or 2 to 4 teaspoons of calorie-reduced salad dressing in a small separate bowl. Dip your fork into the dressing first and then into the salad for flavor with minimal fat.

Alternative low-calorie salad dressings include vinegar or lemon juice with or without a sprinkling of pepper. Also, try topping the salad with flavor-intense vegetables such as tomatoes, peas, mushrooms or grated carrots. At salad bars, when the choice is available, choose a small dish for your salad. The large plate encourages selecting too much. Remember, you can overstuff yourself on a salad. Too much salad consumption can easily be carried over to other food choices. All

Author's Note: The author appreciates the input of both Mary Hoettels, R.D., M.S., and Joan Pleuss, R.D., M.S., C.D.E., in the planning of chapter 22.

things, including salads, should be enjoyed in moderation!

Look at the following examples to see how a salad can add up in calorie content.

## Salads without Toppings

*Salad Ia:* Basic Salad, No Dressing

| | |
|---|---|
| 1 cup iceberg lettuce | 75 calories |
| 2 T. diced green pepper | 13 g carbohydrates |
| ½ cup sliced tomato | 4 g protein |
| ¼ cup sliced mushrooms | 7% fat |
| | 47 mg sodium |
| ¼ cup broccoli flowerets | 0 mg cholesterol |
| ¼ cup raw cauliflowerets | |
| ¼ cup shredded carrot | |
| 2 T. green peas | |
| ¼ cup alfalfa sprouts | |

*Salad Ib:* Basic Salad, Low-Calorie Italian Dressing

| | |
|---|---|
| Same raw ingredients as basic | 107 calories |
| Salad Ia + 2 T. low-calorie Italian salad dressing | 14 g carbohydrates |
| | 4 g protein |
| | 30% fat |
| | 283 mg sodium |
| | 2 mg cholesterol |

*Salad Ic:* Basic Salad, Regular Italian Salad Dressing

| | |
|---|---|
| Same raw ingredients as basic | 217 calories |
| Salad Ia + 2 T. regular Italian salad dressing | 16 g carbohydrates |
| | 4 g protein |
| | 62% fat |
| | 281 mg sodium |
| | 0 mg cholesterol |

## Basic Salads and Combination Salads with Toppings

*Salad IIa:* Basic Salad, Low-Calorie Salad Dressing with Toppings

| | |
|---|---|
| Same raw ingredients as basic | 341 calories |
| Salad Ia + 2 T. low-calorie Italian salad dressing | 21 g carbohydrates |
| | 26 g protein |
| | 45% fat |
| | 1,036 mg sodium |
| + 1 T. grated cheese | 30 mg cholesterol |
| + ½ cup 2% cottage cheese | |
| + 1 T. bacon bits | |
| + 1 T. sunflower seeds | |

*Salad IIb:* Basic Salad, Low-Calorie Italian Salad Dressing with Toppings and Three Combination Salads

| | |
|---|---|
| Same raw ingredients as basic | 534 calories |
| Salad Ia + 2 T. low-calorie Italian salad dressing | 41 g carbohydrates |
| | 29 g protein |
| | 48% fat |
| | 1,332 mg sodium |
| + same toppings as IIa | 30 mg cholesterol |
| + ¼ cup 3-bean salad | |
| + ¼ cup coleslaw | |
| + ¼ cup carrot-raisin salad | |

## Chef Salads

*Salad IIIa:* Chef-Type Salad, No Dressing

| | |
|---|---|
| 2 cups iceberg lettuce | 505 calories |
| ½ cup diced green pepper | 11 g carbohydrates |
| | 52 g protein |
| ½ cup sliced tomato | 50% fat |
| 1 T. green onions | 1,053 mg sodium |
| 2 oz. turkey, light meat, roasted | 398 mg cholesterol |
| 2 oz. 5% fat roast ham | |
| 1 oz. American cheese | |
| 1 oz. Swiss cheese | |
| 1 medium-hard cooked egg | |

*Salad IIIb:* Chef-Type Salad, Regular French Salad Dressing

| | |
|---|---|
| Chef salad ingredients as listed in salad IIIa + 2 oz. (1 ladle) French dressing | 754 calories |
| | 20 g carbohydrates |
| | 52 g protein |
| | 61% fat |
| | 1,830 mg sodium |
| | 431 mg cholesterol |

*Salad IIIc:* Chef-Type Salad, Blue Cheese Salad Dressing

| | |
|---|---|
| Chef salad ingredients as listed in salad IIIa + 2 oz. (1 ladle) blue cheese salad dressing | 796 calories |
| | 15 g carbohydrates |
| | 55 g protein |
| | 65% fat |
| | 1,052 mg sodium |
| | 848 mg cholesterol |

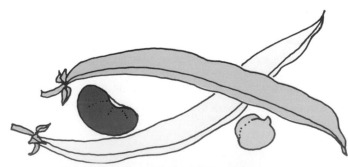

The previous analyses illustrate how a person may consume as little as 75 calories and as much as 800 calories after eating a single salad. It all relates to the kinds of salad dressings, toppings and other combinations added to it.

TOPS members who are on 1,200-, 1,500- or 1,800-meal plans can enjoy a good salad without going overboard. Most should restrict their choice to a basic salad with low-calorie dressings (salads such as Ia, Ib and Ic).

## Other Suggestions for Fast Food Selections

The saying, Good things come in small packages, is a good guideline when making your menu selections. Large portions in the fast food area mean undesired calories, fat, sugar and salt.

- Look for items that are described as broiled, dry broiled or grilled, steamed or poached in its own juice, or garden fresh. (Do check to make sure sulfites are not being used in salads.)
- Skip items that are described as follows: double or triple, whopper or grand deluxe, super or supreme, extra crispy, fried, braised, sauteed, topped with sauce of any kind, topped with bacon, cheese/sausage, deep dish, au gratin or scalloped, or breaded.

Here are some recommendations by menu item.

*Beverages*—2% or skim milk, unsweetened juices, plain coffee or tea (regular or decaffeinated), diet sodas, sparkling water, ice water that is plain or with a twist of lemon for added sparkle

*Soups*—cup portion only of broth-based soup

*Breakfast Entrees*—cereal without added sugar, English muffins or plain toast with margarine or butter on side, plain pancakes (if possible, ask for low-calorie syrup or bring it from home), a single order of scrambled eggs

*Other Entrees*

Beef—roast beef sandwich, single hamburger patty on bun (Note: Skip the sauces, mayonnaise, toppings.) Add flavor with condiments such as mustard or added vegetable. Ask for a dry bun without spread.

Chicken—breast or wing portion (Note: Baked or broiled.) If fried is the only option, choose regular or original recipes, remove skin and breading. Use a plain napkin to pat off fat.

Fish—Baked or broiled is preferred. Skip the tartar sauce, thereby reducing the percentage of calories from fat from almost 60% to about 30%. Blot fish with a napkin to remove excess fat.

Pizzas—Select thin crust with green pepper, mushrooms and onion, and top with mozzarella cheese (particularly skim milk mozzarella if available). If you must have a meat topping, ham is the lowest fat choice; otherwise, skip the ground beef, sausage and pepperoni.

Chili—This may be a good choice if no fat is floating on top. A regular or large portion may be selected depending upon your calorie level. (Note the high sodium content: about 1,000 milligrams in a regular serving and about 1,500 milligrams in a large serving.)

Mexican—Chicken or beef fajitas are your lowest fat choice. A taco salad is an option if you substitute plain beans for the refried variety. Request the meat and condiments on the side so you can control the amount. Substitute salsa or picante sauce for salad dressing. Do not eat the fried tortilla shell used to hold the salad. Choose the soft, unbuttered tortillas instead for your starch choice.

*Side Dishes*

(1) Coleslaw is an option if you eat the cabbage and leave the dressing.
(2) Corn-on-the-cob is a relatively low-fat choice as long as you don't add any more butter.
(3) Baked potatoes are a great, very low fat choice. Be aware that the standard fast food potato is about three starches. Split one with a friend for a more manageable portion, and skip the toppings.
(4) French fried potatoes, whether prepared in animal fat or vegetable oil, are high-fat items. Split a regular order and you only have to count it as one starch and one fat exchange.
(5) Mashed potatoes are a good choice when you don't add any more fat (such as butter or gravy). Limit to ⅓-cup portion.
(6) Potato salad may be a good change of pace when you limit the intake to ½ cup, which is equivalent to one starch and one fat exchange.

*Desserts*

Most baked items are very high in fat and sugar content. For an occasional treat, choose a vanilla soft serve cone (in a cake cone). The companies use an ice milk base, which is a lower fat option. One cone equals 1½ starch plus one fat exchange with only 33% of calories from fat. (Regular ice cream cones may have up to 60% of calories from fat.)

*To lower sodium intake:*

- Skip the sauces, dressings and condiments. Season salads with lemon juice or vinegar or your own low-sodium salad dressing from home.
- Order sandwiches without pickles, pickle relish or cheese.
- Look for low- or no-sodium diet sodas.
- Patronize places which offer fresh meat, fish or poultry. Restructured products and cured meats are higher in sodium.
- Omit breakfast sausage (patties or links), ham, bacon and biscuits.
- Ask for items to be prepared without added salt.

156

- Skip the salt shaker; use herb replacement from home.

*To lower sugar intake:*
- Limit use of ketchup, sweet pickle relish, jelly, honey, syrups and BBQ sauces.
- Choose diet soda, milk, juice or water.
- Avoid sweetened fresh or canned fruits. Look for plain fresh fruit—or bring a fruit from home.
- Avoid gelatin salads.
- Skip desserts.

*To increase fiber intake:*
- Order from a salad bar, emphasizing dark green, leafy or deep yellow vegetables.
- Order sandwiches with tomato and lettuce.
- Select whole grain buns, if available.
- Order a baked potato, but skip the toppings.

*Condiments*

The last comment is on condiment selection. These foods can add zip to lower-fat food items. Some, however, need to be selected with caution due to their calorie, fat* and/or sodium content. Look at the following chart for this information.

| Condiment (1 T.) | Calories | Fat (g) | Sodium (mg) |
|---|---|---|---|
| Chili sauce | 16 | trace | 201 |
| Chutney, tomato | 41 | trace | 34 |
| Cocktail sauce, Heinz Seafood | 20 | trace | 160 |
| Ketchup | 16 | 0.1 | 170 |
| Mayonnaise | 99 | 11 | 78 |
| Mayonnaise, imitation | 35 | 2.9 | 75 |
| Mustard | 11 | 0.1 | 188 |
| Pickle relish, sweet | 21 | 0.1 | 107 |
| Soy sauce | 11 | 0 | 1,029 |
| Steak sauce | 18 | trace | 149 |
| Sweet and sour sauce | 32 | trace | 320 |
| Tartar sauce | 75 | 8 | 182 |
| Teriyaki sauce | 15 | 0 | 690 |
| Worcestershire sauce | 12 | 0 | 147 |

*To find out the number of fat calories, multiply the number of grams of fat by nine.

## Organization of the Tables

The tables that are included in this chapter do not identify a specific fast food restaurant or brand name of food they prepare. The most important reason for doing this is to encourage you to think about what you are eating in a broad, generic way regardless of what restaurant you visit. The second, practical reason is that many foods are similar in preparation, calories and nutrient content. The various burgers, sandwiches, French fries, beverages, salads, breakfast items, etc., are not very different from one restaurant to another and need not be repeated several times in the tables if they are considered generically rather than by fast food choice.

Each table provides information about serving size, calories, carbohydrate, protein, fat, cholesterol and sodium as well as percentage of total calories as fat.

## How To Use the Tables

It is best to plan your meal in a fast food restaurant ahead of time. Begin by examining your allowable exchanges for given meal (breakfast, lunch or supper). On a 1,200-calorie meal plan there is very little room for excessive numbers of starch/bread and fat exchanges. This will demand a very conservative selection of fast foods. There is more leeway for 1,500-, 1,800- or weight-maintenance plans (see chapters 15 and 18, respectively).

Every effort should be made to keep the fast food meal as close to the number of allowable exchanges as possible for a given meal on your diet. Don't overeat fast food and then skip other meals to make up for it. This will result in overeating generally and in excessive intake of calories.

Many fast foods are high in hidden fat calories and are not suitable for a person on a weight-reduction diet. They are included in the tables to provide a point of comparison. If the fast food meal exceeds the number of fat calories to a slight extent, fat exchanges should be removed from other meals to compensate. If the fast food meal is below the number of exchanges for a given item (fruit, milk, etc.), this can be added as a snack or added to the next meal when it is convenient.

# FAST FOOD—BREAKFAST ITEMS

| ITEM AND AMOUNT | CALORIES | EXCHANGES | SODIUM (milligrams) | CHOLESTEROL (milligrams) | FAT |
|---|---|---|---|---|---|
| Biscuit, plain (1 biscuit = 74 g) | 276 | 2 starch, 2 fat | 584 | 5 | 42% |
| Biscuit with egg (1 biscuit = 136 g) | 315 | 1½ starch, 1 meat, 2½ fat | 655 | 232 | 57% |
| Biscuit with egg and bacon (1 biscuit = 150 g) | 458 | 2 starch, 1½ meat, 4 fat | 999 | 353 | 61% |
| Biscuit with egg and ham (1 biscuit = 192 g) | 442 | 2 starch, 2 meat, 3 fat | 1,381 | 299 | 55% |
| Biscuit with egg and sausage (1 biscuit = 180 g) | 582 | 3 starch, 1½ meat, 5 fat | 1,142 | 302 | 60% |
| Biscuit with egg and steak (1 biscuit = 148 g) | 474 | 2½ starch, 1½ meat, 3½ fat | 888 | 272 | 53% |
| Biscuit with egg, cheese and bacon (1 biscuit = 144 g) | 477 | 2 starch, 1½ meat, 4 fat | 1,261 | 261 | 58% |
| Biscuit with ham (1 biscuit = 113 g) | 387 | 3 starch, ½ meat, 2½ fat | 1,433 | 25 | 42% |
| Biscuit with sausage (1 biscuit = 124 g) | 485 | 2½ starch, ½ meat, 5½ fat | 1,071 | 34 | 59% |
| Biscuit with steak (1 biscuit = 141 g) | 456 | 3 starch, ½ meat, 4 fat | 795 | 26 | 51% |
| Croissant with egg and cheese (1 croissant = 127 g) | 369 | 1½ starch, 1 meat, 3½ fat | 551 | 216 | 61% |
| Croissant with egg, cheese and bacon (1 croissant = 129 g) | 413 | 1½ starch, 1½ meat, 4 fat | 889 | 215 | 61% |
| Croissant with egg, cheese and ham (1 croissant = 152 g) | 475 | 1½ starch, 2 meat, 4½ fat | 1,080 | 213 | 64% |
| Croissant with egg, cheese and sausage (1 croissant = 160 g) | 524 | 1½ starch, 2 meat, 5 fat | 1,115 | 216 | 65% |
| Danish pastry, cheese (1 pastry = 91 g) | 353 | 2 starch, 4½ fat | 320 | 20 | 64% |
| Danish pastry, cinnamon (1 pastry = 88 g) | 349 | 2 starch, 1 fruit, 3 fat | 326 | 28 | 44% |
| Danish pastry, fruit (1 pastry = 94 g) | 356 | 2 starch, 1 fruit, 3 fat | 333 | 19 | 56% |
| Eggs, scrambled (2 eggs = 94 g) | 200 | 2 meat, 1 fat | 211 | 400 | 68% |
| English muffin with butter (1 muffin = 63 g) | 189 | 2 starch, 1 fat | 386 | 13 | 28% |
| English muffin with cheese and sausage (1 muffin = 115 g) | 394 | 2 starch, 3 fat, 1½ meat | 1,036 | 58 | 55% |
| English muffin with egg, cheese and Canadian bacon (1 muffin = 146 g) | 383 | 2 starch, 2 meat, 1½ fat | 785 | 234 | 47% |

## FAST FOOD—BREAKFAST ITEMS (continued)

| ITEM AND AMOUNT | CALORIES | EXCHANGES | SODIUM (milligrams) | CHOLESTEROL (milligrams) | FAT |
|---|---|---|---|---|---|
| English muffin with egg, cheese and sausage (1 muffin = 165 g) | 487 | 2 starch, 2 meat, 4 fat | 1,135 | 274 | 57% |
| French toast with butter (2 slices = 135 g) | 356 | 2 starch, ½ meat, ½ fruit,* 3 fat | 513 | 117 | 48% |
| French toast sticks (5 sticks = 141 g) | 479 | 3 starch, 5 fat | 499 | 74 | 54% |
| Pancakes with butter and syrup (3 cakes = 232 g) | 519 | 3 starch, 3 fruit,* 2 fat | 1,103 | 57 | 24% |
| Potatoes, hashed brown (½ cup = 72 g) | 151 | 1 starch, 1½ fat | 290 | 9 | 54% |
| Sausage patty (1 patty = 27 g) | 100 | 1 meat, ½ fat or 1 high-fat meat | 349 | 22 | 76% |

*Fruit exchange used to express sugar content of syrup.

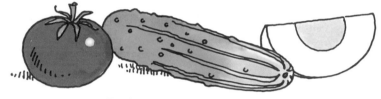

## FAST FOOD—SALADS

| ITEM AND AMOUNT | CALORIES | EXCHANGES | SODIUM (milligrams) | CHOLESTEROL (milligrams) | FAT |
|---|---|---|---|---|---|
| Salad, vegetable, tossed, without dressing (1½ cups) | 32 | 1½ vegetable | 53 | 0 | 4.5% |
| Salad, vegetable, without dressing, with added cheese and eggs (1½ cups) | 102 | 1 meat, 1 vegetable | 119 | 98 | 53% |
| Salad, vegetable, tossed, without dressing, with added chicken (1½ cups) | 105 | 2 lean meat, 1 vegetable | 209 | 72 | 17% |
| Salad, vegetable, tossed, without dressing, with added pasta and seafood (1½ cups) | 380 | 1½ starch, 1½ meat, 2 vegetable, 2 fat | 1,572 | 50 | 50% |
| Salad, vegetable, tossed, without dressing, with added shrimp (1½ cups) | 107 | 2 lean meat, 1 vegetable | 487 | 180 | 20% |
| Salad, vegetable, tossed, without dressing, with added turkey, ham and cheese (chef-style = 1½ cups) | 267 | 4 lean meat, 1 vegetable | 744 | 139 | 54% |
| Scallops, breaded and fried (6 scallops = 144 g) | 386 | 2½ starch, 1 meat, 2 fat | 919 | 107 | 44% |
| Shrimp, breaded and fried (6-8 pieces = 164 g) | 454 | 2½ starch, 1½ meat, 2½ fat | 1,447 | 201 | 50% |

# FAST FOOD—SANDWICHES AND BURGERS

| ITEM AND AMOUNT | CALORIES | EXCHANGES | SODIUM (milligrams) | CHOLESTEROL (milligrams) | FAT |
|---|---|---|---|---|---|
| Cheeseburger, regular, single meat patty, plain (1 burger = 102 g) | 320 | 2 starch, 1 fat, 1½ meat | 500 | 50 | 42% |
| Cheeseburger, regular, single meat patty, with condiments (ketchup, mustard, pickles and onion) (1 burger = 113 g) | 295 | 2 starch, ½ fat, 1½ meat, "free condiments" | 616 | 37 | 43% |
| Cheeseburger, regular, single meat patty, with condiments and vegetables (mayonnaise-style dressing, pickles, onions, lettuce and tomatoes) (1 burger = 154 g) | 359 | 2 starch, 2 fat, 1½ meat, 1 vegetable | 976 | 52 | 50% |
| Cheeseburger, regular, double meat patty, plain (1 burger = 155 g) | 457 | 1½ starch, 3½ meat, 1½ fat | 635 | 110 | 55% |
| Cheeseburger, regular, double meat patty, with condiments and vegetables (see above list) (1 burger = 166 g) | 416 | 1½ starch, 3 meat, 1 vegetable, 1 fat | 1,051 | 60 | 45% |
| Cheeseburger, regular, double meat patty, double-decker bun, plain (bun, ground beef, cheese) (1 burger = 160 g) | 461 | 3 starch, 3 meat, 2 fat | 892 | 80 | 43% |
| Cheeseburger, regular, double meat patty, double-decker bun, with condiments and vegetables (see above list) (1 burger = 228 g) | 649 | 3 starch, 3 meat, 1 vegetable, 3½ fat | 920 | 94 | 49% |
| Cheeseburger, large, single meat patty, plain (1 burger = 185 g) | 608 | 2½ starch, 4 meat, 2 fat | 1,589 | 96 | 49% |
| Cheeseburger, large, single meat patty, with bacon and condiments (see above list) (1 burger = 195 g) | 609 | 2½ starch, 4 meat, 2½ fat | 1,044 | 122 | 55% |
| Cheeseburger, large, single meat patty, with condiments and vegetables (see above list) (1 burger = 219 g) | 564 | 2½ starch, 4 meat, 1 vegetable, 2 fat | 1,107 | 88 | 53% |
| Cheeseburger, large, single meat patty, with ham, condiments and vegetables (see above list) (1 burger = 259 g) | 745 | 2½ starch, 5 meat, ½ vegetable, 3½ fat | 1,713 | 122 | 58% |
| Cheeseburger, large, double meat patty, with condiments and vegetables (see above list) (1 burger = 258 g) | 706 | 2½ starch, 4½ meat, 3 fat, 1 vegetable | 1,149 | 141 | 56% |

# FAST FOOD—SANDWICHES AND BURGERS (continued)

| ITEM AND AMOUNT | CALORIES | EXCHANGES | SODIUM (milligrams) | CHOLESTEROL (milligrams) | FAT |
|---|---|---|---|---|---|
| Cheeseburger, large, triple meat patty, plain (1 burger = 309 g) | 796 | 2½ starch, 6½ meat, 3 fat | 1,211 | 161 | 58% |
| Chicken fillet sandwich, plain (1 sandwich = 182 g) | 515 | 2½ starch, 2½ meat, 3 fat | 957 | 60 | 51% |
| Chicken fillet sandwich with cheese (1 sandwich = 228 g) | 632 | 2½ starch, 4 meat, 3 fat | 1,238 | 76 | 56% |
| Egg and cheese sandwich (1 sandwich = 146 g) | 340 | 1½ starch, 2 meat, 1½ fat | 804 | 291 | 50% |
| Fish sandwich with tartar sauce (1 sandwich = 158 g) | 431 | 2½ starch, 2 meat, 2 fat | 615 | 55 | 48% |
| Fish sandwich with tartar sauce and cheese (1 sandwich = 183 g) | 525 | 3 starch, 2 meat, 3 fat | 939 | 68 | 49% |
| Hamburger, regular, single meat patty, plain (1 burger = 90 g) | 275 | 2 starch, 1 meat, 1 fat | 387 | 36 | 39% |
| Hamburger, regular, single meat patty, with condiments (1 burger = 113 g) | 275 | 2 starch, 1 meat, 1 fat | 564 | 43 | 33% |
| Hamburger, regular, single meat patty, with condiments (see above list) (1 burger = 110 g) | 280 | 2 starch, 1 meat, 1 fat, "free condiments" | 504 | 26 | 42% |
| Hamburger, regular, double meat patty, plain (1 burger = 176 g) | 544 | 3 starch, 3 meat, 2 fat | 554 | 99 | 46% |
| Hamburger, regular, double meat patty, with condiments (see above list) (1 burger = 215 g) | 576 | 2½ starch, 4 meat, 2 fat | 742 | 102 | 50% |
| Hamburger, large, single meat patty, plain (1 burger = 137 g) | 400 | 2 starch, 2 meat, 2 fat | 474 | 71 | 52% |
| Hamburger, large, single meat patty, with condiments and vegetables (see above list) (1 burger = 218 g) | 511 | 2½ starch, 3 meat, 2 fat | 825 | 86 | 48% |
| Hamburger, large, double meat patty, with condiments and vegetables (see above list) (1 burger = 226 g) | 540 | 2½ starch, 4 meat, 1 fat, ½ vegetable | 791 | 122 | 44% |
| Hamburger, large, triple meat patty, with condiments (see above list) (1 burger = 259 g) | 693 | 2 starch, 6 meat, 2 fat | 713 | 142 | 53% |
| Ham and cheese sandwich (1 sandwich = 146 g) | 353 | 2 starch, 2 meat, 1 fat | 772 | 58 | 38% |

| ITEM AND AMOUNT | CALORIES | EXCHANGES | SODIUM (milligrams) | CHOLESTEROL (milligrams) | FAT |
|---|---|---|---|---|---|
| Ham, egg and cheese sandwich (1 sandwich = 143 g) | 348 | 2 starch, 2 meat, 1 fat | 1,005 | 245 | 41% |
| Hotdog, plain (1 hotdog = 98 g) | 242 | 1 starch, 1 meat, 2 fat | 671 | 44 | 54% |
| Hotdog with chili (1 hotdog = 114 g) | 297 | 2 starch, 1 meat, 1½ fat | 480 | 51 | 39% |
| Hotdog with corn flour coating, corndog (1 hotdog = 175 g) | 460 | 3½ starch, 1 meat, 2 fat | 972 | 79 | 37% |
| Roast beef sandwich, plain (1 sandwich = 139 g) | 346 | 2 starch, 2 meat, 1 fat | 792 | 52 | 36% |
| Roast beef sandwich with cheese (1 sandwich = 176 g) | 402 | 2 starch, 3 meat, ½ fat | 1,634 | 77 | 40% |
| Steak sandwich (1 sandwich = 204 g) | 459 | 3 starch, 3 meat | 798 | 73 | 27% |
| Submarine sandwich with cold cuts (includes lettuce, cheese, salami, ham, tomato, onion, oil) (1 sandwich = 228 g) | 456 | 3 starch, 2 meat, 1 vegetable, 2 fat | 1,650 | 35 | 37% |
| Submarine sandwich with roast beef (1 sandwich = 216 g) | 411 | 3 starch, 2½ meat, "free" vegetable | 845 | 73 | 28% |
| Submarine sandwich with tuna salad (1 sandwich = 256 g) | 584 | 3½ starch, 3 meat, 2 fat | 1,295 | 47 | 43% |

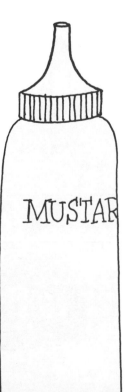

# FAST FOOD—SIDE DISHES

| ITEM AND AMOUNT | CALORIES | EXCHANGES | SODIUM (milligrams) | CHOLESTEROL (milligrams) | FAT |
|---|---|---|---|---|---|
| Coleslaw (¾ cup = 99 g) | 147 | 2½ vegetable, 2 fat | 267 | 5 | 67% |
| Corn-on-the-cob with butter (1 ear = 146 g) | 155 | 2 starch | 30 | 6 | 17% |
| Hush puppies (5 pieces = 78 g) | 256 | 2 starch, 2 fat | 965 | 135 | 40% |
| Onion rings, breaded and fried (8-9 rings = 83 g) | 275 | 1½ starch, 1 vegetable, 3 fat | 430 | 14 | 52% |
| Potato, baked and topped with cheese sauce (1 potato = 296 g) | 475 | 3 starch, 1 meat, 4 fat | 381 | 19 | 55% |
| Potato, baked and topped with cheese sauce and bacon (1 potato = 299 g) | 451 | 3 starch, 1 meat, 3 fat | 973 | 30 | 52% |
| Potato, baked and topped with cheese sauce and broccoli (1 potato = 339 g) | 402 | 2½ starch, ½ meat, 3 fat, 1½ vegetable | 484 | 20 | 47% |
| Potato, baked and topped with cheese sauce and chili (1 potato = 395 g) | 481 | 3½ starch, 2 meat, 1½ fat | 701 | 31 | 41% |
| Potato, baked and topped with sour cream and chives (1 potato = 302 g) | 394 | 3 starch, 3½ fat | 182 | 23 | 50% |
| Potato, French fried, regular order (20-25 strips, 1″- 2″ length = 76 g) | 237 | 2 starch, 2 fat | 124 | 13 | 46% |
| Potato, French fried, large order (30-40 strips, 1″- 2″ length = 115 g) | 358 | 3 starch, 3 fat | 187 | 20 | 46% |
| Potato, mashed (⅓ cup = 80 g) | 66 | 1 starch | 182 | 2 | 14% |
| Potato chips (10 chips = 20 g) | 105 | ¾ starch, 1 fat | 94 | 0 | 60% |
| Potato chips (1-oz. bag) | 148 | 1 starch, 2 fat | 133 | 0 | 61% |
| Potato salad (⅓ cup = 95 g) | 108 | 1 starch, 1 fat | 312 | 57 | 50% |

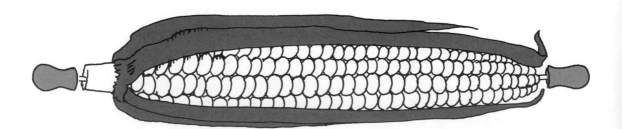

# FAST FOOD—ENTREES

| ITEM AND AMOUNT | CALORIES | EXCHANGES | SODIUM (milligrams) | CHOLESTEROL (milligrams) | FAT |
|---|---|---|---|---|---|
| Chicken, breaded and fried, dark meat (drumstick or thigh) (2 pieces = 148 g) | 430 | 1 starch, 4 meat, 1 fat | 756 | 165 | 56% |
| Chicken, breaded and fried, light meat (breast or wing) (2 pieces = 163 g) | 494 | 1 starch, 5 meat, 1 fat | 975 | 149 | 54% |
| Chicken, breaded and fried, boneless pieces, plain (6 pieces = 102 g) | 290 | 1 starch, 2 meat, 1½ fat | 542 | 62 | 56% |
| Chicken, breaded and fried, boneless with barbecue sauce (6 pieces = 130 g) | 330 | 1 starch, 2 meat, ½ fruit,* 1½ fat | 830 | 61 | 49% |
| Chicken, breaded and fried, boneless with honey (6 pieces = 115 g) | 329 | 1 starch, 2 meat, 1 fruit,* 1 fat | 537 | 61 | 49% |
| Chicken, breaded and fried, boneless with mustard sauce (6 pieces = 130 g) | 323 | 1 starch, 2 meat, ½ fruit,* 1½ fat | 791 | 62 | 50% |
| Chicken, breaded and fried, boneless with sweet-and-sour sauce (6 pieces = 130 g) | 346 | 1 starch, 2 meat, 1 fruit,* 1½ fat | 677 | 61 | 47% |
| Chili con carne (8-fl. oz. cup = 253 g) | 254 | 1½ starch, 3 lean meat | 1,008 | 133 | 28% |
| Clams, breaded and fried (¾ cup = 115 g) | 451 | 2½ starch, 1 meat, 4 fat | 833 | 87 | 52% |
| Crab, baked (1 cake = 60 g) | 88 | 2 lean meat | 303 | 101 | 10% |
| Crab, soft-shell, fried (1 crab = 125 g) | 325 | 2 starch, 1 meat, 2 fat | 1,118 | 45 | 50% |
| Crab cake (1 crab = 109 g) | 290 | ½ starch, 1 fat, 2½ meat | 893 | 149 | 59% |
| Fish fillet, battered or breaded, fried (1 fillet = 91 g) | 211 | 1 starch, 1 meat, 1 fat | 484 | 31 | 47% |
| Oysters, battered or breaded, fried (6 oysters = 139 g) | 368 | 2½ starch, 1 meat, 2 fat | 677 | 109 | 44% |
| Pizza with cheese (2 slices = ¼ of a 12″ diameter pizza = 98 g) | 218 | 2 starch, 1 lean meat | 522 | 14 | 21% |
| Pizza with cheese, meat and vegetables (2 slices = ¼ of 12″ diameter pizza = 130 g) | 304 | 2 starch, 2 meat | 630 | 34 | 24% |
| Pizza with pepperoni (2 slices = ¼ of 12″ diameter pizza = 106 g) | 270 | 2 starch, 1½ meat | 398 | 22 | 33% |

*Fruit exchange used to express hidden sugar content.

# FAST FOOD—MEXICAN FOODS

| ITEM AND AMOUNT | CALORIES | EXCHANGES | SODIUM (milligrams) | CHOLESTEROL (milligrams) | FAT |
|---|---|---|---|---|---|
| Burrito with beans (2 burritos = 217 g) | 448 | 4½ starch, 2 fat | 986 | 5 | 27% |
| Burrito with beans and cheese (2 burritos = 186 g) | 377 | 3½ starch, ½ meat, 1 fat | 1,166 | 27 | 29% |
| Burrito with beans and chili peppers (2 burritos = 204 g) | 413 | 4 starch, ½ meat, 1½ fat | 1,043 | 33 | 33% |
| Burrito with beans and meat (2 burritos = 231 g) | 508 | 4½ starch, 1 meat, 1½ fat | 1,335 | 48 | 32% |
| Burrito with beans, cheese and beef (2 burritos = 203 g) | 331 | 2½ starch, ½ meat, 1½ fat | 990 | 125 | 35% |
| Burrito with beans, cheese and chili peppers (2 burritos = 336 g) | 663 | 5½ starch, 2 meat, 1½ fat | 2,060 | 158 | 31% |
| Burrito with beef (2 burritos = 220 g) | 523 | 4 starch, 2 meat, 1½ fat | 1,492 | 65 | 36% |
| Burrito with beef and chili peppers (2 burritos = 201 g) | 426 | 3 starch, 1½ meat, 1 vegetable, 1 fat | 1,116 | 54 | 35% |
| Burrito with beef, cheese and chili peppers (2 burritos = 304 g) | 634 | 4 starch, 4 meat, 1 vegetable | 2,091 | 170 | 35% |
| Burrito with fruit, small (apple or cherry) (1 small burrito = 74 g) | 231 | 1 starch, 1½ fruit,* 1½ fat | 211 | 3 | 37% |
| Burrito with fruit, large (apple or cherry) (1 large burrito = 155 g) | 484 | 2 starch, 3 fruit,* 3½ fat | 443 | 7 | 37% |
| Chimichanga with beef (1 chimichanga = 174 g) | 425 | 2½ starch, 1½ meat, 1 vegetable, 2 fat | 910 | 9 | 42% |
| Chimichanga with beef and cheese (1 chimichanga = 183 g) | 443 | 2½ starch, 1½ meat, ½ vegetable, 2½ fat | 956 | 51 | 47% |
| Chimichanga with beef and red chili peppers (1 chimichanga = 190 g) | 424 | 3 starch, 1½ meat, 1½ fat | 1,169 | 9 | 40% |
| Chimichanga with beef, cheese and red chili peppers (1 chimichanga = 180 g) | 364 | 2½ starch, 1 meat, 2 fat | 784 | 44 | 43% |
| Enchilada with cheese (1 enchilada = 163 g) | 320 | 2 starch, ½ meat, 3 fat | 784 | 44 | 53% |
| Enchilada with cheese and beef (1 enchilada = 192 g) | 324 | 2 starch, 1 meat, 2 fat | 1,320 | 40 | 49% |
| Enchirito with cheese, beef and beans (1 enchirito = 193 g) | 344 | 2½ starch, 1½ meat, 1 fat | 1,251 | 49 | 42% |

| ITEM AND AMOUNT | CALORIES | EXCHANGES | SODIUM (milligrams) | CHOLESTEROL (milligrams) | FAT |
|---|---|---|---|---|---|
| Frijoles with cheese (8-oz. cup = 167 g) | 226 | 2 starch, ½ meat, ½ fat | 882 | 36 | 31% |
| Nachos with cheese (6-8 nachos = 113 g) | 345 | 2 starch, ½ meat, 3 fat | 816 | 18 | 50% |
| Nachos with cheese and jalapeno peppers (6-8 nachos = 204 g) | 607 | 4 starch, 1 meat, 5 fat | 1,736 | 83 | 57% |
| Nachos with cheese, beans, ground beef and peppers (6-8 nachos = 255 g) | 568 | 3½ starch, 1 meat, 1 vegetable, 4½ fat | 1,800 | 21 | 49% |
| Nachos with cinnamon and sugar (6-8 nachos = 109 g) | 592 | 4 starch, 6 fat | 439 | 39 | 55% |
| Taco, small (1 small taco = 171 g) | 370 | 2 starch, 2 meat, 1 fat | 802 | 57 | 50% |
| Taco, large (1 large taco = 263 g) | 569 | 2½ starch, 3½ meat, 2 fat | 1,234 | 87 | 51% |
| Taco salad (lettuce, tomato, chili sauce, ground beef, cheese, taco shell) (1½ cups lettuce = 198 g) | 279 | 1½ starch, 1 meat, 1½ fat, ½ vegetable, "free vegetable" | 763 | 44 | 48% |
| Taco salad with chili con carne (chili con carne, lettuce, tomato, cheese, taco shell) (1½ cups lettuce = 261 g) | 288 | 1½ starch, 2 meat, ½ vegetable, "free vegetable" | 886 | 4 | 41% |
| Tostada with beans and cheese (1 tostada = 144 g) | 223 | 1½ starch, ½ meat, 1 vegetable, 1 fat, "free vegetable" | 543 | 30 | 40% |
| Tostada with beans, beef and cheese (1 tostada = 225 g) | 334 | 2 starch, 1½ meat, 1½ fat, "free vegetable" | 870 | 75 | 46% |
| Tostada with beef and cheese (1 tostada = 163 mg) | 315 | 1½ starch, 2 meat, 1 fat, "free vegetable" | 896 | 41 | 46% |
| Tostada with guacamole (2 tostadas = 261 g) | 360 | 2 starch, 1 meat, 3 fat, "free vegetable" | 798 | 39 | 58% |

*A portion of fruit exchange used to express hidden sugar content.

# FAST FOOD—CONDIMENTS

| ITEM AND AMOUNT | CALORIES | EXCHANGES | SODIUM (milligrams) | CHOLESTEROL (milligrams) | FAT |
|---|---|---|---|---|---|
| Butter (1 packet = ½ oz.) | 100 | 2 fat | 116 | 31 | 100% |
| Half-and-half (1 packet = ½ oz.) | 18 | ⅓ fat | 6 | 5 | 80% |
| Honey (1 packet = ½ oz.) | 43 | ¾ fruit | 1 | 0 | 0 |
| Jelly (1 packet = ¾ oz.) | 58 | 1 fruit | 4 | 0 | 0 |
| Ketchup (1 packet = ¼ oz.) | 3 | free | 50 | 0 | 20% |
| Lemon (1 packet = ½ oz.) | 3 | free | 0 | 0 | 0 |
| Lettuce (2 leaves = 2 oz.) | 2 | free | 0 | 0 | 0 |
| Mayonnaise (1 packet = ⅖ oz.) | 81 | 2 fat | 64 | 6 | 100% |
| Mustard (1 packet = ⅕ oz.) | 4 | free | 45 | 0 | 0 |
| Non-dairy creamer (1 packet = ⅖ oz.) | 55 | ½ fruit,* ½ fat | 18 | 0 | 57%** |
| Onions (2 slices = ⅔ oz.) | 7 | free | 1 | 0 | 10% |
| Pickles (2 slices = ½ oz.) | 2 | free | 203 | 0 | 0 |
| Salad dressing, blue cheese (1 packet = 2½ oz.) | 342 | 1 vegetable, 7 fat | 760 | 31 | 91% |
| Salad dressing, French (1 packet = 2 oz.) | 228 | ¾ fruit,* 4 fat | 680 | 0 | 81% |
| Salad dressing, Italian (1 packet = 2 oz.) | 326 | ½ vegetable, 7 fat | 502 | 14 | 94% |
| Salad dressing, low-calorie (1 packet = 2 oz.) | 50 | 1 vegetable, ½ fat | 300 | 0 | 41% |
| Salad dressing, oriental (1 packet = 2 oz.) | 102 | 1½ fruit,* ¼ fat | 552 | 0 | 9% |
| Salad dressing, thousand island (1 packet = 2½ oz.) | 396 | ½ fruit,* 8 fat | 600 | 48 | 90% |
| Sugar (1 packet = 6 g) | 25 | ½ fruit* | 0 | 0 | 0 |
| Syrup (1 packet = 1½ oz.) | 122 | 2 fruit* | 19 | 0 | 0 |
| Tartar sauce (1 packet = ½ oz.) | 74 | 1½ fat | 182 | 4 | 99% |
| Tomato (1 slice = 1 oz.) | 5 | free | 2 | 0 | 0 |

*Fruit exchange used to express sugar content.

**All fat is saturated in nature.

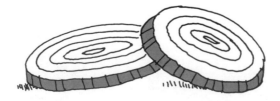

# FAST FOOD—DESSERTS

| ITEM AND AMOUNT | CALORIES | EXCHANGES | SODIUM (milligrams) | CHOLESTEROL (milligrams) | FAT |
|---|---|---|---|---|---|
| Brownie (1 brownie = 60 g) (4 t./26% sugar) | 243 | 1 starch, 1½ fruit,* 1½ fat | 153 | 9 | 38% |
| Cookies, animal crackers (1 box = 67 g) (3¾ t./20% sugar) | 299 | 1½ starch, 2 fruit,* 1½ fat | 274 | 11 | 27% |
| Cookies, chocolate chip (1 box = 55 g) (3½ t./24% sugar) | 233 | 1 starch, 1½ fruit,* 2 fat | 188 | 12 | 46% |
| Fried pie, fruit (apple, cherry or lemon) (1 pie = 85 g) (2½ t./34% sugar) | 266 | 1 starch, 1 fruit,* 2½ fat | 325 | 13 | 47% |
| Ice milk, vanilla, soft serve with cone (1 cone = 103 g) (4½ t./44% sugar) | 164 | 1½ starch, 1 fat | 92 | 28 | 33% |
| Sundae, caramel (1 sundae = 155 g) (10 t./51% sugar) | 303 | 1 starch, ½ milk, 1½ fruit,* 1½ fat | 195 | 25 | 27% |
| Sundae, hot fudge (1 sundae = 158 g) (10 t./56% sugar) | 284 | 1 starch, ¼ milk, 2 fruit, 1½ fat | 182 | 21 | 27% |
| Sundae, strawberry (1 sundae = 153 g) (10⅓ t./62% sugar) | 269 | 1 starch, ½ milk, 1 fruit, 1½ fat | 92 | 21 | 27% |

*Fruit exchange used to express sugar content.

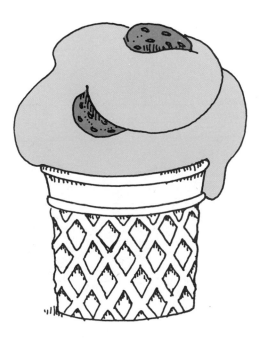

# FAST FOOD—BEVERAGES

| ITEM AND AMOUNT | CALORIES | EXCHANGES | SODIUM (milligrams) | CHOLESTEROL (milligrams) | FAT |
|---|---|---|---|---|---|
| Hot chocolate (6 fl. oz. cup = 206 g) | 103 | 1 fruit,* ½ skim milk | 149 | 0 | 9% |
| Juice, grapefruit (6 fl. oz. cup) | 78 | 1¼ fruit | 0 | 0 | 0 |
| Juice, orange (6 fl. oz. cup) | 84 | 1½ fruit | 0 | 0 | 0 |
| Juice, tomato, regular (6 fl. oz. cup) | 32 | 1 vegetable or ½ fruit | 658 | 0 | 0 |
| Lemonade (8 fl. oz. cup) (5¾ t./91% sugar) | 100 | 1½ fruit* | 8 | 0 | 0 |
| Orange drink (6 fl. oz. cup) (4¾ t./81% sugar) | 94 | 1½ fruit* | 31 | 0 | 0 |
| Shake, chocolate (10 fl. oz. cup) (9 t./41% sugar) | 360 | 3 fruit,* 1 milk, 2 fat | 273 | 37 | 26% |
| Shake, strawberry (10 fl. oz. cup) (10 t./50% sugar) | 319 | 3 fruit,* 1 milk, 1½ fat | 234 | 31 | 23% |
| Shake, vanilla (10 fl. oz. cup) (9 t./47% sugar) | 314 | 2½ fruit,* 1 milk, 1½ fat | 232 | 32 | 23% |
| Regular cola (12 oz.) | 150 | 2½ fruit | 12 | 0 | 0 |
| Other sweetened carbonated drinks (12 oz.) | 125-180 | 2-3 fruit | 10-50 | 0 | 0 |
| Diet cola (12 oz.) | 2 | free | 12 | 0 | 0 |
| Other diet carbonated drinks (12 oz.) | 2 | free | 10-50 | 0 | 0 |
| Tea, instant, sugar-sweetened, lemon-flavored, prepared with water (12 fl. oz. cup) (8¼ t./100% sugar) | 132 | 2 fruit* | 0 | 0 | 0 |

*Fruit exchange used to express sugar content.

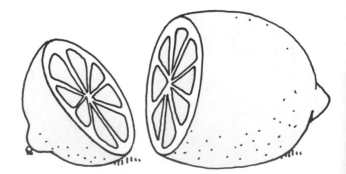

# Chapter 23: Convenience Foods

All of us use convenience foods in our daily life. This chapter will help you learn how to include them into your eating plan. Let's take a look first at some guidelines for determining which of these products would be considered healthy food.

## Fat

Most nutrition experts recommend that the diet of Americans contain less than 30% of the calories as fat. When selecting convenience foods to put into your shopping cart, do a little quick math first.

Example: Glazed Chicken Breast Frozen Dinner

| | |
|---|---|
| Servings per container | 1 |
| Calories | 270 |
| Protein | 26 g |
| Carbohydrate | 27 g |
| Fat | 6 g |

6 grams of fat x 9 (number of calories per gram of fat) = 54 fat calories

54 fat calories ÷ 270 (total calories) x 100 = 20%

This product contains less than 30% fat and thus could be recommended.

## Salt

Many of the convenience foods are also high in salt. Salt is 40% sodium. Look for the sodium content on the label and select those products that will not add up to more than 1,000 milligrams per meal.

## Other Label Information

You may find other information on the label which may be confusing to you. Some of those items are explained below.

Diet, Dietetic—These foods may be lower in sodium or calories. If it is "diet" or "dietetic" because the sodium is lower, then it might not be low calorie. If it is "diet" or "dietetic" because the calories are reduced, then it must either have no more than 40 calories per serving *or* have one-third fewer calories than the regular product. For example, ½ cup of regular ice cream has 130 calories. If it is labeled "dietetic" or "diet," it might still contain 87 calories, which is one-third fewer.

Reduced Calorie—If the food comes under FDA regulation, it must have one-third fewer calories than the regular product. If it comes under USDA regulation, it would be 25% lower in calories.

Low-Calorie—These foods cannot have more than 40 calories per serving. There is no regulation defining what a serving is, however.

Sodium-Free—Less than 5 milligrams of sodium per serving.

Very Low Sodium—No more than 35 milligrams of sodium per serving.

Low-Sodium—No more than 140 milligrams of sodium per serving.

Reduced Sodium—The sodium content of these foods is reduced by at least 75%.

Low-Salt—Foods with labeling or the terms "no added salt," "no salt," "unsalted," "salt-free," etc., may still contain large amounts of sodium. There are many different ingredients besides salt which contain sodium that are added for flavor, preservation, etc.

Low-Fat—Meats which have no more than 10% fat by weight. This also applies to milk, yogurt and cottage cheese which have between .5% and 2% fat. (Whole milk has 3.3% fat.)

Lean—Meat and poultry must have no greater than 10% fat by weight to carry this term. Extra lean meat cannot have more than 5% fat. If lean is part of the brand name, then it is not required to meet these percentages.

Light or Lite—There is no regulation for these terms. It can mean lighter in color or texture, or less sodium, fat or calories.

## Breakfast Items

Following are some of the convenience foods which are not included in the basic exchange lists.

*Cereals*—Hot and cold cereals appearing in the following list were selected because the sugar content is 6 grams or less and the fat content is below 2 grams per serving size. Please note that many new cereal products are constantly entering the market, and it is difficult to include all of them in this chapter. As a general rule select those products that are less than 100 calories per serving size and in the range of one starch exchange.

*Pancakes, Waffles, French Toast and Syrups*—Several brands of frozen items like this are convenient for breakfast. There are also mixes for those who wish to make their own. The calories and exchanges listed are average values. Buttermilk, added fruit, like blueberries, etc., add some calories to the product. Be sure to read the label

Author's Note: The author gratefully acknowledges the help of Joan Pleuss, R.D., M.S., C.D.E., in the preparation of chapter 23.

of each purchase and pay attention to serving sizes.

There are three types of syrups one can use: regular, lite and sugar-free. For weight-conscious individuals, lite and sugar-free types are preferred. Sugar-free syrups are best for consumers with diabetes.

*Egg Substitutes*—For those who are trying to lower their blood cholesterol, egg substitutes that are made from egg whites are a good alternative. Only those products that have less than 55 calories per ¼ cup are recommended. Those of higher calorie content usually contain some fat and are considered medium-fat meat substitutes.

*Other Breakfast Items*—Many breads and bakery goods that can be worked into weight-reduction diets are included in the starch/bread exchange lists in chapter 14. At this point it is a good idea for the reader to review the lists of foods to avoid in chapter 13 as well. Many convenience foods that should not be considered for breakfast are discussed there.

There are many quick-and-easy convenience foods for breakfast. They include instant liquid breakfasts and many types of toaster-heated pastries. These also should be excluded because of their relatively high sugar content. Liquid breakfasts also are low in food fiber.

## CEREALS

| PRODUCT | BRAND | SERVING SIZE | CALORIES | EXCHANGES |
| --- | --- | --- | --- | --- |
| 100% Bran with Oat Bran | Nabisco | ½ cup | 80 | 1 starch |
| All Bran Extra Fiber | Kellogg | ⅓ cup | 70 | 1 starch |
| All Bran | Kellogg | ⅓ cup | 70 | 1 starch |
| Alpha Bits, unsweetened | Post | ¾ cup | 80 | 1 starch |
| Apple Cinnamon Squares | Kellogg | ½ cup | 90 | 1 starch |
| Benefit | General Mills | ¾ cup | 90 | 1 starch |
| Bran Chex | Ralston | ½ cup | 70 | 1 starch |
| Bran Flakes | Kellogg | ½ cup | 70 | 1 starch |
| Cheerios | General Mills | 1 cup | 90 | 1 starch |
| Corn Chex | Ralston | ¾ cup | 80 | 1 starch |
| Corn Flakes | Kellogg | ¾ cup | 80 | 1 starch |
| Cream of Rice | Nabisco | ½ cup | 80 | 1 starch |
| Cream of Wheat | Nabisco | ½ cup | 80 | 1 starch |
| Cream of Wheat, quick | Nabisco | ½ cup | 80 | 1 starch |
| Crispix | Kellogg | ¾ cup | 85 | 1 starch |
| Crispy Critters | Post | ¾ cup | 80 | 1 starch |
| Crunchy Bran, plain | Quaker | ½ cup | 75 | 1 starch |
| Double Chex | Ralston | ¾ cup | 80 | 1 starch |
| Fiber One | General Mills | ½ cup | 60 | 1 starch |
| Frosted Mini-Wheats | Kellogg | 3 biscuits | 80 | 1 starch |
| Fruit & Fibre Tropical Fruit | Post | ⅓ cup | 70 | 1 starch |
| Fruit & Fibre Wheat & Bran | Post | ⅓ cup | 70 | 1 starch |
| Fruit & Fibre Date, Raisin, Nut | Post | ⅓ cup | 90 | 1 starch |
| Fruit Wheats | Nabisco | ½ cup | 80 | 1 starch |
| Grape Nuts | Post | 3 T. | 80 | 1 starch |
| Heartwise | Kellogg | 1 cup | 90 | 1 starch |
| Honey Bunches of Oats | Post | ½ cup | 85 | 1 starch |

| PRODUCT | BRAND | SERVING SIZE | CALORIES | EXCHANGES |
|---|---|---|---|---|
| Instant Cream of Wheat | Nabisco | ½ cup | 80 | 1 starch |
| Instant Grits | Quaker | ½ cup | 80 | 1 starch |
| Instant Oatmeal, regular flavor | Quaker | 1 pkg. | 90 | 1 starch |
| Just Right Nuggets & Flakes | Kellogg | ½ cup | 75 | 1 starch |
| Kix | General Mills | 1 cup | 70 | 1 starch |
| Life Cinnamon | Quaker | ½ cup | 90 | 1 starch |
| Life | Quaker | ½ cup | 90 | 1 starch |
| Malto-Meal Tasty O's | Malto Meal | 1 cup | 90 | 1 starch |
| Malto-Meal | Malto Meal | ½ cup | 80 | 1 starch |
| Malto-Meal, with cocoa | Malto Meal | ½ cup | 80 | 1 starch |
| Natural Bran Flakes | Post | ½ cup | 65 | 1 starch |
| Nutri-Grain | Kellogg | ½ cup | 70 | 1 starch |
| Oat Bran High Oat Fiber RTE (biscuits) | Quaker | ½ cup | 65 | 1 starch |
| Oat Ban | Quaker | ⅓ cup raw | 90 | 1 starch |
| Oat Flakes | Post | ½ cup | 80 | 1 starch |
| Oat Squares | Quaker | ⅓ cup | 65 | 1 starch |
| Product 19 | Kellogg | ¾ cup | 65 | 1 starch |
| Puffed Rice | Quaker | 1¼ cup | 70 | 1 starch |
| Puffed Wheat | Quaker | 1¼ cup | 70 | 1 starch |
| Purina | Pillsbury | ⅔ cup cooked | 80 | 1 starch |
| Quaker Oats Oatmeal | Quaker | ⅓ cup uncooked | 100 | 1 starch |
| Raisin Squares | Kellogg | ½ cup | 90 | 1 starch |
| Regular Grits | Quaker | ½ cup cooked | 75 | 1 starch |
| Rice Chex | Ralston | ¾ cup | 75 | 1 starch |
| Rice Krispies | Kellogg | ¾ cup | 85 | 1 starch |
| Shredded Wheat | Nabisco | 1 biscuit | 85 | 1 starch |
| Shredded Wheat and Bran | Nabisco | ¾ cup | 80 | 1 starch |
| Shredded Wheat, spoon size | Nabisco | ¾ cup | 80 | 1 starch |
| Special K | Kellogg | 1 cup | 85 | 1 starch |
| Strawberry Squares | Kellogg | ½ cup | 90 | 1 starch |
| Team Flakes | Nabisco | ¾ cup | 85 | 1 starch |
| Total | General Mills | ¾ cup | 75 | 1 starch |
| Total Oatmeal, regular | General Mills | ½ cup | 80 | 1 starch |
| Wheat Chex | Ralston | ½ cup | 75 | 1 starch |
| Wheaties | General Mills | ¾ cup | 75 | 1 starch |

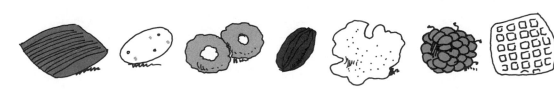

# OTHER BREAKFAST FOODS

| PRODUCT | SERVING SIZE | CALORIES | EXCHANGES |
|---|---|---|---|
| **Pancakes, Waffles and French Toast:** | | | |
| Pancakes, frozen | 3 (4″) | 260 | 3 starch, ½ fat |
| Waffles, frozen | 1 waffle | 85 | 1 starch |
| Pancake and waffle mixes (prepared) | 2 (4″) | 170 | 2 starch, 1 fat |
| French toast | 2 slices | 170 | 2 starch, 1 fat |
| **Syrup:** | | | |
| Regular | 2 T. | 100 | 2 fruit |
| Lite | 2 T. | 60 | 1 fruit |
| Sugar-free | 2 T. | 20 | free |
| **Egg Substitutes:** | | | |
| Plain | ¼ cup | 25 | ½ lean meat |

**Bakery Goods** (See starch/bread exchange lists in chapter 14.)

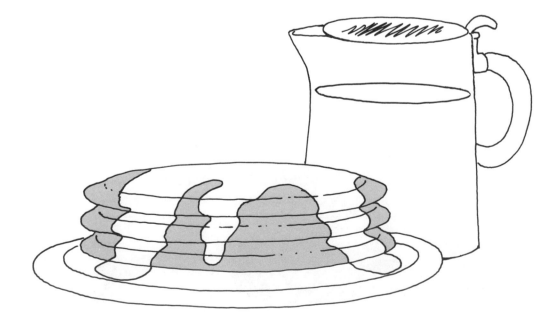

## Microwave and Frozen Entrees

Here are some guidelines when selecting frozen entrees. If you can answer yes to the following questions, then go ahead and purchase the item.

(1) Can this entree be eaten alone (does it provide the meat, starch and vegetable?), or if not, can other foods be added without the meal becoming high calorie?
(2) Does it provide 300 calories or less?
(3) Does it have less than 10 grams of fat?

The entree will also be healthier for you if it has less than 1,000 milligrams of sodium.

Below are listed the calories and exchange values for some of the brands of lower calorie frozen entrees on the market. These are the average values for the brands listed. On reading the labels, you may find that the calories and exchange values are slightly different. Use them if you need to be more exact in your diet.

Remember, these values are for only those entrees which have 300 calories or less and which have less than 10 grams of fat. Be sure to check the label, because some of the varieties packaged by these companies do not fit these criteria. It is emphasized that several other brands that are similar in composition to those listed below may be available in your area. These are examples to guide you in your purchases.

### Pizza

Pizza is a cherished food for most individuals. Unfortunately it is a calorie-dense food with a high fat content. It should not be eaten frequently by anyone on weight-reduction meal plans. Occasional consumption in small amounts should be the rule. It is recommended that vegetarian styles are selected whenever possible. Pizzas without added sausage, pepperoni or other meats are also lower in calories and fat.

Brands that indicate on their labels that each serving size contains no more than 10 grams of fat (two fat exchanges) are preferred. Examples of pizza that meet this restriction are listed below. Again, this is not a comprehensive list but will help TOPS members with their selections for occasional use.

## MICROWAVE AND FROZEN ENTREES

| ENTREE | CALORIES | EXCHANGES |
|---|---|---|
| Armour Dinner Classics Lite | 270 | 2 starch, 2 lean meat |
| Budget Gourmet Slim Selects | 275 | 2 starch, 2 lean meat |
| Con Agra Healthy Choice Dinners | 275 | 2 starch, 1 vegetable, 2 lean meat |
| Le Menu Light Style | 250 | 2 starch, 2 lean meat |
| Stouffer's Lean Cuisine | 260 | 1½ starch, 2½ lean meat |
| Stouffer's Right Choice | 285 | 2 starch, 1 vegetable, 2 lean meat |

## PIZZA

| PRODUCT | SERVING SIZE | CALORIES | EXCHANGES |
|---|---|---|---|
| Celeste | ½ small | 290 | 2 starch, 2 fat, 1 meat |
| Totino's Party | ½ pizza | 323 | 2 starch, 1 vegetable, 1 meat, 2 fat |
| Totino's Pan | ⅙ pizza | 320 | 2 starch, 1 vegetable, 1 meat, 2 fat |
| Totino's Mexican Classic Deluxe | ⅙ pizza | 245 | 1½ starch, 1 meat, 1 fat |
| Totino's Temptin' Toppings | ¼ pizza | 210 | 1 starch, 1 vegetable, ½ meat, 2 fat |
| Totino's Microwave | 1 small | 290 | 2 starch, 2 fat, ½ meat |
| Pillsbury Microwave | ½ pizza | 285 | 2 starch, 2 fat, 1 meat |
| Jeno's Crisp 'N Tasty | ½ pizza | 280 | 2 starch, 2 fat, 1 meat |
| Fox Deluxe | ½ pizza | 250 | 2 starch, 1 fat, ½ meat |
| John's | ½ pizza | 250 | 2 starch, 1 fat, ½ meat |

## Soups

TOPS members often wish to include soup in their meal planning. The exchange lists in chapter 14 are not very detailed in this area. For this reason, a list of commonly purchased soups is included in this section. However, there are so many different brands sold in food stores that not all can be included here. The list is limited to one company's products. If there are soups produced by other companies that are of interest to individuals, seek information from the food label. If this is not sufficient, either contact the company directly or call a registered dietitian in your local hospital or clinic.

Certain types of soup were not included in the list because they contained two or more fat exchanges per serving. As you read through the various kinds of soups, also note the differences in calories in each serving. Individuals who are on lower caloric intakes may prefer the simple condensed soups, because many are below 100 calories for each serving.

# SOUPS

| PRODUCT | SERVING SIZE | CALORIES | EXCHANGES |
|---|---|---|---|
| All soups listed below are the Campbell's brand. | | | |
| **Chunky Style:** | | | |
| Chunky Beef | 1 can (10¾ oz.) | 190 | 1½ starch, 1 meat |
| Chunky Chicken Noodle with Mushrooms | 1 can (10¾ oz.) | 200 | 1 starch, 1 vegetable, 1 lean meat, 1 fat |
| Chunky Old Fashioned Bean 'n Ham | 1 can (11 oz.) | 290 | 2½ starch, 1 meat, ½ fat |
| Chunky Old Fashioned Chicken | 1 can (10¾ oz.) | 170 | 1½ starch, 1 lean meat |
| Chunky Old Fashioned Vegetable Beef | 1 can (10¾ oz.) | 180 | 1 starch, 1 vegetable, 1 meat |
| Chunky Sirloin Burger | 1 can (10¾ oz.) | 220 | 1½ starch, 1 meat, ½ fat |
| Chunky Split Pea with Ham | 1 can (10¾ oz.) | 230 | 2 starch, 1 meat |
| Chunky Chicken Rice | ½ can (9½ oz.) | 140 | 1 starch, 1 meat |
| Chunky Chicken Vegetable | ½ can (9½ oz.) | 170 | 1 starch, 1 vegetable, 1 meat |
| Chunky Chili Beef | ½ can (9¾ oz.) | 260 | 2 starch, 2 lean meat |
| Chunky Clam Chowder (Manhattan style) | ½ can (9½ oz.) | 150 | 1½ starch, ½ fat |
| Chunky Mediterranean Vegetable | ½ can (9½ oz.) | 160 | 1½ starch, 1 fat |
| Chunky Minestrone | ½ can (9½ oz.) | 140 | 1 starch, 1 vegetable, 1 fat |
| Chunky Steak 'n Potato | ½ can (9½ oz.) | 170 | 1½ starch, 1 meat |
| Chunky Turkey Vegetable | ½ can (9⅜ oz.) | 150 | 1 starch, 1 lean meat, ½ fat |
| Chunky Vegetable | ½ can (9½ oz.) | 130 | 1 starch, 1 vegetable, ½ fat |

| PRODUCT | SERVING SIZE | CALORIES | EXCHANGES |
|---|---|---|---|
| **Condensed (as prepared):** | | | |
| Asparagus Cream | 1 cup | 90 | 1 starch, ½ fat |
| Bean with Bacon | 1 cup | 150 | 1½ starch, 1 fat |
| Beef | 1 cup | 80 | 1 starch |
| Beef Noodle | 1 cup | 70 | ½ starch, ½ fat |
| Celery, Cream of | 1 cup | 100 | ½ starch, 1 fat |
| Cheddar Cheese | 1 cup | 130 | ½ starch, 1½ fat |
| Chicken Noodle | 1 cup | 70 | ½ starch, ½ fat |
| Chicken Vegetable | 1 cup | 70 | ½ starch, ½ fat |
| Chili Beef | 1 cup | 130 | 1 starch, 1 fat |
| Clam Chowder, New England (with water) | 1 cup | 80 | 1 starch, ½ fat |
| Green Pea | 1 cup | 160 | 1½ starch, ½ lean meat |
| Minestrone | 1 cup | 80 | 1 starch |
| Mushroom, Cream of | 1 cup | 100 | ½ starch, 1 fat |
| Mushroom, Golden | 1 cup | 80 | 1 starch |
| Oyster Stew (with water) | 1 cup | 80 | ½ starch, 1 fat |
| Potato, Cream of | 1 cup | 70 | ½ starch, ½ fat |
| Split Pea with Ham and Bacon | 1 cup | 160 | 1½ starch, ½ fat |
| Tomato (with water) | 1 cup | 90 | 1 starch |
| Vegetable | 1 cup | 80 | 1 starch |
| Vegetable, Old Fashioned | 1 cup | 60 | 2 vegetable |
| Vegetarian Vegetable | 1 cup | 80 | 1 starch |
| Won Ton | 1 cup | 40 | ½ starch |
| **Semi-Condensed for One (as prepared):** | | | |
| Bean with Ham, Old Fashioned | 11 oz. | 220 | 2 starch, 1 fat |
| Burly Vegetable Beef and Bacon | 11 oz. | 160 | 1 starch, 1 vegetable, 1 fat |
| Clam Chowder, New England (with water) | 11 oz. | 130 | 1 starch, ½ meat |
| Chicken Vegetable, Full Flavored | 11 oz. | 120 | 1 starch, 1 fat |
| Golden Chicken and Noodles | 11 oz. | 120 | 1 starch, ½ meat |
| Tomato Royale | 11 oz. | 180 | 2 starch, 1 vegetable |

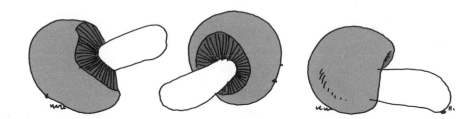

## Frozen Desserts

This chapter has more detailed exchange lists for primarily frozen desserts. Other kinds of desserts can be found at the conclusion of the starch/bread list in chapter 14. Some desserts also are discussed in sections of chapter 22.

*Ice Cream*—All ice creams are high in fat. From the examples given below you will see that your calories will go further if you substitute ice milk or frozen yogurt. Also, the more chocolate, nuts, candy or cake pieces in the ice cream, the higher the calories. For example, the 270 calories listed for Baskin Robbins Deluxe is an average for all their flavors. Very Berry Strawberry is 220 calories for a regular scoop and Rocky Road contains 300 calories, while the international creams are 310.

*Ice Milk*—All brands in ½-cup portions are 125 calories and the equivalent of one starch and one fat exchange.

*Sherbet*—All brands in ½-cup portions are 140 calories and two starch exchanges.

*Dietetic Ice Cream Products*—Several manufacturers have introduced reduced-calorie ice creams that are sweetened with products like Nutrasweet. This will eliminate calories due to added sugar but will not reduce calories that are present as milk carbohydrate, protein or fat.

In the near future ice cream-like desserts will be made with sugar-free fat substitutes. Simplesse, which has the consistency of fat, is actually a protein (see chapter 21). Such products will cut calories from fat by over 50%, and by substituting Nutrasweet for sugar, calories per serving will be even lower. Watch for these new dietetic foods.

*Frozen Yogurt*—Values in the following list are for all flavors. Remember, these values do not include any of the "extras" available at the yogurt shops.

Note: Some frozen yogurts are available in a sugar-free form. This will lower calories per serving. All frozen yogurts, because of their low-fat content, provide an excellent alternative to higher calorie ice creams and frozen custards.

### Frozen Desserts on a Stick and Frozen Bars

Some of the lowest calorie frozen treats are found among these products. Many new types are entering the market to attract people with weight problems. Many are 60 calories or less and are especially useful to individuals on more restricted diets in the range of 1,200 calories.

## ICE CREAM AND YOGURT

| PRODUCT | CALORIES | EXCHANGES |
|---|---|---|
| **Ice Cream** | | |
| Baskin Robbins Deluxe (1 regular scoop) | 270 | 2 starch, 3 fat |
| Baskin Robbins Fat-Free (½ cup) | 100 | 1 fruit, ½ skim milk |
| Baskin Robbins Sugar-Free (½ cup) | 90 | 1 starch |
| Baskin Robbins Light (½ cup) | 130 | 1 starch, 1 fat |
| Ben and Jerry's (½ cup) | 295 | 1½ starch, 3 fat |
| Breyer's (½ cup) | 155 | 1 starch, 2 fat |
| Hagen-Daz (½ cup) | 265 | 1½ starch, 3 fat |
| Sealtest (½ cup) | 150 | 1 starch, 1½ fat |
| Simple Pleasure (½ cup) | 130 | 1 starch, 1 fat |
| **Yogurt** | | |
| Baskin Robbins (½ cup) | 110 | 1½ starch |
| Columbo Lite (½ cup) | 95 | 1 starch |
| Dannon (⅓ cup) | 70 | 1 starch |
| Elan Premium (⅓ cup) | 85 | 1 starch |
| Honey Hill Non-Fat (½ cup) | 80 | 1 starch |
| McDonalds (½ cup) | 90 | 1 starch |
| TCBY (⅓ cup) | 85 | 1 starch |
| Yoplait (⅓ cup) | 85 | 1 starch |

# FROZEN DESSERTS ON A STICK AND FROZEN BARS

| PRODUCT | CALORIES | EXCHANGES |
|---|---|---|
| **Frozen Desserts on a Stick** | | |
| Crystal Light Bar | 14 | free |
| Crystal Light Cool 'N Creamy Frozen Bavarian Bars (orange/vanilla) | 30 | ½ fruit |
| Crystal Light Cool 'N Creamy Frozen Bavarian Bars | 50 | ½ starch |
| Carnation Creamy Lites Frozen Snack Bars | 50 | ½ starch |
| Dannon Frozen Yogurt on a Stick | 50 | ½ starch |
| Dole Fruit and Cream Bar | 90 | 1½ fruit |
| Dole Fruit and Juice Bar | 70 | 1 fruit |
| Dole Fruit 'N Yogurt | 70 | 1 fruit |
| Eskimo Pie Sugar Free | 140 | 1 starch, 2 fat |
| Fudgesicle Fudge Pops Sugar Free | 35 | ½ starch |
| Jello Fruit and Cream Bar | 60 | 1 starch |
| Jello Gelatin Pop | 35 | ½ fruit |
| Jello Pudding Pop | 80 | 1 starch |
| Knudsen Pushups Lowfat Frozen Yogurt | 90 | 1 starch |
| Popsicle Ice Pops Sugar Free | 18 | free |
| Shamitoff's Fruit and Cream Bars | 85 | 1 starch |
| Shamitoff's Natural Fruit Bar | 60 | 1 fruit |
| Welch's Fruit Juice Bar | 45 | 1 fruit |
| Yoplait Soft Frozen Yogurt | 90 | 1 starch |
| **Frozen Bars** | | |
| Dole Fresh Lites | 25 | ½ fruit |
| Dole Fruit and Cream with Chocolate | 160 | 1½ fruit, 2 fat |
| Dole Fruit and Yogurt | 75 | 1 fruit |
| Dole Sun Tops | 40 | ½ fruit |
| Hagen-Daz Ice Cream Bars | 380 | 2 starch, 5 fat |

## Summary

If there is a convenience food that is not included in this chapter or in chapter 14 or chapter 22, you have several alternatives to convert the label to exchanges. You may attempt to calculate it yourself based on food label information (see chapter 19). You may call or write to the company directly to obtain the information, or you may call a registered dietitian in your area for help.

Exchange conversions are also available in books containing analyses of many convenience foods.[1]

# MISCELLANEOUS FOODS

| RECOMMENDED FOOD | CALORIES | EXCHANGES |
|---|---|---|
| Hot cocoa (1 pkg.) | 40 | ½ skim milk |
| Pie crust (⅛ of 2-crust pie) | 375 | 2 starch, 3 fat |
| Regular pudding (½ cup) | 205 | 2 starch, 1 fat |
| Regular pie filling (fruit) (½ cup) | 120 | 2 fruit |
| Dips (2 T.) | 45 | 1 fat |
| Onion rings (2½ oz.) | 195 | 1 starch, 2 fat, 1 vegetable |
| Pasta side dishes (½ cup) | 250 | 2 starch, 2 fat |
| Potato dishes (½ cup) (flavored, dehydrated, frozen) | 125 | 1 starch, 1 fat |
| Rice dishes (½ cup) | 160 | 2 starch |
| Graham cracker crumbs (½ cup) | 285 | 3 starch, 1 fat |
| Soda cracker crumbs (½ cup) | 240 | 3 starch |
| Cornflake crumbs (⅓ cup) | 120 | 1½ starch |
| Bisquick mix (½ cup) | 245 | 2½ starch, 1 fat |

[1]A. Monk and M. Franz, *Convenience Food Facts: Help for the Healthy Meal Planner*, 2nd ed., 1987 (Wellness and Nutrition Library, Diabetes Center, Inc., P.O. Box 739, Wayazata MN).

# Chapter 24: Recipes

Everyone has favorite recipes. Chapter 19 taught you how to convert them to food exchanges, calculate calories and work them into your meal plan. The purpose of this chapter is not to list a large number of additional recipes. Space doesn't permit this. Instead, it provides the reader with a limited number of various types that have been field-tested by a TOPS chapter for ease in preparation and taste appeal. After this was done, one of our dietetic consultants determined their calorie level, exchange equivalents and content of cholesterol and minerals. This team effort resulted in elimination of some recipes that appeared in the first edition of this monograph and the addition of others.

The primary purpose of this chapter is to show the weight-conscious person ways to prepare many favorite foods that are nutritious and reasonably restricted in calories. They should give the reader some ideas about other recipes they might create with similar goals in mind. We hope you enjoy them.

## CHARCOAL TREATS

### OUTDOOR BURGERS

1 lb. lean ground round
¼ cup chopped onion
2 T. finely chopped green pepper
3 T. ketchup
1 T. prepared horseradish
1 t. prepared mustard
Dash of pepper

Combine all ingredients and mix lightly. Shape into four patties about ½″ thick. Broil over hot coals 5 to 8 minutes; turn and broil 3 to 5 minutes or until well cooked. *4 servings. Serving size: 1 patty.*

EXCHANGES: 3 medium-fat meat

CALORIES: 251

73 mg cholesterol
2 mg iron
217 mg sodium

### GRILLED POTATOES

For each serving desired, scrub a 3-oz. baking potato. Wrap in a piece of foil, overlapping ends. Bake 45 to 60 minutes on grill or on top of coals. Turn occasionally. Potato will be pierced easily by a fork when done. Remove foil and serve. Try a butter substitute or herb shake for flavoring. *1 serving. Serving size: one 3-oz. potato.*

EXCHANGES: 1 starch

CALORIES: 93

0 mg cholesterol
1 mg iron
7 mg sodium

### GRILLED TOMATOES

For each serving, select one large ripe tomato. Remove stem; cut in half. Brush each half with ¾ t. low-calorie Italian salad dressing. Add a dash of white pepper with a half pinch of dried basil, if desired, to each half. Place each half, cut side up, on foil pan over hot coals for about 10 minutes or until heated through. Do not invert. Serve hot. *1 serving. Serving size: 2 halves.*

EXCHANGES: 1 vegetable

CALORIES: 25

.5 mg cholesterol
.4 mg iron
66 mg sodium

Author's Note: TOPS #WI 1139, Wauwatosa, (Jacqueline Marks, leader) worked with Mary Hoettels, R.D., M.S., to field test and analyze the recipes in chapter 24. Their efforts are acknowledged and very much appreciated.

# BREAKFAST IDEAS

## FRENCH TOAST

¼ cup egg substitute
2 T. skim milk

2 slices regular or 4 slices lite bread

Beat egg until thick and add milk. Dip bread in egg-milk mixture and brown on nonstick pan. *2 servings. Serving size: 1 slice regular or 2 slices lite bread.*

*EXCHANGES: 1 starch*
*½ lean meat*

*CALORIES: 106*

*.5 mg cholesterol*
*1.2 mg iron*
*250 mg sodium*

## PANCAKES

1 cup flour
2 t. baking powder
Egg substitute equal to 1 egg or 2 egg
   whites

1 cup skim milk
1 T. margarine, melted

Mix and sift dry ingredients into a bowl. Beat egg; add milk. Pour egg-milk mixture slowly into dry ingredients. Beat thoroughly; add melted margarine. Drop spoonfuls on a hot nonstick griddle. When pancakes are puffed and full of bubbles, turn and cook on other side. Serve with sugarless pancake syrup. *7 large or 14 small pancakes. Serving size: 1 large or 2 small pancakes.*

*EXCHANGES: 1 starch*

*CALORIES: 93*

*0 mg cholesterol*
*.15 mg iron*
*118 mg sodium*

## SUGARLESS PANCAKE SYRUP

1 T. cornstarch
2 T. cold water
1 cup boiling water
2 t. butter substitute

¼ t. vanilla
¾ t. maple flavoring
Sugar substitute equal to ½ cup sugar

Blend cornstarch with cold water. Add boiling water and boil for 5 minutes, stirring constantly until smooth. Remove from heat and add butter substitute, vanilla, maple flavoring and sugar substitute. Store in refrigerator. Warm before serving.

*EXCHANGES: Up to 6 T. of syrup is free.*

*CALORIES: 3 per T.*

*0 mg cholesterol*
*0 mg iron*
*trace sodium*

## SANTA FE SCRAMBLED EGGS

2 large eggs plus 4 egg whites
¼ t. parsley flakes
¼ t. oregano
¼ t. salt (optional)
⅛ t. black pepper

¼ cup chopped green pepper
2 green onions, chopped
1 small tomato, chopped
¼ cup shredded mozzarella cheese

In medium bowl blend eggs and spices. Stir in green pepper, onions and tomato. Microwave on high for 3½ to 4 minutes or until soft-set, stirring two or three times during cooking. Stir in mozzarella cheese; cover. Let stand 1 minute or until cheese melts. Serve immediately. *4 servings. Serving size: ¼ of recipe.*

*EXCHANGES: 1 high-fat meat*

*CALORIES: 102*

*146 mg cholesterol*
*.8 mg iron*
*299 mg sodium*

# ENTREES AND CASSEROLES

### BARB'S SPANISH RICE

1 cup uncooked rice
2 T. corn or canola oil
2 1-lb. cans stewed tomatoes

1 medium onion, diced
1 small to medium green pepper, diced
1 pkg. taco seasoning mix

In 2- to 3-qt. saucepan saute rice in oil for 2 to 5 minutes over medium heat until light brown. Add 1 cup water to sauteed rice. Then add tomatoes, onion, green pepper and taco seasoning. Simmer until rice is tender (about 30 to 45 minutes). If a softer rice is desired, add more water and continue cooking until desired consistency is reached. Note: If a sharper taste is desired, add cayenne pepper. To reduce sodium content, substitute chili powder and cumin to taste for taco seasoning. *8 servings. Serving size: ½ cup.*

EXCHANGES: *1½ starch*
*1 vegetable*
*½ fat*

CALORIES: *162*

*0 mg cholesterol*
*1.4 mg iron*
*735 mg sodium (65 mg when chili powder and cumin only used)*

### CHEESY PITA SALAD SANDWICHES

1 medium tomato, coarsely chopped
½ cup sliced cucumber
½ cup alfalfa sprouts
¼ cup chopped sweet red pepper
¼ cup chopped green pepper
¼ cup chopped celery

⅛ t. coarsely ground pepper
¼ cup low-calorie Italian salad dressing
½ cup (2 oz.) shredded Swiss cheese
2 (6") whole wheat pita bread
rounds, cut in half crosswise

Combine first eight ingredients in medium bowl; toss well. Set aside. Divide Swiss cheese evenly into pocket bread halves. Cover with paper towels and microwave on high for 15 to 30 seconds or until cheese melts. Open sandwiches and stuff with equal amounts of vegetable mixture. Serve immediately. *4 servings. Serving size: ½ pita pocket.*

EXCHANGES: *1 starch*
*½ lean meat*
*1 vegetable*
*½ fat*

CALORIES: *158*

*13 mg cholesterol*
*.57 mg iron*
*270 mg sodium*

### FIRST CLASS HASH

¾ lb. lean ground round
12 oz. frozen potatoes O'Brien

¼ cup beef broth

Brown meat in pan, using no fat. Remove meat from pan and add potatoes and broth to pan. Cook according to directions on package of potatoes. Add meat to potatoes and heat until hot. Serve with slice of tomato or serving of egg substitute. *4 servings. Serving size: approx. 1 cup.*

EXCHANGES: *1 starch*
*2 medium-fat meat*

CALORIES: *238*

*56 mg cholesterol*
*2.2 mg iron*
*77 mg sodium*

## CHICKEN CACCIATORE

2 medium whole chicken breasts, boned,
   skinned, halved (2 lbs. raw breast meat)
¾ cup sliced fresh mushrooms
1 14½-oz. can tomatoes, cut up, drained
½ cup chopped green pepper
¼ cup chopped onion
½ cup chopped celery (optional)

3 T. dry red wine
1 clove garlic, minced
½ t. dried leaf oregano
¼ t. dried leaf thyme
Dash of pepper
2 t. cornstarch
2 T. cold water

Place chicken in 1½-qt. micro-proof utility dish or an 8″ square dish. In medium bowl, combine mushrooms, tomatoes, green pepper, onion, celery (if using), wine, garlic, oregano, thyme, salt and pepper. Pour over chicken. Cover with vented plastic wrap. Microwave on high for 14 to 17 minutes or until chicken is cooked through. Remove chicken to serving plate. Cover; keep warm. Combine cornstarch and water. Add to liquid in utility dish. Microwave on high for 1½ to 3½ minutes or until mixture is thickened and bubbling, stirring one to two times. Serve sauce over chicken. *8 servings. Serving size: 3 oz. meat plus ½ cup vegetable mixture.*

EXCHANGES: 3 lean meat
                         1 vegetable

CALORIES: 167

72 mg cholesterol
1.5 mg iron
368 mg sodium

## CHICKEN CHOP SUEY

1 large whole chicken breast, skinned
¾ cup uncooked white rice
½ cup celery, thinly cut slantwise

½ cup finely chopped onion
2 T. lite soy sauce
Dash of white pepper

Steam chicken breast until done, reserving cooking liquid. Remove meat and cut into cubes. Cooked chicken should weigh 8 oz. Add water to broth to make 2 cups. Add uncooked rice, celery and onion to broth-water mixture. Add pepper to taste. Bring to a boil; turn heat to low; cover and simmer about 20 minutes or until rice is tender. Add cooked chicken, soy sauce and dash of white pepper if desired. *4 servings. Serving size: ¼ of recipe.*

EXCHANGES: 2 starch
                         2 lean meat

CALORIES: 240

48 mg cholesterol
1 mg iron
569 mg sodium

## CHICKEN CASSEROLE

1 10½-oz. can cream of chicken soup
½ cup skim milk
½ cup cooked carrots
½ cup cooked string beans
1½ cups cooked noodles

8 oz. cooked diced chicken breast
1 T. minced onion
¼ t. pepper or to taste
½ cup bread crumbs

Blend soup and milk in casserole dish. Mix remaining ingredients, except crumbs, together with blended soup mixture. Top with crumbs. Bake at 400° for 25 minutes. *4 servings. Serving size: ¼ of recipe.*

EXCHANGES: 3 low-fat meat
                         2 starch

CALORIES: 310

74 mg cholesterol
1.9 mg iron
655 mg sodium

## SWEDISH MEAT BALLS WITH ONION SAUCE

1 lb. lean ground round
1 T. fresh parsley
2 egg whites or ¼ cup egg substitute
¼ t. Worcestershire sauce
1 T. olive or canola oil

2 medium onions, peeled and sliced
(about 1 cup)
¼ lb. fresh mushrooms, sliced
1 cup regular or salt-free beef broth

Mix together meat, parsley, egg whites or substitute, and Worcestershire sauce. Divide mixture into 12 equal portions and shape each into a ball. In nonstick skillet or using nonstick spray on a pan, brown the meatballs on medium heat. Remove meatballs from skillet and place on white paper towels to drain. Remove excess fat from pan. Return meatballs to skillet; add onions, mushrooms and broth. Cover and simmer until vegetables are tender and meatballs are cooked through. *4 servings. Serving size: 3 meatballs plus ¼ cup of sauce.*

EXCHANGES: *3 medium-fat meat*
*1 vegetable*
*1 fat*

CALORIES: *266*

*74 mg cholesterol*
*2.7 mg iron*
*436 mg sodium (regular broth)*
*112 mg sodium (salt-free
broth)*

## SCALLOPED POTATOES AND HAM

1 10½-oz. can cream of celery soup
½ cup skim milk
Generous dash of pepper
3 cups thinly sliced potatoes

3 cups diced cooked ham
½ cup thinly sliced onion
Generous dash of paprika

Combine soup, milk and pepper. In 1½-qt. casserole arrange alternate layers of potatoes, meat, onion and soup mixture. Cover and bake at 375° for 1 hour. Uncover and sprinkle with paprika. Bake 15 minutes longer or until potatoes are tender. *6 servings. Serving size: approx. 1 cup.*

EXCHANGES: *1 starch*
*2 lean meat*
*1 vegetable*

CALORIES: *218*

*43 mg cholesterol*
*1.6 mg iron*
*1,243 mg sodium*

## SPINACH-MUSHROOM QUICHE IN RICE CRUST

1½ cups cooked brown rice
1 cup shredded low-salt, low-fat Swiss
cheese, divided
¾ cup egg substitute, divided
¼ T. curry powder
1 pkg. (10 oz.) frozen chopped spinach,
cooked, drained

1 cup evaporated skim milk, undiluted
½ cup sliced fresh mushrooms
2 T. chopped onion
¼ t. garlic powder
⅛ t. pepper

In small mixing bowl, combine rice, ½ cup cheese, ¼ cup egg substitute and curry powder. Press into bottom and sides of 9″ or 10″ glass pie plate. Microwave on high for 4 to 5 minutes or until firm. In medium mixing bowl combine remaining ingredients. Pour into cooked crust. Microwave on medium (50%) for 20 minutes or until knife inserted in center comes out clean. *6 servings. Serving size: ⅙ of pie.*

EXCHANGES: *1 starch*
*1 lean meat*
*½ milk*

CALORIES: *163*

*7 mg cholesterol*
*1.85 mg iron*
*565 mg sodium*

## BEEF TACOS

1 lb. lean ground round
1 t. taco seasoning
10 taco shells
2 cups shredded lettuce

1 large tomato, diced
1 medium onion, chopped
Taco sauce

Brown meat in a nonstick skillet or in microwave. Place meat in paper towel-lined colander and press out remaining fat with back of spoon. Use a pie plate underneath colander to catch fat. Place meat in bowl and add taco seasoning; mix well. Place taco shells in 250° oven for 5 minutes or microwave according to directions. Fill each heated shell with 2 T. meat mixture. Top with some shredded lettuce, diced tomato and onion. Serve immediately. Use taco sauce as desired. *5 servings. Serving size: 2 tacos.*

EXCHANGES: *1 starch*
*2 meat*
*½ vegetable*
*2 fat*

*59 mg cholesterol*
*2.4 mg iron*
*216 mg sodium*

CALORIES: *316*

Variation: Substitute 1 lb. ground turkey meat for beef. Follow above directions.

EXCHANGES: *1 starch*
*2 meat*
*½ vegetable*
*1 fat*

*47 mg cholesterol*
*2 mg iron*
*208 mg sodium*

CALORIES: *237*

## CHILI CON CARNE

1½ cups dry red or kidney beans
1 large onion, sliced
1 green pepper, chopped
1 lb. lean ground round
4 cups (2 1-lb. cans) canned tomatoes

1 T. chili powder (to taste)
1 bay leaf
Dash of paprika
Dash of cayenne powder

Rinse beans and add to 1½ qts. cold water. Let stand overnight. Drain. Cover and simmer until tender (about 1 hour). Drain, reserving bean liquid. Brown onion, green pepper and meat in a little hot fat. Drain off excess fat. Add beans, tomatoes, chili powder, bay leaf, dash of paprika and cayenne. Cover and simmer for 1½ hours, adding reserved bean liquid or water if needed. *6 servings. Serving size: ⅙ of recipe.*

Variation: To save cooking time, use two 1-lb. cans red or kidney beans (4 cups) instead of dry beans. Drain beans and add to meat mixture with tomatoes.

EXCHANGES: *2 starch*
*2 meat*
*2 vegetable*
*1 fat*

*49 mg cholesterol*
*6 mg iron*
*421 mg sodium*

CALORIES: *365*

Variation: Substitute ground turkey for beef. Follow directions above.

EXCHANGES: *2 starch*
*1½ lean meat*
*1½ vegetable*

*39 mg cholesterol*
*6 mg iron*
*325 mg sodium*

CALORIES: *292*

## EASY SAUERBRATEN

2 lbs. beef arm chuck steak
Freshly ground black pepper
1 cup water
1 cup cider vinegar

1 medium onion, sliced (about 1 cup)
2 bay leaves
16 gingersnaps, finely ground

Season steak with pepper. Place in nonstick Dutch oven and roast uncovered at 475°
until both sides are browned (about 5 minutes on each side), turning once. Remove from
oven and pour vinegar and water over steak. Arrange onion slices on top. Add bay leaves
to the liquid. Cover and return to oven, reducing heat to 350°. Cook 1½ to 2 hours or
until tender. Add gingersnap crumbs; replace cover and cook ½ hour longer. Additional
water may be added to thin gravy. Remove meat from gravy; slice thin. Weigh out meat.
Serve with red cabbage and applesauce. *9 servings. Serving size: 3 oz. cooked.*

EXCHANGES: 3 medium-fat meat

CALORIES: 254

76 mg cholesterol
3.4 mg iron
109 mg sodium

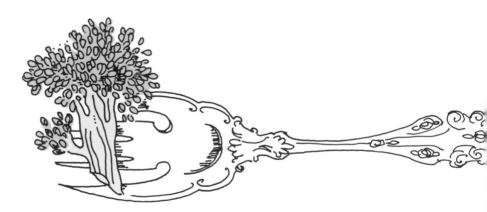

# *APPETIZERS*

Fresh raw vegetables make excellent appetizers. These are some suggestions. Serve these
vegetables with a low-calorie dip or the Chili Sauce Dip recipe listed.

Asparagus spears
Broccoli florets
Green onions
Carrot strips
Celery sticks
Turnip wedges
Green pepper sticks

Cauliflower florets
Radish roses
Kohlrabi wedges
Cucumber slices
Cherry tomatoes
Green beans
Zucchini

# TEMPTING SALADS AND SOUPS

## CRUNCHY WALDORF SALAD

2 cups diced red delicious apples
1 cup seedless grapes
1 t. lemon juice
¼ cup chopped walnuts

½ cup plain nonfat yogurt or ½ cup
    sugar-free pineapple yogurt
4 lettuce cups
4 thin lemon slices

Gently combine all ingredients except lettuce and lemon slices. Chill until serving time. Spoon 1 cup of salad mixture into each lettuce cup. Garnish with lemon slice. *4 servings. Serving size: 1 cup.*

EXCHANGES:  1 fruit
              1 fat

CALORIES: 121

.5 mg cholesterol
0 mg iron
51 mg sodium

## TOMATO-ONION SALAD

1 clove garlic, minced
Sugar substitute equal to 2 t. sugar
½ cup low-calorie Italian salad dressing

½ t. chopped parsley
6 tomatoes, wedged (3 cups)
1 onion, thinly sliced (½ cup)

Combine garlic and sugar substitute in small bowl. To salad dressing add parsley. Pour over tomatoes and onions. Chill. This salad can be made and placed in thermos container and taken to any picnic. *6 servings. Serving size: ½ cup.*

EXCHANGES:  1 vegetable

CALORIES: 22

0 mg cholesterol
.29 mg iron
4 mg sodium

## FOUR FRUIT SALAD

½ of a half water-packed peach
½ of 1 ring of water-packed pineapple
½ of a half of water-packed pear

3 water-packed cherries
½ cup cottage cheese

Arrange fruit on crisp salad greens and top with cottage cheese. *1 serving.*

EXCHANGES:  1 fruit
              2 lean meat

CALORIES: 160

9 mg cholesterol
.97 mg iron
464 mg sodium

## MEAL IN A SALAD BOWL

½ cup cooked green beans
¼ cup diced celery
½ cup raw Chinese cabbage
½ cup diced cooked carrots

1 oz. cooked lean ham, cut in strips
1 oz. part skim mozzarella cheese
¼ cup herb vinegar

Combine ingredients except vinegar and chill thoroughly for 1 to 2 hours. Just before serving add herb vinegar and serve immediately on bed of lettuce. Garnish with radish rose. *1 serving.*

EXCHANGES:  2 lean meat
              2 vegetable

CALORIES: 165

31 mg cholesterol
1.96 mg iron
580 mg sodium

## PICNIC POTATO SALAD

12 small (1-oz.) potatoes, boiled and
  chilled
¼ cup finely chopped onion
¼ cup chopped celery

Pepper to taste
¼ cup low-calorie mayonnaise or
  nonfat yogurt

Dice potatoes and mix other ingredients. Chill before serving. *4 servings. Serving size:*
*¼ of recipe.*

With mayonnaise:
EXCHANGES: 1 starch
          ½ fat

CALORIES: 102

*12 mg cholesterol*
*5 mg iron*
*43 mg sodium*

With yogurt:
EXCHANGES: 1 starch

CALORIES: 78

*.26 mg cholesterol*
*5 mg iron*
*29 mg sodium*

## SAUERKRAUT SALAD

Liquid sugar substitute equal to 1 cup
  sugar
½ cup vinegar
1 16-oz. can sauerkraut
1 green pepper, finely chopped

1 onion, finely chopped
1 stalk celery, finely chopped
1 pimento, finely chopped
1 16-oz. can bean sprouts

Combine sugar substitute and vinegar. Pour over rest of ingredients. Chill at least overnight. Will keep a week or longer and be delicious. *10 servings. Serving size: ½ cup.*

EXCHANGES: 1 vegetable

CALORIES: 25

*0 mg cholesterol*
*1.1 mg iron*
*358 mg sodium*

## QUICK VEGETABLE-BEEF SOUP

½ lb. ground chuck
¼ cup chopped green pepper
¼ cup chopped onion
1 14½-oz. can stewed tomatoes,
  undrained

1 cup frozen mixed vegetables
1 cup water
¼ t. dried whole basil
⅛ t. garlic powder
½ t. freshly ground pepper

Combine meat, green pepper and onion in 2-qt. casserole. Cover with heavy-duty plastic
wrap and microwave on high for 4 minutes or until meat is no longer pink, stirring after
2 minutes. Drain well in a colander, and pat dry with paper towels. Wipe casserole dry
with a paper towel. Return drained meat mixture to casserole. Add remaining ingredients
to meat mixture. Cover and microwave on high for 9 to 10 minutes, stirring every 3 minutes.
Ladle into individual serving bowls. Serve hot. *4 servings. Serving size: 1 cup.*

EXCHANGES: 1½ medium-fat meat
          1 starch

CALORIES: 190

*38 mg cholesterol*
*2.3 mg iron*
*313 mg sodium*

# STARCH/BREAD GROUP

## CRUSTY HERB BUNS

2 pkg. active dry quick-rise yeast
3 cups all-purpose flour
1 t. onion powder
1 t. celery seed
½ t. garlic powder
½ t. oregano

1 t. salt
1 egg, beaten
1 cup skim milk
2 T. olive or corn oil
1 egg white beaten with 1 t. water

Combine yeast, 1½ cups flour, herbs and salt. Heat milk until 120 to 130°. Add milk with the oil to dry ingredients; beat for 2 minutes. Add beaten egg and 1 cup flour; beat for 2 minutes until soft dough is formed. Knead, using remaining ½ cup flour until smooth and satiny (8 to 10 minutes). Cover with plastic wrap and let rise in warm place until doubled in bulk (about 45 to 60 minutes). Punch down; divide dough into 24 pieces and shape into balls. Place on nonstick cookie sheet. Let rise 30 minutes. Brush each bun with egg white-water mixture. Bake at 375° for 20 to 25 minutes or until golden brown. *24 servings. Serving size: 1 bun.*

EXCHANGES: 1 starch

CALORIES: 73

12 mg cholesterol
.8 mg iron
103 mg sodium

## OVEN-BAKED POTATO STRIPS

1 3-oz. raw potato
1 t. corn or olive oil

1 t. Parmesan cheese

Scrub potato; cut lengthwise into strips about ½ " inch thick. Pat strips dry with paper towel. Toss strips with oil in bowl. Spread strips in a single layer on a cookie sheet and bake for 30 to 35 minutes at 450°. Turn strips every 5 to 6 minutes during cooking process to allow for even browning. Toss with Parmesan cheese. *1 serving. Serving size: one 3-oz. potato.*

EXCHANGES: 1 starch
            1 fat

CALORIES: 141

1.3 mg cholesterol
1.1 mg iron
38 mg sodium

## PINEAPPLE BREAD

2 cups sifted all-purpose flour
1 t. baking soda
Sugar substitute equal to ½ cup
  sugar
2 egg whites or ¼ cup egg substitute

2 T. corn or canola oil
1 t. vanilla
1 cup crushed pineapple packed in its
  own juice (Do not drain)
1 cup raisins

Sift flour with baking soda and sugar substitute into mixing bowl. Combine egg, oil and vanilla; add to dry ingredients along with pineapple, stirring just until ingredients are moistened. Fold in raisins. Spread evenly in 8½ x 4½ " loaf pan sprayed with nonstick spray. Bake at 350° for 45 minutes or until loaf tests done. Cool 10 minutes in pan; remove to rack to finish cooling. Store overnight in refrigerator. Cut into 16 ½ " thick slices. *16 servings. Serving size: ½ " slice.*

EXCHANGES: 1 starch
            1 fruit

CALORIES: 130

0 mg cholesterol
.8 mg iron
59 mg sodium

## STUFFED BAKED POTATO

4 small (3-oz.) potatoes, skins on
¼ t. white pepper
1 t. grated onion

¾ to 1 t. butter-flavored substitute
1 egg white, beaten stiff
Paprika

Scrub potatoes; pierce skins with fork. Bake at 400 to 425° until tender, or microwave on high according to manufacturer's directions until tender. Remove when done. Slice thin top from each potato, lengthwise. Remove potato from skins, leaving ¼ " thick shell. Mash potato, adding pepper, onion and butter substitute. Fold in egg white. Pile potato mixture evenly back into potato shells. Sprinkle with paprika. Return to oven or microwave to reheat to serving temperature. *4 servings. Serving size: one 3-oz. potato.*

EXCHANGES: 1 starch

CALORIES: 99

0 mg cholesterol
1.3 mg iron
19-35 mg sodium

# DESSERTS AND COOKIES

## BAKED GRAPEFRUIT

2 grapefruit
8 t. low-sugar strawberry spread

4 whole fresh strawberries (optional)

Cut grapefruit in half. Loosen each section. Top halves with strawberry spread. Microwave on high for 4 to 6 minutes or until grapefruit are very hot, rotating after half the time. Top each half with strawberry in center. *4 servings. Serving size: ½ grapefruit with topping.*

EXCHANGES: 1 fruit

CALORIES: 56

0 mg cholesterol
118 mg iron
15 mg sodium

## CARROT BRAN MUFFINS

1 cup 40% bran flakes
¾ cup skim milk
2 cups finely shredded carrot
1 cup whole wheat flour
2 T. brown sugar
2 T. vegetable oil

1 T. lemon juice
1 t. baking powder
½ t. baking soda
¼ to ½ t. cinnamon
1 whole egg or 2 egg whites, slightly beaten

Combine bran, milk and carrot; let stand 5 minutes. Add remaining ingredients, stirring until particles are moistened. Line each muffin or custard cup with two paper liners; fill half full. Microwave on high as directed below or until top springs back when touched, rotating and rearranging after half the time.

1 muffin . . . . . . . . . . . . . . . . ¼ to ¾ minute
2 muffins . . . . . . . . . . . . . . . ½ to 2 minutes
4 muffins . . . . . . . . . . . . . . 1 to 2½ minutes
6 muffins . . . . . . . . . . . . . . 2 to 4½ minutes

*12 servings. Serving size: 1 muffin.*

EXCHANGES: 1 starch

CALORIES: 76

20 mg cholesterol with whole egg (trace cholesterol with egg whites)
1.2 mg iron
87 mg sodium

## CREAM PUFFS

½ cup water
1 T. shortening
½ t. salt

½ cup cake flour
2 eggs

Combine water, shortening and salt. Bring to a boil. Reduce to low heat and add flour. Beat until mixture forms a smooth, compact ball and cleans sides of pan. Remove from heat and beat in eggs thoroughly, one at a time. Beat mixture until smooth and velvety. Drop by spoonfuls onto ungreased cookie sheet. Bake at 375° for about 40 minutes or until golden brown and almost dry. Serve with whipped topping made from nonfat dry milk and flavored with vanilla. *6 servings. Serving size: 1 cream puff.*

EXCHANGES: ½ starch
                    1 fat

CALORIES: 94

91 mg cholesterol
.4 mg iron
207 mg sodium

## SUNSHINE CAKE

1 cup sifted cake flour
1½ t. baking powder
¼ cup cooking oil
1 egg yolk and 2 egg whites
½ cup unsweetened frozen orange
    juice concentrate

⅓ cup fructose
4 egg whites
¼ t. cream of tartar

Sift flour and baking powder together into a bowl. Make a well in center of dry ingredients and add, in order, cooking oil, unbeaten egg yolk, 2 egg whites, orange juice concentrate and fructose. Beat until smooth. Add cream of tartar to egg whites and beat until stiff. Add egg yolk mixture to beaten egg whites and gently fold in until blended. Do not over-mix. Pour into 9″ tube pan. Bake at 325° for 35 minutes. Serve plain, with fruit sauce or as shortcake with fresh fruit. *10 servings. Serving size: ¹/₁₀ of cake.*

EXCHANGES: 1 starch
                    1 fat

CALORIES: 132

27 mg cholesterol
.17 mg iron
76 mg sodium

## CHOCOLATE CHIP COOKIES

⅓ cup softened margarine
½ cup granulated sugar substitute
    equal to ¾ cup sugar
2 T. water
1 t. vanilla

Egg substitute equal to 1 egg
1 cup plus 2 T. flour
½ t. baking soda
½ cup finely chopped nuts
½ cup miniature chocolate chips

Cream margarine. Mix in sugar substitute, water and vanilla. Add egg substitute to mixture. Sift dry ingredients; stir into mixture. Mix in chocolate chips and nuts. Drop on cookie sheet sprayed with nonstick spray and bake at 375° for 10 to 12 minutes. *4 dozen cookies. Serving size: 2 cookies.*

EXCHANGES: ½ starch
                    1 fat

CALORIES: 84

0 mg cholesterol
.26 mg iron
55 mg sodium

## LEMON FLUFF

¼ cup cornstarch
1½ cups water
Sugar substitute equal to ½ cup sugar
⅓ cup unsweetened lemon juice

2 eggs, separated
1 t. grated lemon rind
1 3-oz. pkg. Neufchatel cheese

In 1½-qt. saucepan combine cornstarch, water, sugar substitute and lemon juice. Cook over medium heat, stirring constantly, until mixture boils. Boil 1 minute. Stir about ½ cup of hot mixture into egg yolks; add to hot mixture in saucepan. Cook and stir until mixture is thick. Remove from heat. Blend in cheese and lemon rind. Cool slightly. Beat egg whites until stiff. Blend in lemon mixture on low speed of mixer. Spoon into six parfait glasses. Chill until firm. Garnish with twists of lemon peel. *6 servings. Serving size:* ⅙ *of recipe.*

EXCHANGES: ½ starch
½ meat
½ fat

102 mg cholesterol
14 mg iron
80 mg sodium

CALORIES: 86

## LEMON CAKE-CUSTARD

3 eggs, separated
¼ t. salt
Sugar substitute equal to 2 T. sugar
⅓ cup lemon juice

2 T. butter or margarine, melted
1½ cups skim milk
5 T. flour

Beat egg whites until soft peaks form. Add salt and sugar substitute. Beat egg yolks slightly and add lemon juice, melted butter and milk. Add egg yolk mixture to flour slowly; then beat until smooth. Fold in egg whites. Pour into greased 1-qt. casserole. Set casserole in pan of warm water. Bake at 350° for 1 hour and 10 minutes. *8 servings. Serving size:* ⅛ *of custard.*

EXCHANGES: ½ starch
1 fat

CALORIES: 90

103 mg cholesterol
145 mg iron
153 mg sodium

## MAPLE MERINGUE ORANGE CUPS

2 large navel oranges
2 T. reduced-calorie maple syrup, divided
2 egg whites

⅛ t. cream of tartar
⅛ t. ground nutmeg
Orange rind strips

Cut oranges in half crosswise. Clip membranes and remove pulp, being careful not to puncture bottom. Coarsely chop pulp; mix with 1 T. maple syrup. Spoon pulp mixture into orange cups. Place in microwave-safe 8″ cake dish. Microwave, uncovered, on high for 2 to 2½ minutes. Beat egg whites (at room temperature) and cream of tartar until foamy. Gradually add remaining syrup, beating until stiff peaks form. Spread meringue over top of each shell; seal edges. Microwave, uncovered, on high for 1 to 1½ minutes or until meringue is set. Sprinkle with nutmeg. Garnish with orange rind strips. *4 servings. Serving size: 1 orange cup.*

EXCHANGES: 1 fruit

CALORIES: 52

0 mg cholesterol
.1 mg iron
7 mg sodium

## MICROWAVE PEAR CRUNCH

2 t. slivered almonds
3 medium ripe pears, chopped
2 t. lemon juice
¼ t. almond extract

1 T. all-purpose flour
1 T. firmly packed dark brown sugar
1 T. margarine
2 T. regular oats, uncooked

Place almonds in a custard cup. Cover with heavy-duty plastic wrap and microwave on high for 1 to 1½ minutes or until almonds are toasted; set aside. Combine pears, lemon juice and almond extract in a medium bowl, tossing well. Divide among four 6-oz. custard cups or individual baking dishes; set aside. Combine flour and sugar; cut in margarine with a pastry blender until mixture resembles coarse meal. Stir in oats and reserved almonds. Divide among custard cups. Microwave on high for 6 minutes or until pears are tender, rotating cups after 3 minutes. *4 servings. Serving size: 1 custard cup.*

EXCHANGES: *1½ fruit*
*1 fat*

CALORIES: *139*

*0 mg cholesterol*
*.6 mg iron*
*36 mg sodium*

## PERFECT BREAD PUDDING

2¼ cups milk
1 slightly beaten egg plus 2 egg whites
2 cups day-old bread cubes
½ cup granulated sugar substitute
    equal to ½ cup brown sugar

½ t. cinnamon
1 t. vanilla
½ cup seedless raisins

Combine milk and eggs; pour over bread cubes. Stir in remaining ingredients. Pour mixture into 8″ round baking dish. Place in shallow pan on oven rack; pour hot water around it 1″ deep. Bake at 350° for about 45 minutes or until knife inserted halfway between center and outside comes out clean. *8 servings. Serving size: ⅛ of pudding.*

EXCHANGES: *1 starch*
*1 fruit*
*½ skim milk*

CALORIES: *176*

*70 mg cholesterol*
*1.2 mg iron*
*180 mg sodium*

## STRAWBERRY LAYER DESSERT

1½ cups sliced fresh or sugar-free
    frozen strawberries
1 envelope low-calorie strawberry gelatin
1½ cups hot water

1 cup low-calorie nondairy whipped
    topping
1 10″ tube angel food cake (1 lb.)

Slice strawberries; set aside. Dissolve gelatin in hot water. Chill until partially set. Beat mixture until light and fluffy. Fold in nondairy whipped topping. Chill until of spreading consistency. Transfer 1½ cups of mixture to small bowl; fold in strawberries. Split cake crosswise, making three equal layers. Fill between layers with strawberry mixture. Frost top and sides of cake with remaining whipped topping mixture. Chill until serving time. Garnish with fresh strawberries. *16 servings. Serving size: ¹⁄₁₆ of cake.*

EXCHANGES: *1 starch*
*½ fruit*

CALORIES: *112*

*0 mg cholesterol*
*33 mg iron*
*101 mg sodium*

## PUMPKIN PIE

**Pie Shell:**

1⅓ cups all-purpose flour
¼ t. salt

¼ cup corn or canola oil
3 to 4 T. ice water

Combine flour and salt. Stir in oil and add water until a ball can be formed. Roll between two sheets of lightly flour waxed paper. Fit into 9″ pie plate.

**Filling:**

Sugar substitute equal to ¾ cup sugar
  (white or brown)
⅔ cup instant nonfat dry milk solids
1¼ cups water
1 15-oz. can (1¾ cups) canned pumpkin

Egg substitute equal to 3 whole eggs
1¼ t. cinnamon
½ t. nutmeg
¼ t. allspice
⅛ t. cloves

Combine all ingredients by hand or in a food processor until well blended. Pour into pie shell. Bake at 400° for 15 minutes; reduce heat to 350° and bake an additional 35 to 45 minutes or until knife inserted midway between center and edge comes out clean. Cool. *8 servings. Serving size: ⅛ of pie.*

*EXCHANGES: 1 starch*
          *½ milk*
          *1½ fat*

*1.2 mg cholesterol*
*1.4 mg iron*
*135 mg sodium*

*CALORIES: 188*

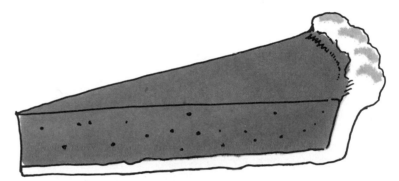

## REFRIGERATOR COOKIES

1½ cups sifted flour
1½ t. baking powder
½ cup corn oil margarine

⅓ cup creamed cottage cheese
Sugar substitute equal to 3 T. sugar
1½ t. lemon extract

Sift flour with baking powder. Cream margarine in mixing bowl. Add remaining ingredients. Beat well. Blend in sifted dry ingredients gradually. Place on waxed paper and shape into a roll 9″ long. Wrap in waxed paper. Chill at least 2 hours. Cut into ¼″ slices; place on greased cookie sheets. Bake at 350° for 12 to 15 minutes until lightly browned. *3 dozen cookies. Serving size: 2 cookies.*

*EXCHANGES: ½ starch*
          *1 fat*

*.3 mg cholesterol*
*0 mg iron*
*49 mg sodium*

*CALORIES: 92*

## PEANUT CRUNCHIES

Cream ⅓ cup crunchy peanut butter with margarine in recipe for Refrigerator Cookies. Omit 3 T. sugar. Use sugar substitute equal to ⅓ cup. *3 dozen cookies. Serving size: 2 cookies.*

*EXCHANGES: ½ starch*
          *1½ fat*

*.3 mg cholesterol*
*.14 mg iron*
*108 mg sodium*

*CALORIES: 116*

## CHERRY PUFF

1 No. 2 can (2½ cups) unsweetened
   pitted tart red cherries, drained
½ cup liquid from cherries
Sugar substitute equal to ½ cup sugar
2 T. quick-cooking tapioca
2 egg whites

Dash of salt
¼ t. cream of tartar
2 egg yolks
⅓ cup granulated sugar substitute
   equal to ⅓ cup sugar
⅓ cup sifted cake flour

Chop cherries; add cherry liquid, sugar substitute and tapioca. Simmer mixture 5 minutes, stirring constantly. Beat egg whites until foamy; add salt and cream of tartar. Beat stiff. Beat egg yolks until thick and lemon-colored; add granulated sugar substitute gradually. Beat thoroughly. Fold egg yolks into whites. Sift flour over, folding in. Pour cherry mixture into 8 x 8 x 2″ baking dish sprayed with nonstick spray. Pour batter on top. Bake at 325° for 30 to 35 minutes. Serve warm. You may garnish with 2 T. nondairy whipped topping, which is free. *6 servings. Serving size: ⅙ of recipe.*

EXCHANGES: ½ meat
               1 fruit

CALORIES: 93

90 mg cholesterol
1.8 mg iron
34 mg sodium

## CHERRY COBBLER

1 1-lb. can (2 cups) water-packed cherries
¾ t. cornstarch
1 t. lemon juice
⅛ t. almond flavoring
Sugar substitute equal to 1 T. sugar
½ cup sifted cake flour

¾ t. baking powder
1 T. margarine or butter
½ egg (or about 2 T. blended)
2 T. skim milk
Sugar substitute equal to 2 T. sugar

Drain cherries, reserving ⅔ cup juice. Place drained cherries in 8″ pie pan or shallow cake pan. Combine juice drained from cherries, cornstarch, lemon juice and almond flavoring in saucepan. Heat until slightly thickened. Pour over cherries. Mix together dry ingredients. Cut in butter until mixture is almost granular. Add milk and sugar substitute to egg. Stir into dry ingredients. Drop onto cherries, making four biscuits. Bake at 425° for about 25 to 30 minutes. Serve warm. *4 servings. Serving size: 1 biscuit and ½ cup sauce.*

EXCHANGES: ½ starch
               1 fruit
               ½ fat

CALORIES: 130

34 mg cholesterol
1.8 mg iron
102 mg sodium

## JOYCE'S GRANOLA

4 cups oatmeal
⅓ cup coconut
2 T. raisins
¼ cup wheat germ

¼ cup walnuts or sunflower seeds
¼ cup honey
¼ cup oil
1 t. vanilla

Combine all ingredients. Microwave on high for 5 to 7 minutes, stirring every 1½ to 2 minutes. *Yield: About 6 cups. 18 servings. Serving size: ⅓ cup.*

EXCHANGES: 1 starch
               1 fat

CALORIES: 134

0 mg cholesterol
.8 mg iron
6 mg sodium

# SAUCES AND TOPPINGS

## BARBECUE SAUCE

2 T. chopped onion
½ cup ketchup
¼ cup water
2 T. lemon juice
1 T. vinegar

¾ t. prepared mustard
Sugar substitute equal to 2 T. sugar
Dash of pepper
1½ T. Worcestershire sauce
½ t. liquid smoke (optional)

Combine all ingredients in small saucepan and simmer 20 minutes or microwave on high for 4 to 5 minutes. Store unused sauce in refrigerator. Use rather sparingly on chicken, hamburger or pot roast. *Yield: 1 cup.*

EXCHANGES: Up to 2 T. is free

CALORIES: 23 per 2 T.

0 mg cholesterol
.3 mg iron
216 mg sodium

## CHERRY SAUCE

1 1-lb. can sour pie cherries
2 T. cornstarch
1 t. grated orange rind
½ cup unsweetened orange juice

Sugar substitute equal to 1 T. sugar
1 stick cinnamon
5 whole cloves
⅛ t. red food coloring (optional)

Drain cherries, reserving liquid. Blend liquid with remaining ingredients. Cook mixture over medium heat, stirring constantly until thick. Stir in cherries. *8 servings. Serving size: ¼ cup.*

Serving suggestions: Serve over angel food cake, frozen vanilla yogurt or sugar-free pudding.

EXCHANGES: 1 fruit

CALORIES: 70

0 mg cholesterol
.9 mg iron
5 mg sodium

## WHIPPED TOPPING

½ cup instant nonfat dry milk
½ cup ice water

1 to 2 T. unsweetened lemon juice
Sugar substitute equal to 2 T. sugar

Combine ingredients in small mixing bowl. Beat with mixer at high speed until stiff peaks form, scraping sides of bowl often. Serve immediately. Use as topping for desserts, cakes or salads. *3 to 4 servings. Serving size: 1 cup.*

EXCHANGES: Up to ¼ cup is free. ½ cup equals ½ fruit exchange.

CALORIES: 17 per 4 T.

0 mg cholesterol
0 mg iron
16 mg sodium

## CHILI SAUCE DIP

1 12-oz. bottle of chili sauce
2 T. horseradish
3 to 4 drops Tabasco sauce

2 T. lemon juice
¼ cup finely chopped celery
1 T. minced parsley

Combine ingredients. Chill and serve with crisp raw vegetables. *Yield: 1½ cups.*

EXCHANGES: Up to 2 T. is free.

CALORIES: 8 per T.

0 mg cholesterol
.39 mg iron
24 mg sodium

# BEVERAGES

### COCOA MIX

⅓ cup nonfat dry milk
2½ to 3 t. powdered unsweetened
    cocoa

1 to 2 packets granulated artificial
    sweetener

Mix ingredients thoroughly. For camping or traveling, seal in a plastic bag. Add ¾ cup hot or cold water to dry mix, which is approximately 6 T. *1 serving. Serving size: 1 cup.*

*EXCHANGES: 1 skim milk*

*CALORIES: 98*

*4 mg cholesterol*
*.6 mg iron*
*125 mg sodium*

Note: 1 serving also provides 289 mg calcium.

### MULLED CRANBERRY DRINK

2 cups low-calorie cranberry juice
    cocktail
½ cup unsweetened grapefruit juice
Sugar substitute equal to ⅓ cup sugar

1½ cups water
¼ t. cinnamon
¼ t. cloves
⅛ t. allspice

Combine ingredients in saucepan. Heat to boiling. Pour into mugs. *Yield: 1 quart. 4 servings. Serving size: 1 cup.*

*EXCHANGES: ½ fruit*

*CALORIES: 37*

*4 mg cholesterol*
*.16 mg iron*
*47 mg sodium*

### LOW-CALORIE PUNCH

2 cups low-calorie cranberry juice
½ cup grapefruit juice

½ cup orange juice
1 16-oz. bottle of sugar-free white soda

Mix all ingredients together and add ice. *12 servings. Serving size: 1 cup.*

*EXCHANGES: 1 fruit*

*CALORIES: 70*

*0 mg cholesterol*
*.16 mg iron*
*28 mg sodium*

### TOMATO COCKTAIL

2½ cups tomato juice
1 t. celery powder
2 t. unsweetened lemon juice
Sugar substitute equal to 2 t. sugar

⅛ t. onion powder
⅛ t. Worcestershire sauce
1 bay leaf
Dash of cayenne

Combine ingredients. Let stand 15 minutes. Remove bay leaf. Chill. *4 servings. Serving size: ⅔ cup.*

*EXCHANGES: 1 vegetable*

*CALORIES: 29*

*0 mg cholesterol*
*1.1 mg iron*
*563 mg sodium*

# Chapter 25: Alcoholic Beverages

Counting calories in alcoholic beverages is necessary and should always be included in the total exchanges of any meal plan when they are consumed. As a general rule, weight-conscious individuals should keep alcohol intake to a minimum.

Alcohol calories are usually counted as fat exchanges. Carbohydrate ingredients in addition to alcohol are expressed as starch/bread or fruit exchange equivalents. The term "proof" refers to the relative alcohol content of distilled liquors, such as gin, rum, vodka, bourbon, brandy, whiskey and cognac. Lower proof liquors have lower alcohol content and calories.

Alcoholic beverages have a wide range of calories depending on the type of drink and the brand of ingredient. For this reason the calories and exchange values of the various types of beverages shown in table 19 are estimations that are suitable for daily meal planning. The table is by no means complete. Only some of the more common drinks are included.

## Some Suggestions on How To Hold Alcohol Calories Down

*Time your consumption.* Alcoholic beverages tend to stimulate appetite. When in a restaurant, it is best to order your meal first and have a drink with the meal. This cuts down on the time available for cocktails. In a similar way, social hours before banquets and other parties may lead to more drinking than planned. In this situation learn to sip your drink slowly. Have more ice added when it is half finished. Another way to limit yourself is to arrive at the social hour closer to dinner time. Learn to say "no" if the number of beverages brought to you is excessive for your needs.

*Select your cocktail sensibly.* For those of you who want to socialize without alcohol, there are several ways to do it without anyone knowing. There are many low-calorie or no-calorie beverages that can be dressed with ice and a twist of lemon or lime that resemble an alcohol drink. These include diet sodas, mineral water, club soda, seltzer and even plain water. Others may choose low-calorie beverages such as tomato juice on the rocks. If extra fruit exchanges can be worked into the social setting on your meal plan, fruit juices on ice may be selected.

Calories in individual cocktails containing alcohol also can be controlled. Avoid mixed drinks that are prepared with a great deal of sugar. This can be done by using the low-calorie or no-calorie mixers described above as the main ingredient with a limited amount of distilled liquor. If beer is drunk, order the "light" or "extra light" variety.

## Allowances for Alcoholic Beverages in Your Meal Plan

It is best to plan ahead if an alcoholic beverage is going to be drunk between, before or with meals. Select the type of drink in advance and determine how many fat, starch/bread or fruit exchanges are contained in one serving (see table 19). Serving size is important. The exchange lists in the table are for beverages with volumes between 1 and 12 ounces. Know how to estimate the number of ounces that apply to a specific drink. Once the exchanges have been determined, they are subtracted from the meal plan. It is best to make the subtraction from the meal that is associated with it or closest to it in time. This will highlight the need to account for the calories in the beverage and is less likely to be forgotten or ignored.

Those of you who are following weight-reduction diets in the range of 1,200 to 1,500 calories per day (see chapter 15) have very little leeway for alcoholic beverages. Lunch and supper plans have a total of only one to two fat exchanges, two fruit exchanges and two to three starch/bread exchanges for the two meals. One 12-ounce serving of regular beer would use up one starch/bread and two fat exchanges. Two 4-ounce servings of wine cooler are equivalent to one fruit and two fat exchanges. In other words, there is little left for regular food because of the relatively high-calorie content of alcoholic beverages. Higher calorie meal plans can accommodate alcohol-containing drinks to some extent. However, it is still at the expense of regular food that has better nutritive value than the empty calories of these beverages. For these reasons, regular consumption of alcoholic drinks is discouraged if weight loss is to be achieved without sacrificing good nutrition.

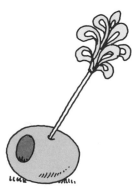

## TABLE 19: CALORIE CONTENT AND FOOD EXCHANGES IN COMMON ALCOHOL-CONTAINING BEVERAGES

| BEVERAGE | CALORIES | EXCHANGES |
|---|---|---|
| Beer | | |
|     Regular, 12 fl. oz. | 150 | 1 starch, 2 fat |
|     Light beer, 12 fl. oz. | 90-100 | 2 fat |
|     Extra light beer, 12 fl. oz. | 70 | 1½ fat |
|     Near beer, 12 fl. oz. | 40-65 | 1 fruit |
| | | |
| Table Wine | | |
|     Red or rose, 4 fl. oz. | 85 | 2 fat |
|     Dry wine, 4 fl. oz. | 80-91 | 2 fat |
|     Sweet wine, 4 fl. oz. | 102 | ⅓ fruit, 2 fat |
|     Light wine, 4 fl. oz. | 53 (avg.) | 1 fat |
|     Wine cooler, 4 fl. oz. | 61 | ½ fruit, 1 fat |
| | | |
| Dessert Wine | | |
|     Sherry, 2 fl. oz. | 84 | 2 fat |
|     Sherry, sweet, 2 fl. oz. | 95 | 2 fat |
|     Port, muscatel, 2 fl. oz. | 95 (avg. of 2) | ½ starch, 1½ fat |
| | | |
| Champagne, domestic, 4 fl. oz. | 84 | 2 fat |
| | | |
| Distilled liquor, 86 proof, 1½ fl. oz. | | |
|     Gin, rum, vodka, bourbon, brandy, scotch, whiskey, cognac | 105 | 2 fat |
| | | |
| Vermouth | | |
|     Dry, 3½ fl. oz. (French) | 105 | 2 fat |
|     Sweet, 3½ fl. oz. (Italian) | 167 | 1 starch, 2 fat |
| | | |
| Mixed Drinks | | |
|     Bloody Mary, 5 fl. oz. | 56 | 1 starch |
|     Dacquiri, 3 fl. oz. | 122 | ½ fruit, 2 fat |
|     Manhattan, 3 fl. oz. | 164 | ½ fruit, 3 fat |
|     Margarita, 3 fl. oz. | 105 | 1 fruit, 1½ fat |
|     Martini, 3 fl. oz. | 140 | 3 fat |
|     Pina colada, 3 fl. oz. | 240 | 2 starch, 2 fat |
|     Screwdriver, 3 fl. oz. | 111 | 1 starch, 1 fat |
|     Tom Collins, 10 fl. oz. | 180 | 1 fruit, 3 fat |
|     Whiskey sour, 3 fl. oz. | 120 | 1 starch, 1 fat |
| | | |
| Liqueurs | | |
|     Flavored brandy, 1 fl. oz. | 96 | ½ fruit, 1½ fat |
|     Creme de cacao, 1 fl. oz. | 106 | 2 fat |
|     Creme de menthe, 1 fl. oz. | 101 | ½ fruit, 1½ fat |
|     Peppermint schnapps, 1 fl. oz. | 115 | 1 fruit, 1½ fat |
|     Benedictine, 1 fl. oz. | 106 | 2 fat |
| | | |
| Hard cider, 6 fl. oz. | 71 | 2 fat |

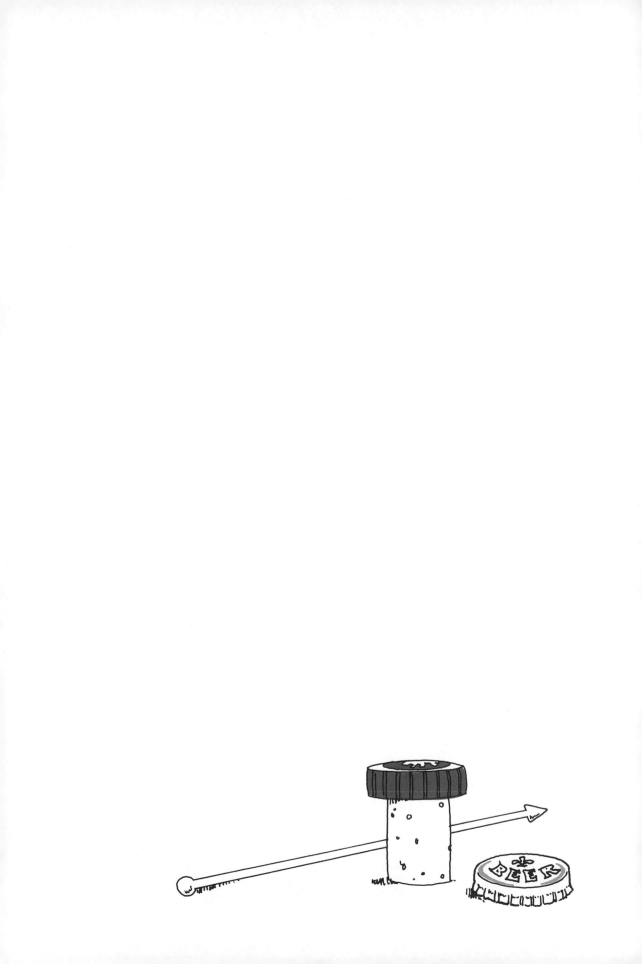

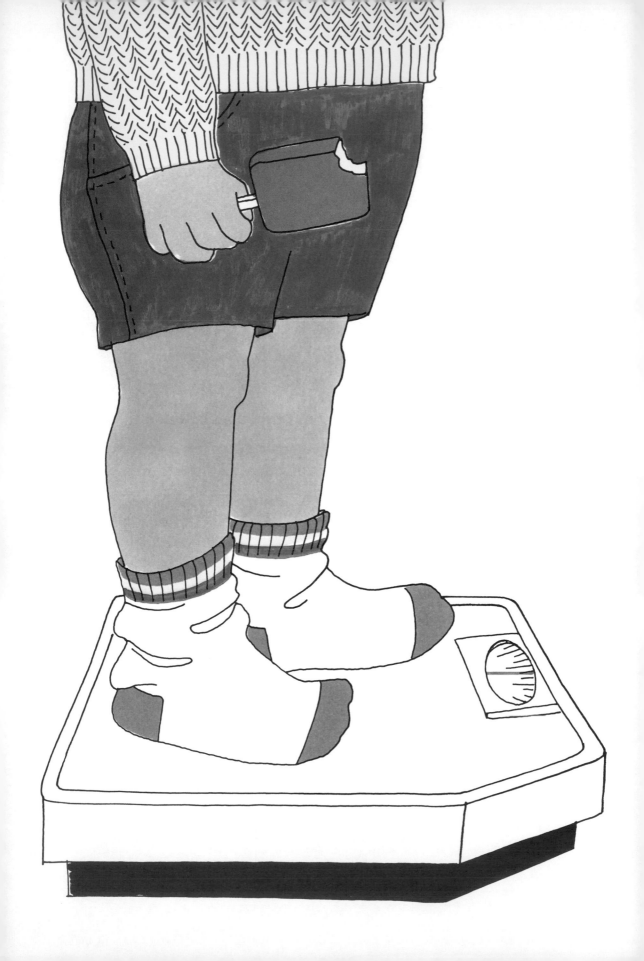

# PART NINE:
# Special Problems


Chapter 26: Obesity and Diabetes Mellitus

Chapter 27: Obesity and High Blood
Pressure

Chapter 28: Obesity in Children and
Adolescents

Chapter 29: Obesity and Pregnancy

Chapter 30: Obesity and Blood Cholesterol

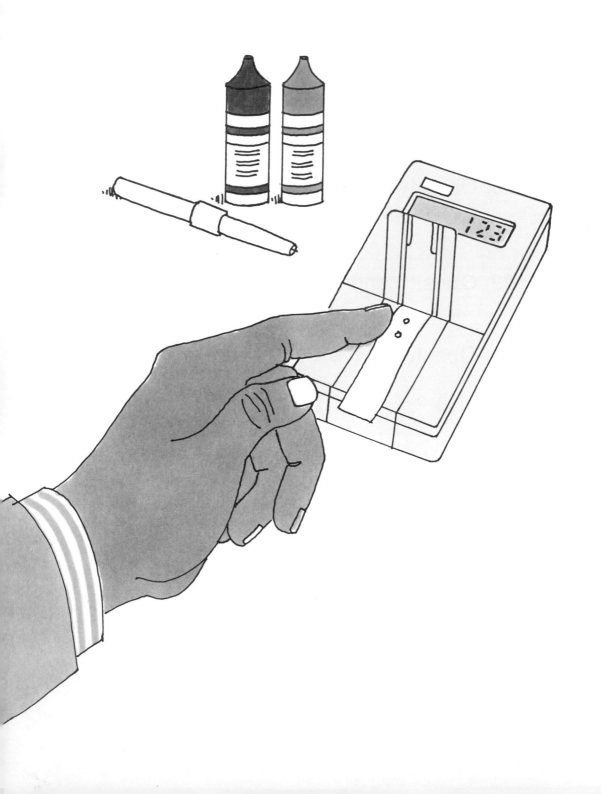

# Chapter 26: Obesity and Diabetes Mellitus

## What Is Diabetes?

Diabetes mellitus exists when blood sugar is abnormally and chronically elevated. There are two kinds of diabetes mellitus that occur spontaneously in human subjects. Type I or insulin-dependent diabetes mellitus (IDDM) usually has its onset in children and young adults and requires a diet and insulin injections for control of blood sugar. Type II or noninsulin-dependent diabetes mellitus (NIDDM) is most often diagnosed after the age of 40. Blood sugar is commonly controlled with diet alone or diet in combination with oral medications. Occasionally insulin also may be required.

In 1985 there were approximately 6 million cases of known diabetes in the United States. Of these, less than 10% were Type I and over 90% were Type II. It is also estimated that there are a significant number of undiagnosed Type II diabetic individuals in the United States and that as many as 25% of the American population carry genes for diabetes. Inheritance of Type I diabetes is much less strong than the Type II variety. Experts estimate that because familial transmission is so important in Type II diabetes, its prevalence in America will double every 15 years.

## What Causes Diabetes Mellitus?

In insulin-dependent or Type I diabetes, the primary cause is progressive destruction of insulin-producing beta cells in the pancreas. The process is actually an abnormal immune (allergic-like) response in which the body fails to recognize beta cells as normal tissue and takes steps to destroy them as if they were foreign to the body and should not be there. The scientific term is autoimmunity. Pancreatic beta cell destruction eventually causes insulin deficiency to occur. This hormone must be replaced by daily insulin injections.

Type II or noninsulin-dependent diabetes is caused primarily by resistance to one's own insulin. In other words, more insulin than normal must be released by the pancreas to drive glucose (sugar) out of the blood and into cells. There is often an associated sluggish pancreatic secretion of insulin during the initial hour or two following a meal that may contribute to elevated blood sugar levels. In this much more common form of diabetes, therapy is directed at reducing insulin resistance and increasing pancreatic insulin secretion. Insulin injections are usually not necessary.

## How Is Diabetes Diagnosed?

Diabetes in adults is diagnosed in two ways. If glucose (in milligrams per 100 milliliters of serum or plasma) is 140 or higher after an overnight fast on two or more occasions, diabetes is present and no further testing is required. For lower levels of fasting (morning) glucose, a two-hour oral glucose tolerance test is done. After a 75-gram glucose mixture is drunk, 1-, 1½- and 2-hour blood samples are obtained. Diabetes is diagnosed if the 1- and/or 1½-hour values are equal to 200 or more and the two-hour level is also 200 or more.

## How Does Obesity Affect Diabetes?

Obesity, like Type II diabetes, also causes resistance to one's own insulin. Blood concentrations of insulin before and after meals are higher in obese subjects and become progressively higher as more weight is gained. This means that more insulin is needed to keep blood sugar levels normal. If obesity is present in subjects with Type II diabetes, insulin resistance will be much greater and blood sugar levels are higher than they are at a normal weight or after weight reduction.

Our research survey has documented that within the TOPS membership, the incidence of Type II diabetes rises steadily with increasing obesity levels (see chapter 2). It is of interest that as many as 50% of all Type II diabetic individuals are also obese. In patients who have insulin-requiring (Type I) diabetes, excessive body fat also increases the need for greater dosages of insulin. Weight loss reduces insulin requirements.

From these facts it is obvious that obesity has bad effects on diabetes. It may hasten its onset and severity among those who have the inherited tendency to develop diabetes. Once diabetes is established in a person, obesity makes it more difficult to control the disease, since it promotes more insulin resistance and higher blood sugar levels. In Type II diabetic patients who do not reduce their weight, the added strain on the pancreas may cause exhaustion of insulin reserve and the need to add insulin injections.

## How Do I Know If I Have Diabetes?

Classic symptoms usually occur only in Type I diabetes. Because of severe insulin deficiency, blood sugar is usually quite high. This causes excessive urination, thirst, weakness, weight loss and craving for food. However, in Type II diabetes, symptoms may not be that obvious, because blood sugar levels are frequently only mildly to moderately increased. Weight gain and excessive obesity may continue in the presence of diabetes.

All individuals should have blood test screening

for diabetes at least once a year. Some people should be watched especially carefully. They include those with a family history of diabetes and severe obesity. Women who have had heavy babies (over 9 pounds), unexplained stillborns and other abnormal obstetrical histories also are more vulnerable. Middle-aged men with impotence also have a higher incidence of diabetes and should be checked. Any adult who has had a stroke, heart attack or who develops other forms of vascular disease also needs evaluation. Frequently a complete oral glucose tolerance test is necessary to establish the diagnosis.

## How Is Diabetes Mellitus Managed?

The most important component of diabetes management is the diet. All the exchange system meal plans in this monograph are approximately the same as those recommended for patients with diabetes. If obesity is present, a weight-reduction plan is selected (see chapters 14 to 16). If desirable weight is present, weight-maintaining diets are prescribed (see chapter 18). Your physician and dietitian will help you choose the right meal plan and provide instruction.

Your doctor will also refer you to a nurse-specialist who can educate you on all aspects of self-care. These include the proper use of medications, including insulin, if necessary; recognition of low and high blood sugars; how to monitor blood sugar control at home; how to deal with infection; foot and skin care; emergencies and other complications. More than ever, a sensible program of exercise is essential, not only for losing weight but for improving blood sugar levels. Guidelines for these are similar to those described in chapters 10 and 11 and should be approved by a physician.

Home blood glucose monitoring deserves special emphasis. The patient can be taught how to obtain drops of blood from the finger tips with little discomfort with special equipment. The blood is placed on a paper strip with chemical reagents on it. The color developed on the strip indicates the blood sugar value. This can be read from a color chart or inserted directly into equipment that gives a direct reading on a meter. In this way, your doctor can determine whether your blood sugar control before and after meals is in the right range. If not, adjustments of diet and medications can be made.

## Why Is Control of Diabetes Mellitus Important?

If blood sugar concentrations are not well controlled, complications of diabetes often occur earlier and may be more severe. Diabetes is a leading cause of blindness, kidney failure and vascular disease. The latter includes stroke, heart attacks and peripheral vascular disease. If de-

sirable body weight is achieved and maintained and if good nutrition and blood sugar levels exist, serious complications can be avoided and a healthy life lies ahead.

## Summary

Diabetes mellitus may have few symptoms when it is the adult, Type II type. Nevertheless, if it is not diagnosed early, serious health complications can result.

Blood sugar screening tests should be included in one's annual physical checkup. A complete oral glucose tolerance test is necessary to make the diagnosis.

Diabetes often has a strong hereditary pattern. If family history is positive, testing for diabetes is very important.

Obesity aggravates diabetes mellitus. Weight reduction and good nutrition bring diabetes under much better control.

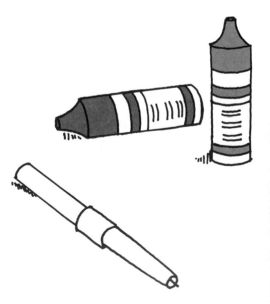

# Chapter 27: Obesity and High Blood Pressure

As discussed in chapter 2, obesity increases the risk of high blood pressure or hypertension. The severity of hypertension often parallels the degree of overweight. Medical science does not understand completely the reasons for this relationship. Obese subjects have a greater blood volume, and the heart must pump harder to maintain proper circulation. Plasma insulin is increased in overweight people, and this hormone is known to promote salt retention. This together with other alterations of salt-retaining hormones may be responsible for the increased blood volume and high blood pressure. There may be other changes in adrenaline-like stress hormones which also influence constriction of blood vessels and boost pressure by increasing resistance to blood flow.

Several research studies also have shown that weight reduction in obese, hypertensive patients lowers blood pressure. For these reasons, health experts advise individuals with elevated blood pressure to achieve body weights that are within 15% of desirable ranges (see chapter 1).

## What Is Hypertension?

High blood pressure in adults is defined as any value equal to or exceeding 140/90. The first number represents *systolic* pressure, measured when the heart contracts. The second number is *diastolic* pressure, measured while the heart relaxes. The most important measurement in medicine is the second number or diastolic pressure. Hypertension is graded according to the range of diastolic values. All measurements are recorded as millimeters (mm) of mercury using a standard mercury column blood pressure cuff.

| Diastolic Blood Pressure | Class |
| --- | --- |
| under 85 | Normal |
| 85-89 | High normal |
| 90-104 | Mild hypertension |
| 105-114 | Moderate hypertension |
| 115 or higher | Severe hypertension |

Physicians also recognize a less serious form of the disorder called *systolic hypertension*. This is diagnosed when the second, diastolic level is normal (less than 90) but the first, systolic value is elevated.

| Systolic Blood Pressure | Class |
| --- | --- |
| under 140 | Normal |
| 140-159 | Borderline systolic hypertension |
| 160 or higher | Isolated systolic hypertension |

Most cases of sustained systolic hypertension occur in elderly subjects. It rarely requires treatment. Healthy people who are exercising or under some emotional or physical stress may also have short-lived elevations of systolic blood pressure. This is a normal response and is not significant medically. Most cases of potentially serious hypertension have elevations of both systolic and diastolic blood pressure. It is emphasized that all blood pressure readings should be taken after at least five minutes of rest, preferably in a doctor's office. Obese individuals should have pressure taken with a large cuff. Normal-sized cuffs may give false elevations of blood pressure. It is also emphasized that two or more elevated blood pressure readings should be obtained on separate days under fairly relaxed conditions before the diagnosis is made.

## What Are Some Important Facts About High Blood Pressure?

It is estimated that 60 million Americans have some form of hypertension. Black populations have a higher incidence than do whites, but it is common in both groups. Elevated blood pressure has serious effects on the cardiovascular system. Even mild forms of hypertension, if untreated, increase the risk of heart attack, stroke and kidney failure. Hardening of the arteries (atherosclerosis) is accelerated.

There are many conditions that increase the risks of high blood pressure complications. These same problems also increase the risk of developing hypertension. They are listed below:

Obesity (discussed earlier)
Diabetes mellitus
Elevated blood cholesterol
Cigarette smoking
Excessive alcohol use
Certain drugs and medicines*

*Review all prescribed and nonprescribed drugs with your physician. Appetite suppressants, cold and sinus remedies, oral contraceptives, cortisone-like drugs, certain arthritis and several antidepressant drugs can aggravate hypertension.

## What Can I Do To Control My Blood Pressure?

(1) If you have hypertension, see your physician as often as necessary. Blood pressure problems can be treated effectively with a wide variety of drugs now available.
(2) If obese, lose weight.
(3) If you have diabetes, make certain it is well controlled.

(4) If blood cholesterol is increased, have a thorough evaluation and follow-up for treatment.

(5) Stop smoking cigarettes.

(6) Avoid alcohol.

(7) Exercise within the guidelines defined by your physician. Exercise relieves tension and can reduce blood pressure.

(8) Avoid excessive stress, if possible.

## Summary

Many health experts look upon high blood pressure as a "silent" killer. If undiagnosed and/or untreated, serious damage to the heart, major blood vessels and kidneys may result.

Blood pressure should be checked often in obese adults, because hypertension is more common in the obese, and the severity of high blood pressure often parallels the degree of overweight.

A major step in controlling high blood pressure is weight reduction. A great number of effective medications also can be used by physicians to treat this condition if necessary. The outlook for a healthy life is good if high blood pressure is discovered early and treated aggressively.

# Chapter 28: Obesity in Children and Adolescents

Today approximately 11 million American children are significantly overweight. Between the mid-1960s and late 1970s the prevalence of obesity increased 54% in children between the ages of 6 and 11 and 39% among adolescents between 12 and 17 years old. This suggests that a major change in lifestyle and environmental factors which are separate and distinct from hereditary influences are contributing to the problem.

## Factors Responsible for the Rising Incidence Of Obesity in Children and Adolescents

### Family

Most authorities on the subject stress the importance of the family in shaping eating patterns in youngsters. Since single parent and working parent families are more common today, there is greater reliance on fast food restaurants and convenience food preparation. Children are given increasing responsibility for preparing or buying their own meals and developing their own eating habits. Often this is done with little input from anyone about what good nutrition really is. This, in turn, leads to an inevitable attraction to tasty, calorie-dense meals and snacks of high sugar, salt or fat content. If parents themselves are obese and eat in the same fashion and have the same lifestyle, attempts to correct obesity in the child are doomed to failure. Often, familial obesity is just as much a product of custom as it is of hereditary factors.

### Mass Media

Mass media contribute to childhood obesity in at least two ways. Youngsters are perpetually bombarded with advertising that promotes high-calorie food consumption as a way of life. Excessive television watching not only provides graphic illustrations of these food products, but it also guarantees physical inactivity and cues to eat while viewing TV.

### School

Kids spend much of their time at school and in school-related activities. Most institutions meet their responsibilities well by teaching what good nutrition is all about, running good school lunch programs and providing broad opportunities in exercise and physical training for the majority of children who are not in competitive sports. Ideally, their facilities for sports and exercise are available during the summer as well.

Unfortunately, these are times of rising education costs and shrinking tax dollar support. Tight budgets may lead to major cutbacks in these important areas. Parents should make their school boards aware of their concerns. Health, physical development and prevention of childhood malnutrition, which includes obesity, should be a joint venture between families and their school districts.

### Peer Pressure

Peer pressure can add to the problem. At certain stages of adolescent development, the child becomes more preoccupied with gaining acceptance and interacting with schoolmates than with his or her own family. There is a quest for independence. Eating out with the gang at fast food restaurants, parties and other functions is a natural form of social expression. The peer group may influence food choices in a major way, and often it may be done to project an image among boys and girls in their age groups. Any food, regardless of quality, that identifies with young children or babies or older adults is frequently avoided. Obese children who have been coached to eat more conservatively and sensibly may have to stop their thrust to lose weight when they are in these situations. Eating differently may be looked upon as not conforming and not being part of the group.

### Psychological and Social Factors

Discrimination against obese children is as prevalent as it is among the adult overweight. This may take the form of needling, teasing and outright social ostracism by schoolmates. The overweight appearance may seriously compromise their ability to achieve recognition, awards, prizes, jobs, college entrance, etc. This may lead to social withdrawal, idleness, boredom, and feelings of futility and inadequacy. Overeating may become more pronounced, and physical activity, more reduced.

The family can accentuate the problem. Permissive, overly protective parents may do little more than offer inappropriately high levels of emotional support that suppress the child's own track towards psychological, social and physical maturity. Negativistic parents can overwhelm the child by being unreasonably critical, inflexible and ashamed. The latter response is especially damaging because there may be no positive source for fostering self-worth or esteem either at home or at school.

### Exercise

Many obese children are exercising little or not at all. Parents should be aware of how many hours per week their children are involved in active exercise at school, after school or on weekends. This should be balanced against the number of hours per week the child is idle and not performing school-related work. A certain amount of free time with rest and relaxation is important. Listening to music, watching television, reading, going to movies, sports events and other social events are important outlets. However, most of these forms of entertainment expend little energy and may be the very situations that lead to overeating.

If there are too many hours spent in an inactive lifestyle and there is not enough involvement in active exercise, this can contribute greatly to the child's weight problem.

## Correcting Childhood Obesity

Strategies for helping your child correct a weight problem are not unlike what was recommended to adults with weight problems in an earlier section (see Part 4). They include:

(1) Taking the child to a physician for a general checkup and defining his or her obesity level

(2) Defining the child's abnormal eating pattern and developing a sensible eating schedule
(3) Teaching the child what foods to restrict or avoid and what foods to consume
(4) Seeking ways to increase exercise and general physical activity

On the other hand, childhood and adolescent obesity requires a different approach than adult obesity in certain important areas.

•Emphasis is not placed on obesity in a direct way. Instead, focus is directed toward changing eating and exercise habits to guarantee better health and well-being. By talking to the child in this way, acceptance of the need to change lifestyle is more likely to occur. He or she must be motivated enough to make the decision and the changes.

•Strict diets, especially fad or crash diets, should never be forced on youngsters. This can seriously impair growth and development. Teenagers who are obese also resist any strict meal planning because of their desire to be independent and make their own food choices.

•Most growing obese kids do not need to lose a

## TABLE 20: WEIGHT AND HEIGHT FOR NORMAL MALES, AGES 2 TO 18 YEARS

| AGE (years) | WEIGHT (pounds) BY PERCENTILE* | | | HEIGHT (inches) BY PERCENTILE* | | |
|---|---|---|---|---|---|---|
| | 5th | 50th | 95th | 5th | 50th | 95th |
| 2 | 23.1 | 27.1 | 34.1 | 32.5 | 34.2 | 37.2 |
| 3 | 26.5 | 32.2 | 39.1 | 35.0 | 37.4 | 40.2 |
| 4 | 30.0 | 36.7 | 44.6 | 37.7 | 40.5 | 43.3 |
| 5 | 33.6 | 41.1 | 50.8 | 40.2 | 43.3 | 46.1 |
| 6 | 37.3 | 45.5 | 58.0 | 42.4 | 45.7 | 48.6 |
| 7 | 41.0 | 50.3 | 66.3 | 44.5 | 47.9 | 51.1 |
| 8 | 44.9 | 55.7 | 75.9 | 46.5 | 50.0 | 53.4 |
| 9 | 49.0 | 61.9 | 87.1 | 48.4 | 52.0 | 55.8 |
| 10 | 53.5 | 69.2 | 99.6 | 50.3 | 54.1 | 58.3 |
| 11 | 59.0 | 77.7 | 113.2 | 52.2 | 56.4 | 61.0 |
| 12 | 65.7 | 87.5 | 127.8 | 54.2 | 58.9 | 63.9 |
| 13 | 74.0 | 98.9 | 143.0 | 56.3 | 61.6 | 66.9 |
| 14 | 84.1 | 111.7 | 158.7 | 58.6 | 64.2 | 69.6 |
| 15 | 94.8 | 124.8 | 174.1 | 61.1 | 66.5 | 71.6 |
| 16 | 105.0 | 136.6 | 188.4 | 63.4 | 68.3 | 73.0 |
| 17 | 113.3 | 145.9 | 200.9 | 64.9 | 69.4 | 73.7 |
| 18 | 118.7 | 151.5 | 210.7 | 65.2 | 69.6 | 73.9 |

*5th percentile: 95% of all males in this age group have weights or heights *above* these values.
50th percentile: Average weight and height for this age group.
95th percentile: 95% of all males in this group have weights or heights *below* these values.

SOURCE: Hamill, P.V.V., et al., "Physical Growth: National Center for Health Statistics Percentiles," *American Journal of Clinical Nutrition* 32 (1979): 607-629. Data from National Center for Health Statistics (NCHS), Hyattsville, Maryland.

great deal of weight. Instead, future rates of weight gain are slowed down relative to gains in height until the two are normal with advancing age. In other words, the youngster "grows" into his or her present weight.

One exception is the obese adolescent who has already reached maximum height in later teens. In this situation, weight reduction is necessary, but the meal plan should always be nutritious and prescribed by a physician with instruction and guidance by a registered dietitian.

Another special case is the extremely obese child regardless of age. It is best to begin with a thorough evaluation by a physician with the understanding that treatment may require an intense effort by health professionals.

## Physician Input and Defining Obesity Level

Obesity level should not be determined by the parents. A pediatrician or family physician who is familiar with patterns of childhood development should make this assessment. As a matter of good preventive medicine, a child should be seen an-

nually by a physician so that all aspects of health are evaluated.

Tables 20 and 21 give average heights and weights (50th percentile) for boys and girls between the ages of 2 and 18. The 5th and 95th percentiles also are given. These charts are adapted from the National Center for Health Statistics and are based on measurements of large populations of children. Health professionals use these charts to determine in what percentile the child is for both weight and height.

A young person who is below the 50th percentile for height but significantly above it in weight is very likely to be obese. On the other hand, those who are above average for height but below average for weight may be substantially underweight. The physician can record these values annually from early childhood on and, together with a physical examination, determine when any significant deviations from normal are occurring. If a physician is not seen at regular intervals, progress cannot be followed adequately. Possible nutritional, endocrine or other medical illnesses that affect

## TABLE 21: WEIGHT AND HEIGHT
## FOR NORMAL FEMALES, AGES 2 TO 18 YEARS

| AGE (years) | WEIGHT (pounds) BY PERCENTILE* | | | HEIGHT (inches) BY PERCENTILE* | | |
|---|---|---|---|---|---|---|
| | 5th | 50th | 95th | 5th | 50th | 95th |
| 2 | 21.9 | 26.0 | 31.1 | 32.1 | 34.2 | 36.9 |
| 3 | 25.5 | 31.0 | 37.9 | 34.8 | 37.0 | 39.6 |
| 4 | 28.8 | 35.1 | 43.8 | 37.4 | 40.0 | 42.6 |
| 5 | 32.0 | 38.9 | 49.8 | 39.8 | 42.7 | 45.5 |
| 6 | 35.3 | 42.9 | 56.7 | 42.0 | 45.1 | 48.3 |
| 7 | 39.0 | 48.0 | 65.3 | 44.0 | 47.5 | 51.0 |
| 8 | 43.2 | 54.6 | 76.4 | 46.0 | 49.8 | 53.6 |
| 9 | 48.0 | 62.6 | 89.4 | 48.1 | 52.0 | 56.3 |
| 10 | 53.6 | 71.6 | 103.8 | 50.2 | 54.4 | 58.9 |
| 11 | 59.9 | 81.3 | 118.8 | 52.6 | 57.0 | 61.5 |
| 12 | 67.1 | 91.4 | 133.8 | 55.0 | 59.6 | 64.1 |
| 13 | 75.1 | 101.4 | 148.1 | 57.2 | 61.9 | 66.2 |
| 14 | 83.1 | 110.6 | 160.8 | 58.5 | 63.1 | 67.4 |
| 15 | 90.2 | 118.1 | 171.1 | 59.3 | 63.7 | 68.0 |
| 16 | 95.5 | 123.0 | 178.2 | 59.7 | 63.9 | 68.2 |
| 17 | 98.4 | 124.7 | 181.4 | 60.1 | 64.2 | 68.3 |
| 18 | 99.6 | 124.6 | 181.4 | 60.5 | 64.4 | 68.4 |

*5th percentile: 95% of all females in this age group have weights or heights *above* these values.
50th percentile: Average weight and height for this age group.
95th percentile: 95% of all females in this age group have weights or heights *below* these values.

SOURCE: Hamill, P.V.V., et al., "Physical Growth: National Center for Health Statistics Percentiles," *American Journal of Clinical Nutrition* 32 (1979): 607-629. Data from National Center for Health Statistics (NCHS), Hyattsville, Maryland.

210

growth and development may be missed. Obesity is one of them. Early recognition and steps for correction are in the child's best interest.

A word of caution: Estimation of normal weights and heights for individual children can be very difficult at the time of puberty when major growth spurts begin. There are some who enter this stage at an earlier age, and others, somewhat later. "Early bloomers" may be taller and heavier than their peers for a time. "Late bloomers" may be shorter and lighter. Eventually, as adolescence advances, these differences cancel and appropriate heights and weights are achieved.

Another point that deserves emphasis. Children, like adults, come in all sorts of sizes, shapes and physiques. Some aspects of development are determined by heredity that is passed on by parents and other relatives. That is why a physician's input is so important in individual cases.

## Defining Your Child's Abnormal Eating Pattern

Chapter 12 discusses different types of abnormal eating patterns in adults. These also apply to children. The critical thing for parents to estimate is when and where most overeating of calorie-dense foods is taking place. At home? At school? When socializing and eating with friends? Children, like adults, can be heavy snackers at school, after school and at night. They can consistently overeat at meal time. They also can be binge eaters during periods of stress.

Food cues also are part of the problem in childhood obesity, since children also are exposed to vending machines, local stores and fast food restaurants, which are often signals to buy and to eat. In the home, just being in the kitchen, watching television, doing homework or being idle are other potential cues that lead to overeating.

By recognizing when and where the child is overeating, further guidance and solutions can be offered.

## Nutritional Needs of Children

Children and adolescents require more calories and more protein per inch of height or pound of weight than adults because they are growing. Table 22 gives the average calorie and protein requirements at different ages. Note the broad range of caloric needs, which reflects the large variation in physical activity and size within the various age groups.

To assure good nutrition, all children should have at least four servings each of starch/breads, fruits, and vegetables each day. In the 2- to 10-year-old age group, 2 cups of milk products and 3 ounces of meat equivalents are recommended. Between the ages of 11 and 18, 4 cups of milk products and 4 to 5 ounces of meat, poultry, fish and related foods are desirable. Meeting these guidelines on a daily basis will guarantee consumption of important food groups and essential vitamins and minerals. Additional food intake is often required, especially in very active children and adolescents who are athletes or in an active growth spurt.

Good nutrition from this standpoint should be discussed with the child. In a similar way, foods that should be avoided are also reviewed with the child (see chapter 13).

This entire approach by the parents actually involves education of the child about good nutrition. If done in a pleasant, though thorough, way it will eventually give the child a sense of independence in making the right food selections.

If the parents have difficulty understanding what the proper nutritional needs of their child should be, they should seek help from an experienced registered dietitian.

### Setting the Eating Schedule

Stress the importance of three meals each day. Parents should be certain that enough time is allowed for the child to eat and enjoy a good breakfast and evening meal. During the school year

## TABLE 22: AVERAGE NUTRITIONAL NEEDS OF CHILDREN

| GROUP | AGE (years) | CALORIES/DAY | CALORIE RANGE | PROTEIN/DAY (grams) |
|---|---|---|---|---|
| Children | 1-3 | 1,300 | 900-1,300 | 23 |
| | 4-6 | 1,700 | 1,300-2,300 | 30 |
| | 7-10 | 2,400 | 1,650-3,300 | 34 |
| Boys | 11-14 | 2,700 | 2,000-3,700 | 45 |
| | 15-18 | 2,800 | 2,100-3,900 | 56 |
| Girls | 11-14 | 2,200 | 1,500-3,000 | 46 |
| | 15-18 | 2,100 | 1,200-3,000 | 46 |

SOURCE: Recommended Dietary Allowances, revised 1980, Food and Nutrition Board, National Academy of Sciences–National Research Council, Washington, D.C.

lunch can be packed. If there is a lunch program at school, milk, soup and other sensible food choices can supplement the packed lunch. Otherwise, the child will have to select his or her own food for the entire meal if lunch is not carried. The decision to allow eating cafeteria food at school should be based on parents knowing that the quality of meals is good. Often menus for an entire week are available to parents in advance, if desired. This will assure food quality and help the parents and their child make the right food choices.

Most kids are famished after school. A reasonable snack at that time is appropriate. Often a second snack is desired at night before going to bed. There is nothing wrong with snacks provided that the right food is available.

Parents and child should have an understanding about the eating pattern. Once that is established, it should become a matter of routine and not changed. It becomes the first positive step in changing lifestyle. In other words, if everyone agrees on two snacks, one after school and one at night, in addition to the three main meals, it should be a daily occurrence. No eating at other times.

### The Home Example

Parents need to keep calorie-dense foods out of sight and preferably out of the home. Snacks to avoid are difficult to pass by if they are in plain view in the kitchen. Replace such things as salty, starchy junk foods, pastries, cakes and pies, and candy with fresh fruit, whole grain bread, peanut butter, plain popcorn, simple crackers or cookies, cut celery and carrot sticks, milk, etc. The preferred food items for snacking should be what the youngster enjoys and wants. A variety should be available for his or her own choice and in amounts that are learned to be reasonable.

Meal time at home is the most important of all. The family should eat together with plenty of time to enjoy the meal without distractions like television, newspapers and telephone calls. The child should eat slowly and be allowed to pick from the food being served. There should be no pressure to eat this or that, but there also should be no attempt to provide a separate menu. If an important food like vegetables, milk or meat is consistently refused, parents will have to explain their importance for health and encourage at least some consumption.

### Exercise

Physical education programs at school should have the child's full participation. If there is talent for after-school sports, every encouragement is appropriate. Parents can also help their child take advantage of weekend or summer sports offered by schools, churches, the YMCA and other groups.

If there is too much idleness at home, cut back on excessive television viewing and other leisure activities that don't call for physical activity. Putting up basketball hoops and buying a bicycle, tennis racquet or baseball glove are steps in the right direction to get things going. Friends who are active should be invited to play with him or her.

Kids can also expend some energy by helping with the yard work, walking the dog and doing other chores around the house. In fact, family projects are a good way to get everyone exercising. A family outing on bicycles, a hike in the woods or a swim in the lake are examples.

The main goal is to draw the child out of idleness, withdrawal and physical inactivity and into a more active life with the family and peers.

### A Good Feeling with Emotional Support

Kids have to feel positive about themselves. Take an interest in their school work, social life and accomplishments. Help them to feel as secure as possible. An obese child is at a disadvantage because of how he or she looks. For that reason, attempts should be made to improve that appearance: good grooming and clothes that are becoming to him or her. Learning how to respond to peer teasing and jeers over being obese is something parents can help the child develop. This reduces the likelihood of the youngster becoming negative, hostile and defensive in a social setting.

Emotional and social turmoil can aggravate obesity problems. Parents must communicate with their children to find out where potential and actual problems exist. Frequently they center on peer relationships and peer acceptance. They may involve frustrations at school with courses, teachers or various extracurricular activities. It also may be a problem within the family itself where friction exists between brothers and sisters, the parents themselves or other relatives.

By communicating without being intrusive or too overbearing, by listening carefully, the sources of unhappiness can be defined and positive solutions often can be offered. Professional help may be needed.

### Height and Weight Records

As stated earlier, parents have to be careful about not focusing too much attention on obesity in a growing child. Taking weights too often may do just that, especially if little progress is made and each weigh-in becomes a showdown.

Allow the physician to obtain accurate heights and weights in the physician's office. If the doctor is seen relatively infrequently and additional measurements are recommended in the home, they probably should be done no more than three or four times a year. Emphasize the height measurement and take it first. Go to a specific area of the house and have the child stand close to a wall (not against it). Place the edge of a sturdy book or carpenter's square against the wall and slide it down until it comfortably touches the top of the head. Make a pencil mark on the wall and measure the distance between the mark and the floor with a good tape measure or yardstick. A series of marks will accumulate upward as the child grows. Next, take the weight on a quality bathroom scale after setting the zero mark correctly.

Write the heights and weights with dates in a notebook and take the values to your doctor. Remember, growing children may actually gain weight even though they may look thinner. This may simply reflect replacement of body fat weight with developing muscle and a growing skeleton.

Most parents can tell if their child is losing fat by just looking at him or her. This is evident in the face, arms, thighs, and abdomen, and how clothes are fitting.

*The Need for Patience*

All the recommendations in this chapter sound simple and straightforward. However, obesity in children and adolescents can be a frustrating problem to control. Parents have to be patient because there may be setbacks just like those occurring in adults who are overweight. If there is a backslide in weight, decide with the child's input what may have caused it. Make the necessary adjustments together and begin again.

## Summary[1]

Obese children, like obese adults, have to change their lifestyle by correcting bad eating habits and exercising more.

Obese children should not follow rigid diets or meal plans. By changing bad eating habits and exercising more, they grow into their weight as height increases.

All children and adolescents have certain nutritional needs. Educating the child to meet those needs is very important. Equally important is the necessity to teach obese kids what foods to avoid. Examples of good nutrition in the home have to be provided by the parents.

A very positive approach to the problem is essential. Emphasis on changing lifestyle for the sake of good health without a negative emphasis on obesity itself will help the child develop his or her own good eating habits and exercise activities independently.

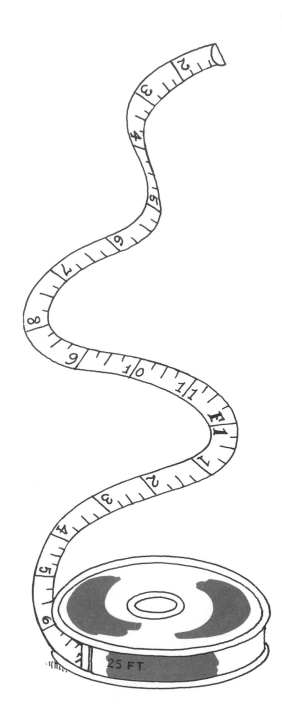

[1]Recommended reading: E. Satter, *How To Get Your Kid To Eat . . . But Not Too Much* (Bull Publishing Co., Palo Alto CA, 1987).

# Chapter 29: Obesity and Pregnancy

Obese pregnant women who have no underlying medical problems usually deliver healthy newborn babies. Newborn fatality rates are no different than in a general population of nonobese women. However, health complications in obese pregnant women are more prevalent. Recent surveys reveal that pregnancy-onset high blood pressure, preeclampsia (high blood pressure with body swelling), blood clots in veins, urinary tract infections and diabetes mellitus are significantly higher in overweight women, and the frequency of these complications is even higher among those who are severely obese. Obese women also tend to have heavier babies. For this and other reasons, the number of Caesarean sections performed on overweight pregnant women is higher than in nonobese subjects.

Obese women should seek care from their personal physician and obstetrician as soon as pregnancy is diagnosed. Ideally, care should be sought before conception takes place so that any medical problems can be treated or controlled ahead of time. Physicians also recommend that attempts at weight reduction should be made before pregnancy occurs. No programs for weight loss should be followed during pregnancy. This can have damaging effects on the baby. Obesity has a number of ailments associated with it (see chapter 2), and in obese individuals of the childbearing age there is a higher incidence of hypertension, diabetes, vein problems, blood cholesterol abnormalities, gallbladder disease, etc. If some of these disorders are not diagnosed and controlled adequately before and throughout pregnancy, complications in the mother as well as in the baby are more frequent than in obese pregnant subjects who have no medical problems.

## Nutrition and Weight Gain during Pregnancy

Proper nutrition for expectant mothers is very important for healthy development of the baby. The total number of calories needed to support pregnancy varies a great deal, depending on the weight level and age of the person just before conception takes place. The information in the paragraphs below indicates the number of calories and recommended weight gains for normal weight, overweight and underweight adults as well as ado-lescents under the age of 20. These recommendations are based on opinions from the National Academy of Sciences–National Research Council (see table 5), a survey of the relationship between weight gain and successful outcome of pregnancy,[1] and certain reviews on nutrition for pregnant women.[2,3]

A normal nonobese nonpregnant adult woman of average physical activity requires about 30 calories per kilogram body weight[1] (13.6 calories per pound) to maintain her weight level. During pregnancy it is estimated that an additional 300 calories per day are needed for development of the baby.[2] However, one group advises that the additional food need not be consumed until after the third month of a normal gestation.[4] Ideal weight gain is in the range of 24 to 27 pounds. During the first three months, 2 to 4 pounds are gained. Thereafter, about 0.9 pound per week is added until delivery.

Juvenile or adolescent girls need about 45 or more calories per kilogram body weight or 20.5 calories per pound per day, because the mothers themselves are growing and developing and require a greater food intake to support their own needs as well as those of the baby. Weight gains of about 30 pounds are suggested.

Underweight women (less than 90% of ideal body weight) have to "catch up" on their own body weight deficit as well as provide nutrition for their babies. Depending on the degree of underweight, total daily caloric intakes range between 36 to 50 calories per kilogram (16.4 to 22.7 calories per pound). Weight gains of 30 pounds or more are necessary for the most successful outcome.

One of the most controversial areas is what the caloric intake of obese pregnant women should be. Much research is being done in this area now. At present, it is recommended that a total weight gain should be in the range of 20 to 22 pounds and meal plans should be approximately 30 calories per kilogram or 13.6 calories per pound per day.

It should be emphasized that these are only initial guidelines. Adjustments upward or downward may have to be made depending on the physical activity of the mother and her general lifestyle.

[1] R.L. Naeye, "Weight Gain and the Outcome of Pregnancy," *American Journal of Obstetrics and Gynecology* 135 (1979):3-9.

[2] R.M. Pitkin, "Nutritional Requirements in Normal Pregnancy," *Diabetes Care* 3 (1980):472-475.

[3] P.K. Schulman et al., "Role of Nutrition in the Management of the Pregnant Diabetic Patient," *Seminars in Perinatology* 2 (1978):353-360.

[4] Food and Nutrition Board, Commission on Life Sciences, National Research Council. *Recommended Dietary Allowances*, 10th ed. (National Academy Press, Washington, D.C., 1989), pp. 33-34.

This is always done under the supervision of a physician or registered dietitian.

## Protein, Vitamins and Minerals

Pregnant women have an increased need for protein, vitamins and minerals. Ten to 30 grams of additional high-quality protein per day normally is advised. The higher value amounts to total daily intakes of 1.3 grams per kilogram (0.6 grams per pound) in adult, mature women. In adolescents these values are increased to 1.5 and 0.7 grams per kilogram and per pound, respectively. Supplements of iron, calcium, and the vitamin folacin as well as other vitamins and minerals are needed. Most prenatal vitamin-mineral preparations that are prescribed by obstetricians meet those requirements. They should be taken daily.

## Developing a Meal Plan

Exchange diets using the system in this monograph are suitable for pregnancy. However, the total number of calories and the amounts of additional protein require the assistance of an experienced registered dietitian. The meal plan should emphasize 50% or more of total calories as carbohydrate predominantly from fruits and vegetables, with approximately 30% fat. The fat content should contain no more than 10% of total calories as saturated fat. Protein allowances are increased to accommodate gestation. Low-calorie and artificial sweeteners should not be used during pregnancy. It is also advisable not to smoke cigarettes or drink alcoholic beverages during pregnancy.

Some women, particularly in early as well as late pregnancy, cannot eat great amounts of food at any single meal. In early stages, it may be trouble with nausea. In late stages, the size of the baby may put pressure on the stomach. The dietitian can make adjustments by allowing smaller main meals with in-between meal snacks at mid-morning and mid-afternoon. It is always a good idea to have a snack before bedtime to ensure adequate nutrient supplies for the baby overnight.

## Medical and Obstetrical Monitoring

After the initial, detailed history and physical examination and baseline laboratory tests, the pregnant obese woman will make regular visits to her physicians. Blood pressure, weight, and occasional blood tests and urinalyses are done commonly along with follow-up examinations.

She may be asked to check urine ketones every morning with a paper reagent strip. Ketones are substances that build up in the urine if there is not enough food intake or if there is stress of some form or another. If ketones appear in the urine,

it should be brought to the attention of the physician and the cause found.

## Screening for Diabetes

It is recommended that all pregnant women be screened for diabetes between the 24th and 28th week of gestation. It is estimated that 2 to 3% of all pregnancies in large medical centers may be complicated by pregnancy-onset (gestational) diabetes mellitus. Obesity may increase the likelihood of developing diabetes. This is most apt to occur after the 24th week when many hormones that promote diabetes in susceptible women are reaching high levels. The usual screening test is done by drinking 50 grams of a glucose solution without regard to time of day or time of the last meal. If a venous plasma glucose, obtained one hour later, is 140 milligrams per deciliter or higher, the screening test is positive, and a complete three-hour oral glucose tolerance test is done. This procedure is performed after an overnight fast when the woman is not ill or stressed and has been eating normally the previous three days. After a baseline plasma glucose determination, a 100-gram solution of glucose is drunk. Additional plasma glucose measurements are done at one, two and three hours later. The upper limits of each value are given in table 23.

If diabetes is diagnosed, the patient should be managed by a physician who is skilled in the field of diabetes and pregnancy.

## TABLE 23:
## CRITERIA FOR DIAGNOSING DIABETES MELLITUS DURING PREGNANCY WITH A 100-GRAM ORAL GLUCOSE TOLERANCE TEST

| TIME (hour) | PLASMA GLUCOSE LEVEL (mg/dl) |
|---|---|
| 0 | 105 |
| 1 | 190 |
| 2 | 165 |
| 3 | 145 |

NOTE: Any two values at or above these limits is positive for gestational diabetes mellitus.

## Obstetrical Monitoring

Obstetricians have many methods in addition to routine physical examinations for monitoring the well-being of the baby. Expectant mothers may be asked to count the number of "kicks" they feel from the baby over a specific time period. This is a way of determining fetal activity and health. In selected cases, baby's heart rate is monitored with a device placed on the abdomen. Changes in rate during movements of the baby (nonstress test) or after administration of a hormone, oxytocin (stress test), provide valuable information about fetal health.

Ultrasound is a way of taking "pictures" of the baby inside the uterus. Growth, size and development can be determined. This may be important to the obstetrician in planning the time and method of delivery.

Amniocentesis is another method for assessing the baby's health. Samples are withdrawn from the sac of fluid surrounding the baby. Fluid analysis and examination of cells floating in it can be used to determine genetic defects in early pregnancy as well as estimate how mature the baby's lungs are in late pregnancy if early delivery is necessary. The ability to breathe air and utilize oxygen by the newborn is critical after birth. Amniocentesis aids the obstetrician in making decisions about timing of delivery without the danger of respiratory distress in the newborn.

## Exercise during Pregnancy

Obese pregnant women, whether physically fit or not, need some exercise. This tones the muscle, increases stamina and provides conditioning that is needed for carrying the baby and eventually giving birth. The obstetrician should be asked what types of exercise are safe. As a general rule, any physical exertion that results in too much jumping, bouncing or twisting movements should be avoided. If aerobic dancing is desired, a low-impact level should be followed. Jogging, skiing, cycling and other sports that could result in stressful movements or a fall and injury are undesirable.

An ideal exercise for expectant mothers is walking. Guidelines for brisk walks are similar to those outlined in chapter 11. A warm-up and cool down period before and after the walks with some stretching exercises is appropriate. A few words of caution for exercising pregnant women: (1) Don't allow your heart rate to exceed 140 beats per minute. (2) Twenty minutes at the higher heart rate is long enough during any exercise session. (3) If weakness, light headedness or other unusual symptoms appear, stop exercising.

Another ideal exercise for pregnant women is swimming. The water "buoys" up the body and relieves the strain of carrying the extra weight of the baby and placenta. This allows the mother to exercise her own body with greater ease. Again, brisk swimming as opposed to light swimming should be limited to 20 minutes without exceeding heart rates of 140 beats per minute. Common

sense should tell the mother how much she can endure comfortably.

Light to moderate housework, outdoor gardening and yard work, shopping and other activities of housewives obviously are other forms of exercise. They do not have to be avoided because of pregnancy unless the physician places limits on some of them.

## After Delivery

### Weight Changes

Congratulations! You are now a proud mother with a newborn baby. Its delivery results in weight losses that average 15 pounds during the first week. This represents losses due to weight of the baby, placenta and fluid. Prepregnancy weight under ideal circumstances is reached between eight and 12 weeks after birth of the newborn. Those women who have gained excessive amounts of weight during pregnancy will be heavier than they were before they conceived. That is why control of weight gain throughout gestation is so important for obese expectant mothers.

### Breastfeeding

Breastfeeding your baby has all sorts of advantages, because human breast milk, in adequate supply, is the best nutrition for newborn infants. To ensure good breast milk flow, a generous fluid intake is necessary. Without it, milk volume will fall significantly. In addition, a well-balanced meal plan is very important to maintain a high quality of nutrients in the breast milk. It is not the time to begin low-calorie diets and a major weight-reduction program.

A good meal plan for nursing mothers is not much different from what was followed during pregnancy. More calories as well as additional protein, vitamins and minerals are necessary. This is especially important during the first four weeks after delivery. The Food and Nutrition Board–National Research Council currently recommends 500 additional calories per day above weight maintenance levels for nonobese breastfeeding mothers. Consult your physician and dietitian for specific guidelines, especially if you are obese.

Those women who cannot breastfeed for personal or medical reasons can usually begin their program of weight loss whenever they are ready (two weeks or more after delivery and upon approval of their physician).

## Summary

Obese women who wish to become pregnant need a thorough medical evaluation before pregnancy occurs. Every attempt should be made to lose as much weight as possible and achieve desirable weight before conception. During pregnancy and the breastfeeding period, no weight-reduction diets and programs for weight loss should be followed.

Excessive weight gain during pregnancy will only result in a higher weight after delivery. Close interactions with the physician, registered dietitian and other health professionals will safeguard the health of the expectant mother and developing baby and guarantee a happy outcome.

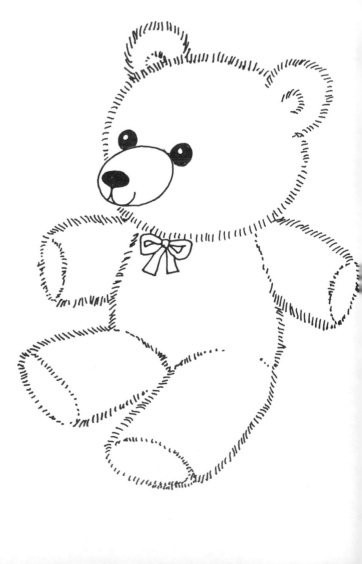

# Chapter 30: Obesity and Blood Cholesterol

The National Heart, Lung and Blood Institute and many professional societies are urging the public and physicians to be more aware of the relationships between plasma cholesterol levels and risks for cardiovascular disease.[1] It is estimated that approximately 25% or one out of every four American adults has a cholesterol problem. Guidelines issued in the report of the expert panel state that total plasma cholesterol levels should not exceed 200 milligrams per deciliter of plasma (200 mg/dl). Borderline values range from 200 to 239, and abnormally high concentrations exceed 240 mg/dl (see table 24).

A variety of population studies as well as animal model research indicates a definite increase in the incidence of cardiovascular disease and mortality when total levels are high. Other risk factors that increase the incidence further are cigarette smoking and hypertension. Obesity and weight gain may also contribute to cholesterol elevations. Diabetes compounds the problem as well.

Many TOPS members also have read about "good" and "bad" cholesterol components. Cholesterol is derived from dietary sources and is also made by a variety of tissues in the body. The liver "packages" cholesterol into lipoproteins, cholesterol-protein complexes, that allow cholesterol to dissolve in blood and be transported to different organs. "Bad" cholesterol is linked to apoprotein B to form low density lipoprotein cholesterol (LDL cholesterol). It is this form that deposits in arteries to the heart, brain and other vital organs and causes arterial hardening or atherosclerosis. Eventually blood flow through the arteries is obstructed, and depending on the site of obstruction, heart attacks, stroke or peripheral vascular accidents may result.

LDL cholesterol also can be measured. Plasma levels should not be above 130 mg/dl (see table 24). If they are above 160, high risks for cardiovascular disease exist. If above 190 mg/dl, a very high risk is diagnosed. Three factors contribute to high total and LDL cholesterol levels: (1) too much saturated fat and cholesterol consumption; (2) exaggerated production of lipoproteins by the liver; (3) impaired peripheral tissue uptake and metabolism of LDL cholesterol. Although dietary sources of cholesterol and fat can be reduced, factors 2 and 3 may be inherited defects or acquired as a result of underlying medical conditions (hypothyroidism, diabetes, and certain chronic kidney and liver ailments). Those athletes who self-administer anabolic steroids or certain susceptible women who take another type of steroid (progestins) may also be at risk for high LDL cholesterol. A variety of other medications may also influence blood cholesterol.

"Good" cholesterol consists of high density lipoprotein or HDL cholesterol. This complex carries cholesterol out of the blood and back to the liver, where it is degraded and excreted with bile to the intestinal tract for elimination. Abnormally low levels are below 35 mg/dl. Factors that raise the concentration include exercise, cessation of smoking, improved diabetic control and correction of obesity.

Physicians frequently monitor plasma triglycerides as well. The source of this blood fat is food as well as the liver. The role of triglycerides in cardiovascular disease is controversial and probably not as important as cholesterol. Nevertheless, certain studies link elevations of plasma triglyceride to cardiovascular disease. Other experts feel that specific protein complexes that carry tri-

## TABLE 24: NORMAL AND ABNORMAL PLASMA TOTAL AND LDL-CHOLESTEROL LEVELS

| PLASMA TOTAL | TOTAL CHOLESTEROL (mg/dl) | LDL-CHOLESTEROL (mg/dl) |
|---|---|---|
| Normal | Less than 200 | Under 130 |
| Borderline high | 200-239 | 130-159 |
| High | 240 or higher | 160 or higher |

NOTES: All values apply to adults. Values are expressed in milligrams per 100 milliliters (deciliter) of plasma (mg/dl).

Note: HDL-cholesterol is abnormally low if less than 35 mg/dl.

[1]National Heart, Blood and Lung Institute, National Institutes of Health, United States Public Health Service, Bethesda, Maryland. January 1988. *National Cholesterol Education Program: Report of the Expert Panel on Detection, Evaluation and Treatment of High Blood Cholesterol in Adults.* N.I.H. publication no. 88-2925.

218

glyceride in the blood also are potential sources of LDL cholesterol. Controlling high levels of triglyceride may indirectly help to control LDL cholesterol.

## Detection and Monitoring of Cholesterol Disturbances

Measurements of plasma or serum cholesterol should be done each year during the annual physical examination by your physician (see chapter 10). If the total cholesterol level is below 200 mg/dl, the nutritional guidelines outlined in this monograph should be followed to ensure a reasonable restriction of dietary fat and saturated fat in the meal plan. This will help to hold down cholesterol levels in the future.

Those who have borderline high (200 to 239 mg/dl) or elevated cholesterol (240 mg/dl or higher) should have the test repeated to confirm the elevation. In addition to total cholesterol, it is recommended that LDL ("bad") and HDL ("good") cholesterol fractions also be measured at that time.

## Dietary Management

### The Step One Diet

To correct abnormal cholesterol elevations, the National Cholesterol Education Program recommends beginning with the Step One Diet. This approach is very similar to the meal plans outlined in this monograph for adults who are overweight (see chapters 15 and 16) and for adults who are at a desirable weight (see chapter 18). It resembles the recommendations for ideal diets for adult Americans described in chapter 6. In other words, carbohydrate is in the range of 50% of total calories consumed and total fat is reduced to approximately 30% or less of total calories. Saturated fat is only 10% of total calories. Thus, emphasis is placed on additional saturated fat restriction and more consumption of unsaturated fat. Dietary cholesterol intake is limited to 300 milligrams per day.

Increasing intake of food fiber (see chapter 5) may also help to lower plasma cholesterol. Soluble food fiber appears to be especially beneficial. Those foods containing higher amounts of soluble food fiber are listed in table 9, chapter 13. That chapter also provides guidelines for what foods to avoid and what foods to consume to maintain a lower fat and saturated fat intake while increasing the proportion of unsaturated fat.

After four to six weeks and again after three months on this meal plan, the total cholesterol level and its LDL and HDL fractions are measured. If the physician feels definite progress is being made, the program is continued. If no lowering of cholesterol occurs, the decision may be made to refer the individual back to a registered dieti-

tian for further instruction. On the other hand, if the diet is being conscientiously followed but cholesterol remains too elevated, the Step Two Diet is advised.

### The Step Two Diet

This diet requires the assistance of a registered dietitian. None of the meal plans in this monograph are this restricted in fat. Saturated fat intake is lowered from 10% to 7% of total calories and dietary cholesterol is reduced from 300 milligrams to only 200 milligrams per day. Although this meal plan can also assure balanced nutrition, it requires more education of the patient and more careful selection of foods that have well-defined amounts of fat content.

Plasma cholesterol concentrations are determined after four to six weeks and three months on the Step Two Diet. If total and LDL cholesterol fractions are not returned to normal by the end of three months, drug therapy is indicated.

### Drug Treatment of Cholesterol Problems

In recent years a variety of medications have become available to broaden the approach physicians may take to control a cholesterol problem. Agents that are prescribed primarily for cholesterol elevations include binding resins (cholestyramine, colestipol), nicotinic acid and lovastatin. Binding resins in the form of powders tie up cholesterol and prevent its absorption in the intestinal tract. Nicotinic acid and the newer drug, lovastatin, have blocking effects on the production of cholesterol in tissues like liver. Drugs that principally lower plasma triglycerides include gemfibrozil and probucol. Often doctors will use drugs in combination to produce a maximum effect. It is not uncommon to reduce cholesterol by 50% with such combinations. Resistant cases may require the additional skills and consultations of specialists experienced in the treatment of these disorders. Patients who take these medications require close supervision in their use and must be followed by their doctor for possible undesirable side effects, including those on intestinal, liver or gallbladder function. Periodic laboratory tests to exclude side effects are often necessary. In the near future, other effective drugs will be approved for use in controlling blood cholesterol problems.

### Summary

There is no question that elevated cholesterol levels in blood promote cardiovascular disease. All individuals should have their plasma cholesterol checked periodically.

Adults with obesity have a greater tendency to have cholesterol problems. Obesity is also an added risk factor for developing cardiovascular disease. Other additional risk factors include hypertension, diabetes and cigarette smoking.

The best way to control cholesterol is to reduce body weight to desirable levels and maintain that weight. This is done with lifelong meal plans that also reduce saturated fat and cholesterol intake. Additional food fiber also helps. Exercise helps by improving circulation, strengthening the heart and increasing HDL (the "good") cholesterol.

Blood pressure control and good control of diabetes, if present, also reduce the risks of cardiovascular disease. Cigarette smoking should cease.

The meal plans outlined in this monograph are a good start and are ideally suited to provide good nutrition and lower weight as well as cholesterol. More severe problems may require additional diet modifications and drug therapy.

# Index

222

Recipe: conversion to exchanges, 139

Recipes, 179-196; beverages, 196; breakfast ideas, 180; charcoal treats, 179; cookies, 189-194; desserts, 189-194; entrees, 181-185; salads, 186-187; sauces, 195; soups, 186-187; starch/bread group, 188-189; toppings, 195

Restaurants, fast food, 153-156

Salt: and convenience foods, 169; spice substitutions for, 147, 148. *See also* Sodium

Sodium, 67-68; excessive intake of, 34

Soups, canned, 174; exchanges for, 174-175

Spices, 147, 148

Starch, 22; sources of, 65

Starch/bread exchanges, 73-74

Sugar: excessive intake of, 33

Sugar substitutes: sugar equivalencies of, 146; types, 145-146

Thyroid: hormone treatment, 43

Triglyceride abnormalities, 16

U.S. Senate Committee on Nutrition and Human Needs: recommendations, 34-35

Vegetable exchanges, 80

Vein disorders, 17

Vitamins, 25-29; A, 25, 28-29; B, 27; C, 27, 28; D, 25, 28-29; E, 25-27; fat-soluble, 25-27; K, 25; recommended dietary allowances, 25, 26; water-soluble, 27

Vitamin supplements, 25, 29

Walking, 57

Weight loss, rate of, 85, 86

Weight maintenance. *See* Maintenance, weight

Weight plateaus, 86

Weight tables: for adults, 13, 14; for children, 208, 209

Yogurt: exchanges for, 176